Tricks and Traps in MRI of the Pituitary Region

Jean-François Bonneville

Tricks and Traps in MRI of the Pituitary Region

Springer

Jean-François Bonneville
Department of Medical Imaging and Endocrinology
Centre Hospitalier Universitaire de Liège
Liége, Belgium

ISBN 978-3-031-64709-3 ISBN 978-3-031-64710-9 (eBook)
https://doi.org/10.1007/978-3-031-64710-9

This Springer imprint is published by the registered company Springer Nature Switzerland AG
The registered company address is: Gewerbestrasse 11, 6330 Cham, Switzerland

To my wife

to my sons

to their children

and their family

to Françoise, Sonia, Véro, Julia

to Jean-Louis

to Albert

Preface

This book is neither a textbook nor an up-to-date work exposing the supposed benefits of the use of radiomics analysis or ChatGPT in the diagnosis of pituitary lesions. It is a compendium of the difficulties of MRIs in the pituitary region and of their remedies collected during a long period of time. It offers simple solutions to overcome pitfalls and traps.

The proposed technical protocols and the general way to go will appear to some readers simplistic or provocative or even outrageous. But the exposed philosophy has been proven efficient for decades and has been shared with endocrinologists and neurosurgeons.

A text full of abbreviations becomes boring, annoying, or even unreadable: I tried to keep them to a minimum and I am sure you will accept RCC for Rathke Cleft Cyst without being upset. However, the World Health Organization has recently changed the classification of pituitary adenomas. This change categorized pituitary adenomas as neuroendocrine tumors and proposed the name to be revised to pituitary neuroendocrine tumor or PitNET. But to be sure to be understood and that their work be recorded, most authors have made the choice to append both denominations in their recent papers, or even to use a triple denomination: "Pituitary neuroendocrine tumor (PitNET)/pituitary adenoma," that is certainly neither economical nor ecological. In this book, I use indifferently either pituitary adenoma or PitNET although the repetitive alternating typing of upper and lower case letters made me at first a little bit upset. At the end, however, I came to find the term PitNET rather pleasant to the eye but nobody knows if it will stand the test of time.

I have adopted CE for Contrast Enhanced in the captions of the figures: after you get to the end of this book, I hope you will remember one of my favorite messages which is that gadolinium is not the universal panacea. If you had the curiosity to count the number of figures with gadolinium, you would see that nonenhanced images, particularly T2W images, far exceeds the enhanced ones.

Lastly, I used a few abbreviations you may never have seen just to intrigue you and get your attention on previously undescribed variations or curiosities such as IUO for Infundibular Unidentified Object.

I wish you a pleasant and instructive reading.

Liége, Belgium — Jean-François Bonneville

Contents

Abbreviations

ACTH	Adrenocorticotropic hormone
AVP	Arginine vasopressin
CE T1WI	Contrast-enhanced T1WI
CP	Craniopharyngioma
CSF	Cerebrospinal fluid
CT	Computed tomography
DWI	Diffusion–weighted image
ENT	Ears, nose, and throat
GE	Gradient echo
GH	Growth hormone
GHRH	Growth hormone-releasing hormone
IGF-1	Insulin-like growth factor 1
IPSS	Interrupted pituitary stalk syndrome
PitNET	Pituitary adenoma
RCC	Rathke cleft cyst
SE	Spin echo
T1WI	T1-weighted image
T2WI	T2-weighted image
TSH	Thyroid-stimulating hormone

1 The (My) Golden Rules

Unless you are practicing in a Pituitary Center, you, my dear colleagues radiologists, you did not manage a pituitary MRI every day and probably not one every week: it is a very special examination with possible crucial issues that require your full attention.

If it is the first pituitary MRI of your patient and not a follow-up, some recommendations are welcome.

- Take a short time to greet your patient and ask a few questions: undoubtedly, you will learn more than what you have read on the MRI prescription.
- You must know what you are looking for—for instance, macro (visual field defect), micro (hyperprolactinemia), or possible picoadenoma (Cushing disease), and you have to adapt your technical protocol.
- The localizer image may sometimes tell you in seconds if there is a mass of the sellar region or not: do not neglect its reading to adapt possibly your protocol (Fig. 1.1).
- Be personally present during the examination to modify, if necessary, the choice of the sequences in real time. For instance, deciding to inject gadolinium (it is not compulsory!); adding an axial T1W or a sagittal T2W sequence to elucidate an unexplained intrasellar image; changing the thickness of the reformat to confirm a tiny lesion or understand an artifact; obtaining an additional FLAIR sequence to precise a liquid-looking image. Your presence during a pituitary MRI may seem like a heavy burden but is for me key to best helping the clinician and the patient.
- Allow at least 15–20 min for a pituitary MRI: again, it could be a complex examination.
- If a brain MRI is also ordered or is considered necessary, it will be scheduled in a different session.

The first MRI could be often the first of many follow-up studies: comparison will be easy and accurate if the same rigorous projections are chosen. We perform all coronal

J.-F. Bonneville, *Tricks and Traps in MRI of the Pituitary Region*,
https://doi.org/10.1007/978-3-031-64710-9_1

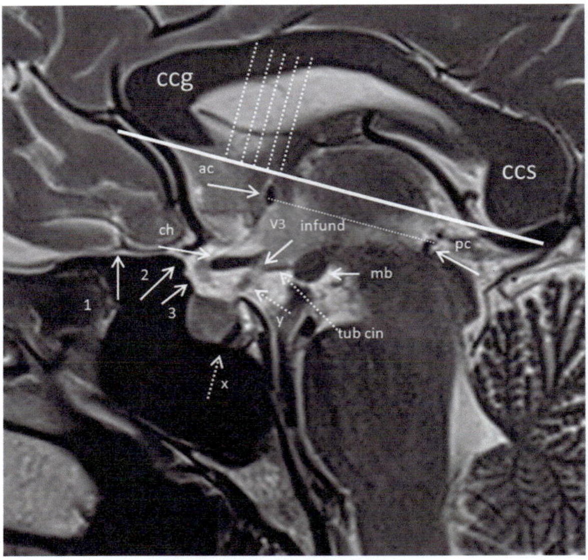

Fig. 1.1 Sagittal T2W image. Main landmarks of the hypothalamic-hypophyseal region. 1: Planum sphenoidale. 2: Tuberculum sellae. 3: Chiasmatic sulcus. x: Pars intermedia/Rathke cleft cyst (anatomical variant). y: Pituitary stalk. *infund* infundibulum, *tub cin* tuber cinereum, *ch* optic chiasm, *ac/pc* anterior and posterior commissures, *ccg/ccs* corpus callosum, genu, and splenium. Coronal sections are obtained perpendicularly to the line joining the inferior border of the genu and of the splenium of the corpus callosum. This line is very close to the classical bicommissural line adopted by the anatomists (thin dotted line), but more easy to draw

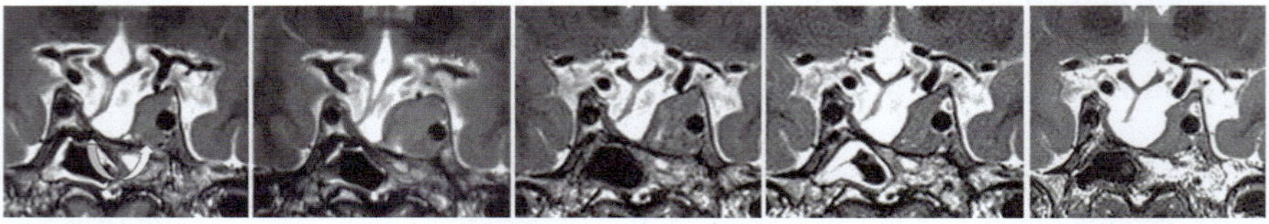

Fig. 1.2 Example of a postoperative MRI follow-up for 10 years. T2W coronal sections according to the subcallosal line

sequences perpendicularly to a line joining the genu and the splenium of the corpus callosum. This line is easier to draw than the classical bicommissural line (Fig. 1.2). Our landmark being distant from the sellar area is immovable at the difference of the sellar floor or the pituitary stalk which could be modified after surgery or medical treatment. It has the advantage to be applicable to any MR scanner whatever the firm.

- The most informative sequence is most of the time T2W, not a gadolinium-enhanced one. Favor a long acquisition time to get the best information.
- Dynamic imaging must never be systematic and reserved for exceptional cases or research purpose.
- Hyperprolactinemia is certainly one of the most frequent indications for pituitary MRI in your practice. Symptomatology is secondary amenorrhea, often after stopping the pill, galactorrhea, or infertility. A lot of "microincidentalomas" can

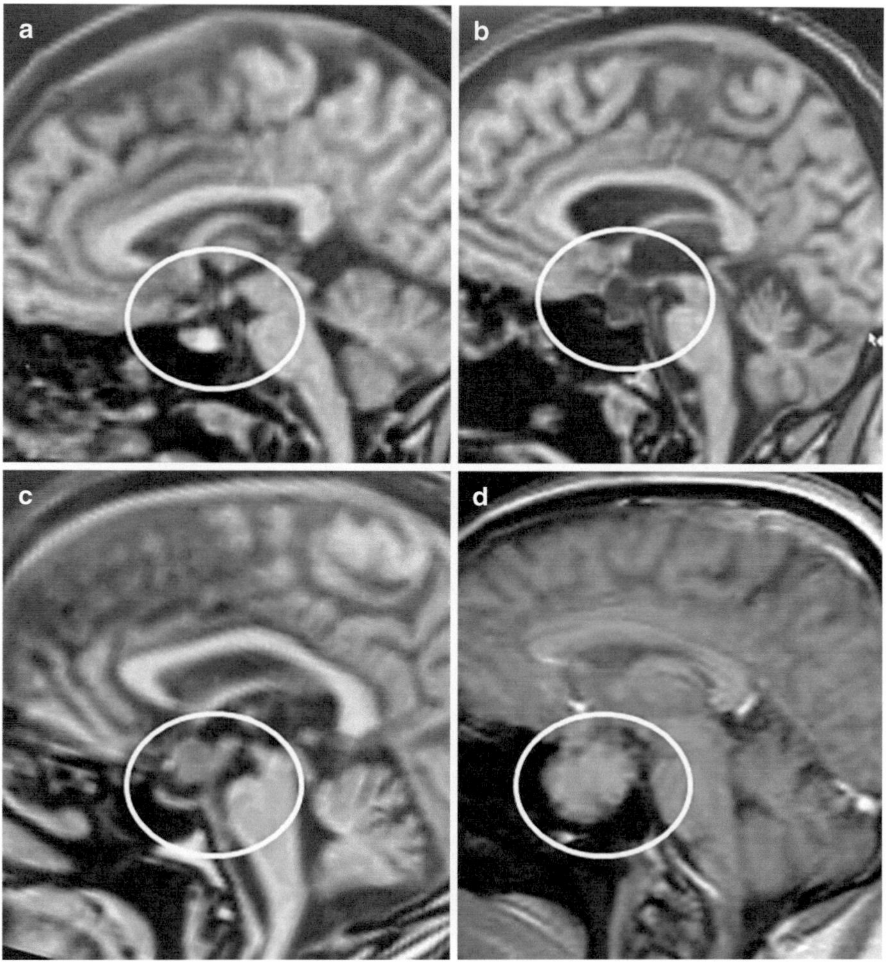

Fig. 1.3 Sagittal localizer images may help to adapt the MRI protocol

mimic microprolactinomas. Fortunately, there is an excellent correlation between prolactin level and pituitary adenoma size—except when the lesion is liquid or hemorrhagic. Most microprolactinomas (less than 10 mm) correspond to a prolactin level between 35 and 120 μg/L, but an intrasellar prolactinoma invading the cavernous sinus can be responsible of a 1000 μg/L prolactinemia. A tiny millimetric image associated with a 100 μg/L prolactin level or more is not a prolactinoma but probably an artifact or an incidentaloma.

- Therefore, knowledge of the prolactin level is essential and must be always requested. If it is not available at the time of the MRI, ask your secretary to call the laboratory.
- Pituitary MRI follow-up is another frequent indication: after medical treatment of prolactinomas, after surgery or radiotherapy, or just for monitoring a nonsecreting adenoma. Tumoral volume and signal changes are well seen on T2WI (Fig. 1.3). Gadolinium injection is usually unnecessary.

T2W MRI: The Master Sequence

2

The T2W MRI sequence largely deserves a dedicated chapter. This sequence is curiously neglected in the scientific literature, particularly the endocrinological and neurosurgical literature. For instance, in a journal specifically devoted to the normal and pathological pituitary gland, about nine out of ten figures are post-gadolinium-enhanced. Moreover, T2W images, when present, are frequently of poor quality (Fig. 2.1). The choice of the parameters of this sequence must be managed by a specialist, ideally by an MR engineer. It is undeniable that the image quality is higher with a 3.0 Tesla scanner, but a 1.5 Tesla MR scanner can give excellent results if the T2 sequence is optimized. A long acquisition time is essential, but an excellent T2 sequence often allows the number of sequences to be reduced, especially those obtained after gadolinium injection.

We will briefly list and illustrate several situations where T2W imaging is at least as informative, or more often more informative, than enhanced T1W sequences (Figs. 2.2, 2.3, and 2.4).

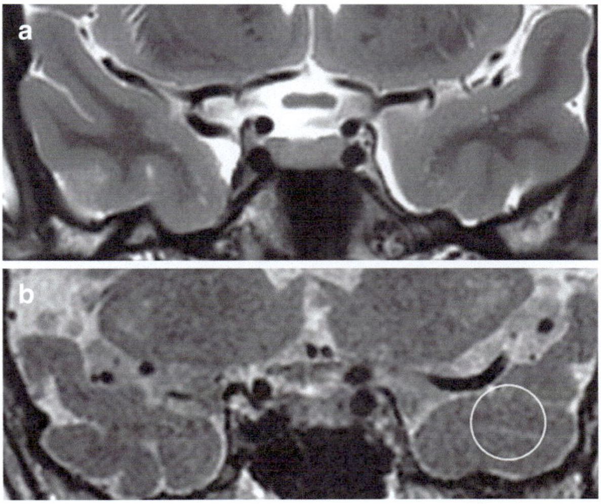

Fig. 2.1 Optimized (**a**) versus unacceptable (**b**) coronal T2WIs. In **b**, the poor signal resolution does not distinguish gray and white matter of the temporal lobe

J.-F. Bonneville, *Tricks and Traps in MRI of the Pituitary Region*,
https://doi.org/10.1007/978-3-031-64710-9_2

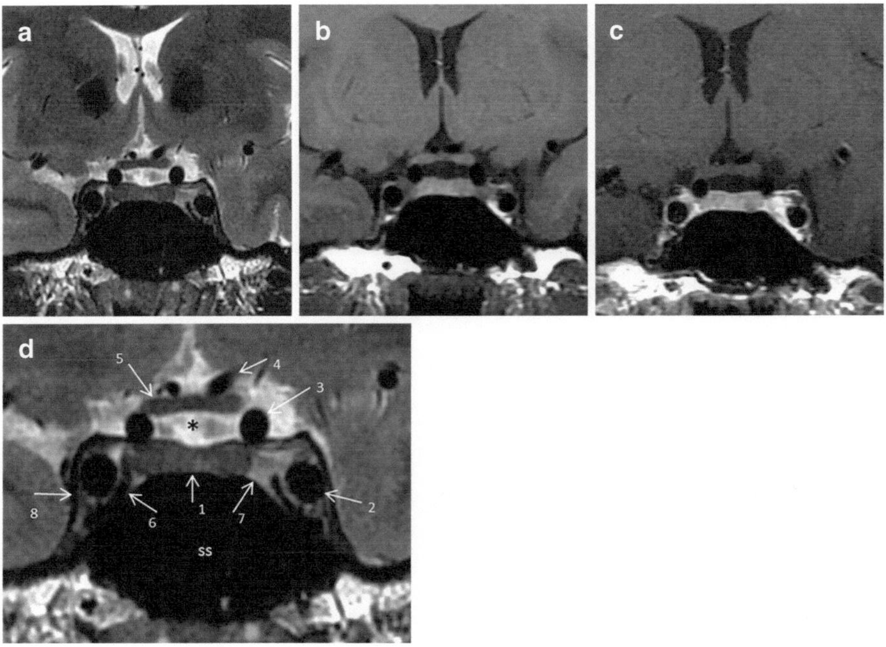

Fig. 2.2 T2W coronal images (**a**, **d**) versus T1W (**b**) and enhanced T1W images (**b**, **c**). 1: Sellar floor. 2: Internal carotid artery. 3: Supra clinoid carotid artery. 4: Anterior cerebral artery. 5: Optic chiasm. 6: Vein of the carotid sulcus. 7: Laterosellar veins. 8: Lateral wall of cavernous sinus

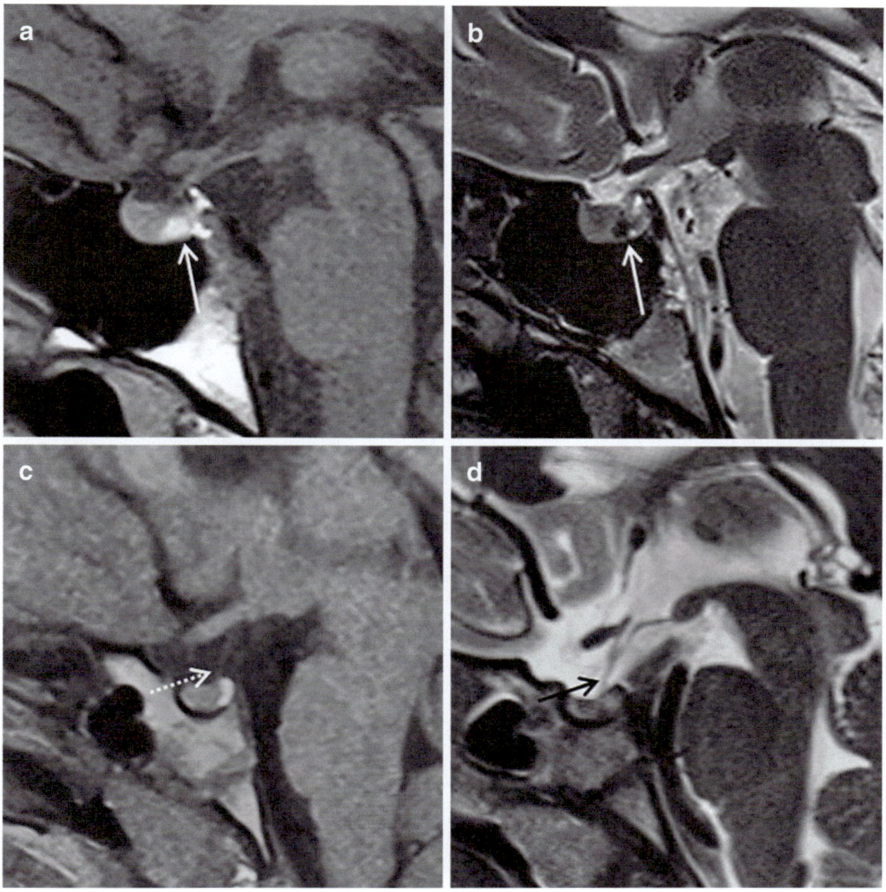

Fig. 2.3 Sagittal unenhanced T1W versus T2WI. (**a**, **b**) The T1W hyperintense nodule (arrow) is not the bright spot of the posterior lobe but a small T2W hypointense Rathke cleft cyst. (**c**, **d**) In this 7-year-old girl with growth hormone deficiency, hypoplasia of the pituitary stalk (arrows) is better shown in **d** T2WI than in **a** sagittal T1WI

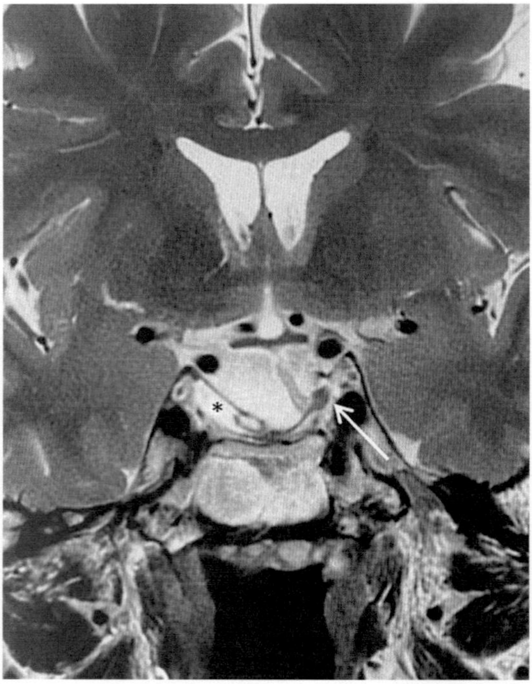

Fig. 2.4 Coronal T2W image 1 year after pituitary surgery. The anterior pituitary is perfectly visible as a small rounded T2 hypointense nodule located at the distal end of the tilted pituitary stalk (arrow). Note that there is no relation between the size of the residual pituitary gland and the severity of a possible deficit. Contralaterally, a triangular T2W hyperintense area (asterisk) reflects here the presence of a sero-hematic residue. Its T2W signal being different from that of the tumor before surgery (not shown) eliminates a tumoral remnant

2.1 Hyperprolactinemia

This is one of the most usual indications of MRI of the pituitary gland. If hyperprolactinemia is symptomatic and greater than 30–35 μg/L, and if macroprolactinemia and an iatrogenic cause have been eliminated, an MRI will show a pituitary adenoma visible from the T2 sequence which must be performed first. Microprolactinomas are more or less hyperintense on T2W images, rarely hypointense or isointense (see Chaps. 12 and 13). The sequences performed after gadolinium injection certainly demonstrate more clearly the contours of the adenoma and allow a more accurate measurement of its diameter or volume. But are these details useful when the treatment is first-line medical? In addition, the enhancement of the surrounding pituitary gland is likely to mask a tiny microadenoma. In my practice, I reserve gadolinium injection to these cases of clear symptomatic hyperprolactinemia when the nonenhanced sequences are negative.

It is common practice to perform a control MRI, in general 6 months after the institution of the treatment by cabergoline. When the treatment is effective, which is the most common case, the adenoma decreases in volume and especially sees its T2W hypersignal more pronounced and thus becomes even more visible. Then, there is no justification for performing a sequence with gadolinium injection in this situation.

2.2 Ratke Cleft Cyst (RCC)

This is one of the most common mistakes: an intrasellar mass discovered by chance is frequently reported as a pituitary adenoma after the reading of T1 and CE T1 WIs when it is a Rathke cleft cyst. However, the coronal T2W sequence will better show a difference of signal between the RCC and the pituitary gland which frequently encircles the cyst bilaterally, what is never the case with PitNET (see Chap. 24). Besides, in more than half of the cases of Rathke cyst, the T2W sequence demonstrates a hypointense intracystic hyperproteinic nodule which is pathognomonic of the diagnosis.

Another frequent mistake in sagittal T1W sequence is the confusion between the bright spot of the posterior lobe and an intrasellar mucoid Rathke cleft cyst; this is immediately clarified by a T2W (Fig. 2.3a, b) or an axial T1W sequence.

2.3 Growth Retardation

The pituitary stalk configuration is an important feature in the setting of growth hormone deficit in children. For decades, gadolinium injection was formally recommended for its precise demonstration. It is today accepted that a high-resolution high contrast millimetric T2W sequence (CISS, FIESTA) is superior to a T1W enhanced sequence to separate total pituitary stalk absence—usually observed in multiple hormone deficit—from hypoplastic or truncated pituitary stalk—usually observed in isolated growth hormone deficit. A 2D 2 mm Fast Spin Echo sagittal sequence gives similar results (Fig. 2.3c, d). In these situations of growth retardation, gadolinium injection must be abolished, making MR examinations quicker, better accepted, without any risk, and less expensive. Unenhanced T1W sequences, sagittal and optionally axial, demonstrate clearly the vasopressin storage in ectopic or eutopic position. A tumoral process can be ruled out without gadolinium injection.

2.4 Diabetes Insipidus and Hypophysitis

Is the pituitary stalk normal, thickened, or atrophic? The question is fundamental when diabetes insipidus or hypophysitis is suspected. In the literature, the diameters of the pituitary stalk have been measured very carefully at the level of the optic chiasma and at the pituitary insertion. The extreme precision of these figures is unfortunately of no help in the borderline cases.

The morphology of the stalk is sometimes more interesting to consider. The pituitary stalk usually has a bulge at the top and tapers below; a cylindrical stalk, of constant thickness from top to bottom, may suggest thickening while the measured diameters are still within the norm. This feature is more obvious on T2W images. Similarly, deepening of the posterior recess of the third ventricle which can mimic a pituitary stalk thickening is better recognized in the same sequence. At last, a previously undescribed T2 hypointense ring, predominant anteriorly, which encircles the upper part of the stalk, constitutes a new landmark undetectable on T1W- and T1W-enhanced MRI (Fig. 5.2).

2.5 Postoperative Pituitary MRI

After pituitary surgery, an MRI follow-up spreads over years or even decades. The use is still to perform these examinations with gadolinium injection. For early controls, at 3 or 6 months after the intervention, the injected sequences are most often illegible and therefore useless due to an undifferentiated enhancement of the sellar content and/or the presence of surgical packing or sero-hematic suffusion (Fig. 36.2). At 1 year, the T2 sequence is the most likely to separate a possible remnant or a recurrence from normal pituitary tissue. Beyond 1 year, the goal of the examination is strictly to look for an increase in size of an adenoma remnant or for a recurrence. The unenhanced T2W sequence easily answers these questions (Fig. 2.4).

Recent papers have proposed to spare gadolinium injection for MRI surveillance of *unoperated* pituitary macroadenoma: for more than a decade, our team has controlled *operated* adenomas without the use of contrast agents.

In summary, the T2W sequences are by far our favorites (Bonneville JF 2019) and they deserve it (Fig. 2.5). We use largely the coronal T2 sequence in all circumstances and particularly for the research of PitNETS and postoperatively and the

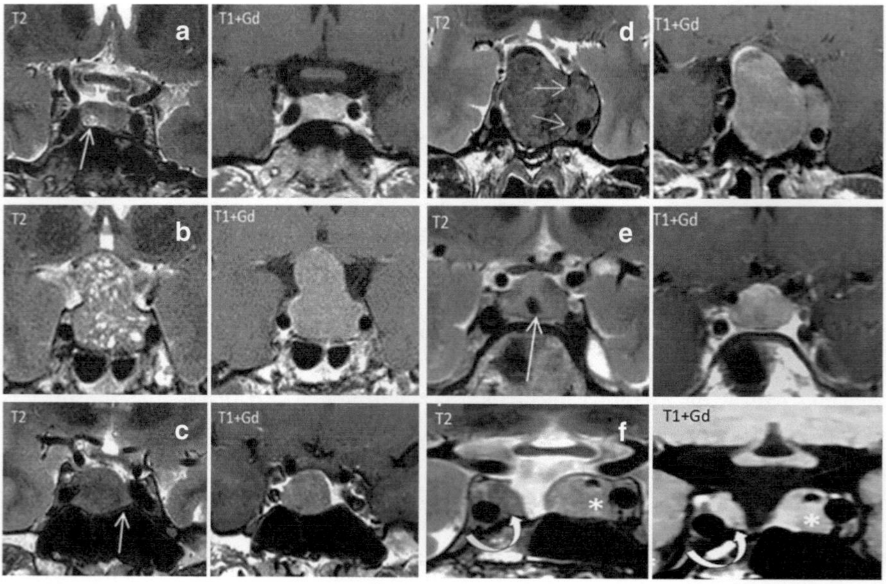

Fig. 2.5 Examples of the efficacy of T2WIs over CE T1W images. (**a**) Microprolactinoma. (**b**) Silent corticotropic adenoma. (**c**) Densely granulated growth hormone-secreting adenoma. (**d**) Invasion of cavernous sinus. (**e**) Hyperproteinic nodule of a Rathke cleft cyst. (**f**) Post-operative tumoral remnant (asterisk) versus normal residual pituitary tissue (arrow)

sagittal T2W sequence systematically in case of diabetes insipidus, in hypogonadotropic hypogonadism, in children with growth retardation or precocious puberty and each time where an optimal image of the hypothalamic-hypophyseal junction is required.

Further Reading

Bonneville JF. A plea for the T2W MR sequence for pituitary imaging. Pituitary. 2019;22(2):195–7. https://doi.org/10.1007/s11102-018-0928-9.

Axial T1: An Underused MRI Sequence

3

An important diagnostic tool for pituitary diseases is incomprehensibly rarely performed in radiologic centers including tertiary centers, the unenhanced axial T1W sequence, preferably with Fat saturation (AxT1W Fatsat). This projection deserves a short but full chapter with convincing illustrations. At the end of this short presentation, you will have at least seven good reasons to keep this weapon ready in your bag.

First, the axial T1W sequence demonstrates at best the vasopressin storage—formerly antidiuretic hormone—stored in the posterior lobe. As the sagittal T1W sequence is said to be unable to detect it in a variable percentage of normal cases, axial T1W Fatsat demonstrates it almost always. The disadvantages of the sagittal sequence for the visualization of vasopressin—anterior concavity, thickness, compact bone or fatty composition of the dorsum sellae—are here eliminated. Thus, AxT1W must be the first sequence to be obtained when a vasopressin deficit is suspected. Fat saturation is highly recommended to avoid chemical shift artifacts from the dorsum (Fig. 3.1).

Second, this statement is even more true in several physiologic or pathologic conditions known to interfere with plasmatic osmolality and then likely to reduce the amount of stored vasopressin, for instance in the elderly, in patients with diabetes mellitus, under dialysis, in stress situation or during pregnancy (Fig. 3.2).

Third, AxT1 is the only sequence able to separate the posterior lobe from an incidental Rathke cleft cyst (RCC). Indeed, the distinction of a normal posterior lobe from a mucinous T1 hyperintense RCC may be impossible on a sagittal view. On AxT1W, the posterior lobe is clearly recognizable as strictly applied to the anterior T1W hypointense surface of the dorsum sellae while an intrasellar mucoid RCC which is usually median is in close contact with the anterior surface of the posterior lobe from which it is separated by a thin line, possibly the wall of the RCC (Fig. 3.3c, d).

Fourth, a lateral imprint of the anterior surface of the posterior lobe, clearly visible on AxT1WI, signals an intrasellar mass effect and can constitute a useful marker, for instance in the presence of an isointense pituitary adenoma (Fig. 3.4).

J.-F. Bonneville, *Tricks and Traps in MRI of the Pituitary Region*,
https://doi.org/10.1007/978-3-031-64710-9_3

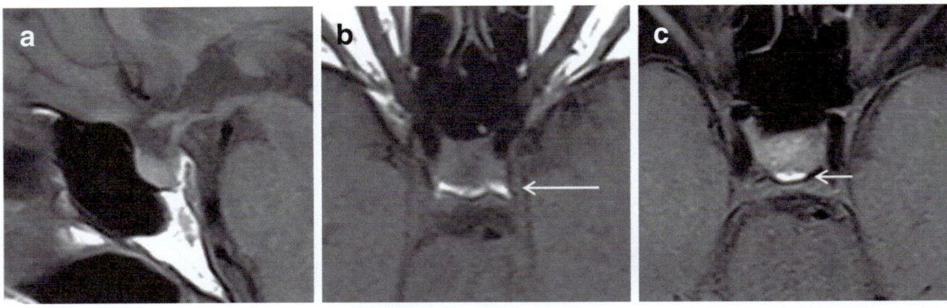

Fig. 3.1 Sagittal T1W (**a**) versus axial T1 (**b**) versus axial T1 Fatsat (**c**) images. The chemical shift artifact from the dorsum (long arrow in **b**) is deleted in **c**. The posterior lobe which is masked in **a** is clearly visible in **c** (short arrow)

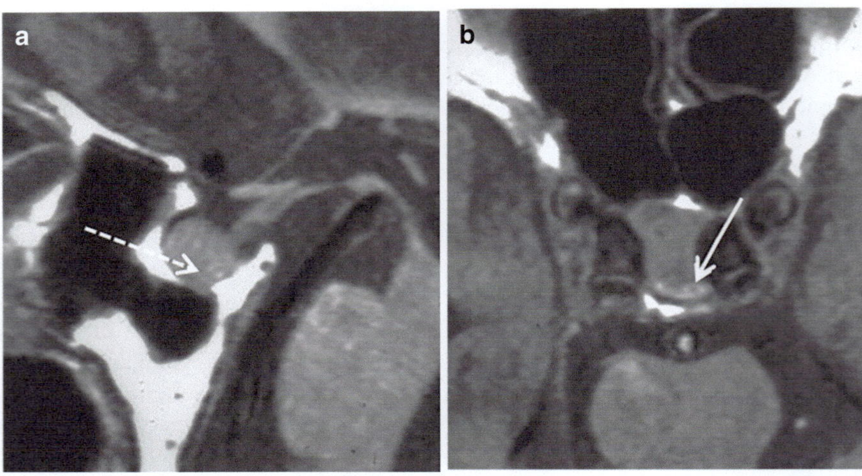

Fig. 3.2 (**a**, **b**) Sagittal and axial T1WIs. The bright spot of the posterior lobe is visible on axial view only in this non symptomatic 75-year-old man

Generally speaking, the research of a mass effect is an important tool to differentiate a pituitary adenoma from a T2W hyperintense cyst. Pituitary adenomas may modify the sellar floor, the upper surface of the gland, the pituitary stalk, the secondary pituitary bed, or the posterior lobe configuration while intrasellar "cysts" whose internal pressure is low do not or less.

Fifth, only axial T1W sequences are able to formally identify posterior lobes cysts (Fig. 3.5 and Chap. 26).

Sixth, in front of a bulging sellar content, visualization of an uncompressed posterior lobe eliminates a mass effect from a sellar mass and permits to refer to an anatomical variant (Fig. 3.6).

Seventh, AxT1W Fatsat, as well as gadolinium enhanced and axial T2W sequences, are very useful for the early diagnosis of a discrete invasion of the posterior part of the cavernous sinus which is illustrated in Chap. 18.

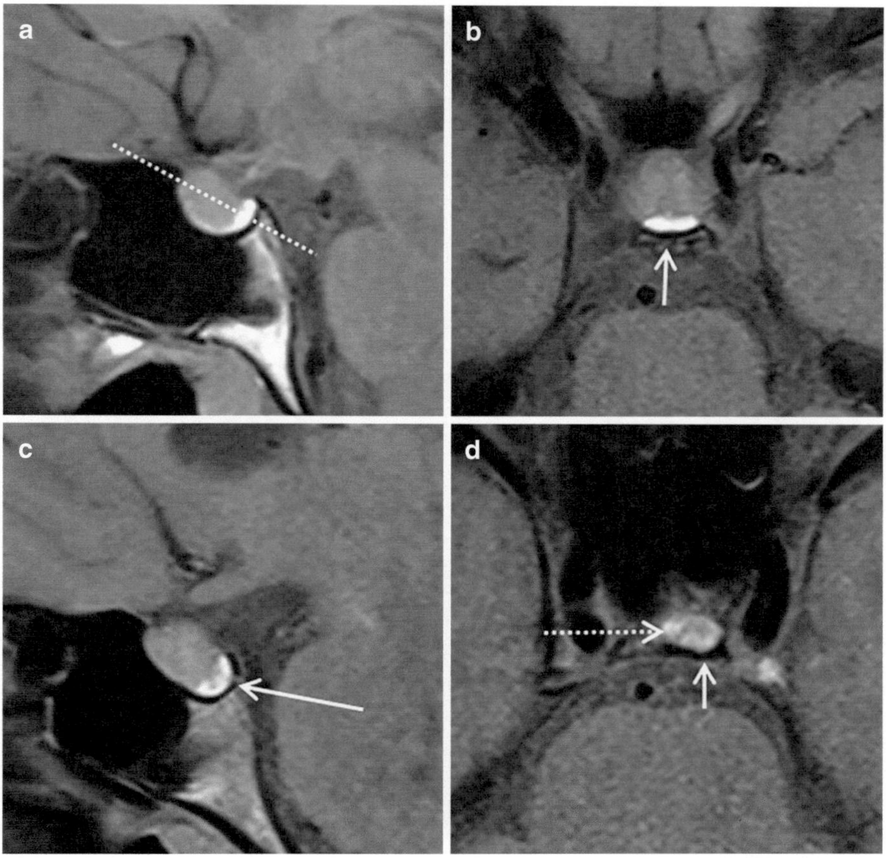

Fig. 3.3 Upper row. Normal posterior lobe on axial T1WI. The orientation of the sequence is marked in **a**. Lower row: Rathke cleft cyst (dotted arrow) separated from the posterior lobe (small arrow) by a thin line in **d**. (**a**, **c**) Sagittal T1WIs. (**b**, **d**) Ax Fatsat T1WIs

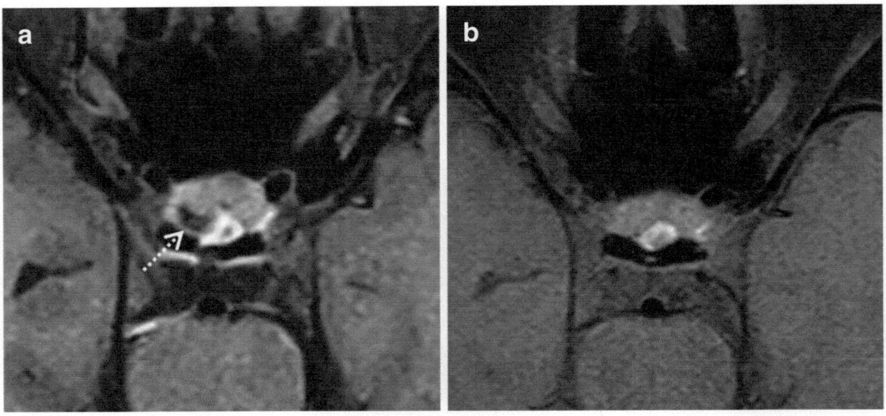

Fig. 3.4 (**a**, **b**) Axial T1W Fatsat images before (**a**) and after medical treatment of a prolactinoma (**b**). In **a**, the T1W hypointense microadenoma (arrow) imprints on the posterior lobe. After pituitary adenoma shrinkage (**b**), compression of the posterior lobe is less pronounced

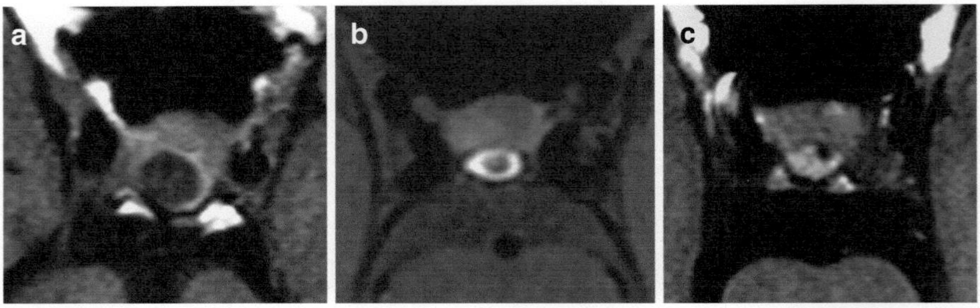

Fig. 3.5 Various cysts of the posterior lobe in axial T1WIs (**a**–**c**). The T1 hypointense cysts are totally surrounded by the T1 hyperintense AVP storage

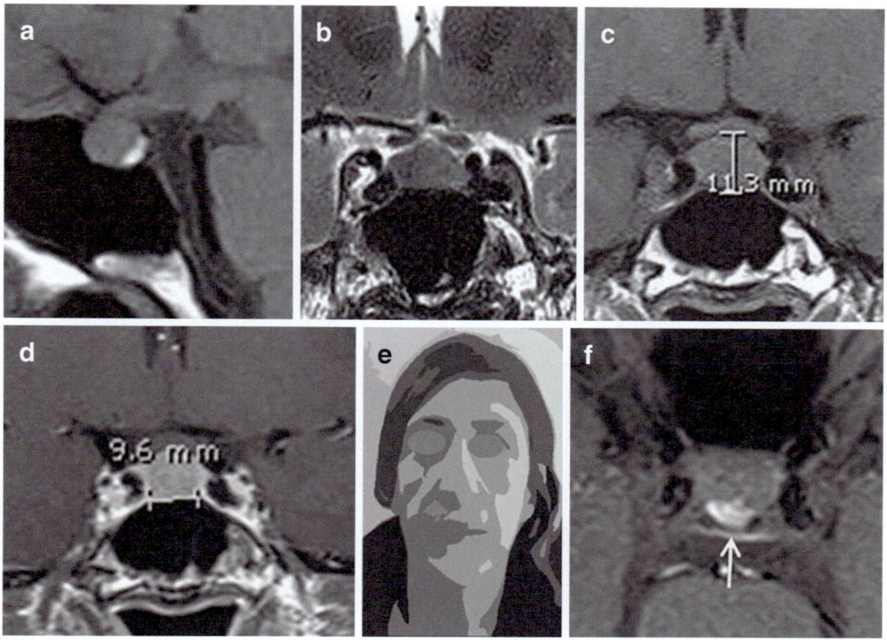

Fig. 3.6 Intriguing 11 mm height pituitary gland in a 42-year-old woman with migraines. Sagittal and coronal T1WIs (**a**, **c**) and coronal T2WI (**b**). An anatomical variant is diagnosed through three arguments. 1: Narrow sellar floor and small sella (**d**). 2: Short transverse diameter of the face and the head (**e**). 3: Non-compressed posterior lobe in axial T1WI (**f**)

4 A Look on Sphenoid Sinus

An assessment of the sphenoid sinus is often neglected during the reading of an MRI of the pituitary region, but its observation may be rewarding in many circumstances.

At birth, the sphenoid bone is not pneumatized and appears on T1W images as hypointense as the red bone marrow. During a short period of time, between 6 and 12 months, the bone marrow turns to yellow and, consequently, the T1W signal of the sphenoid moves from hypo- to hyperintense as does fat; this transient pattern can be disturbing in mimicking an abnormality (Fig. 4.1b). Conversely, the persistence of a T1W hypointensity of the sphenoid bone beyond 2 years of age must draw attention as it can indicate a hematologic disease.

Pneumatization of the sphenoid bone starts between 2 and 4 years at the limit of ethmoid and sphenoid bones and progresses backward until adolescence (Fig. 4.1). It is more or less severely delayed in children with growth retardation. Delayed closure of the spheno-occipital synchondrosis attests to growth hormone deficit (Fig. 11.3).

The final extension of the sphenoid sinus is very variable.

Pneumatization may extend significantly and affect dorsum sellae, clivus, pterygoid process, anterior clinoid process, and the greater wing of the sphenoid.

Excessive pneumatization tends to counteract the increase in the size of the pituitary fossa under the influence of pituitary gland growth. The result may be a short, flat, or narrow sella with a resulting bulging of the pituitary gland mimicking a pathologic gland, especially in adolescent and young females whose pituitary gland is physiologically temporarily enlarged (Fig. 4.2a–c).

In adults, in about one out of three cases, pneumatization stops early, in front of the lowest point of the sellar floor, i.e., the nadir of the sella, and the posterior part of the sphenoid is occupied by cancellous bone. In this situation, a patent inferior intercavernous sinus (IICS) is demonstrated on coronal views, especially on T2W images, as a hyperintense thin band between the pituitary gland and the sphenoid bone (Fig. 7.3). The presence of an IICS has to be known by the surgeon in case of a transsphenoidal approach. The absence of sphenoid pneumatization— named

J.-F. Bonneville, *Tricks and Traps in MRI of the Pituitary Region*,
https://doi.org/10.1007/978-3-031-64710-9_4

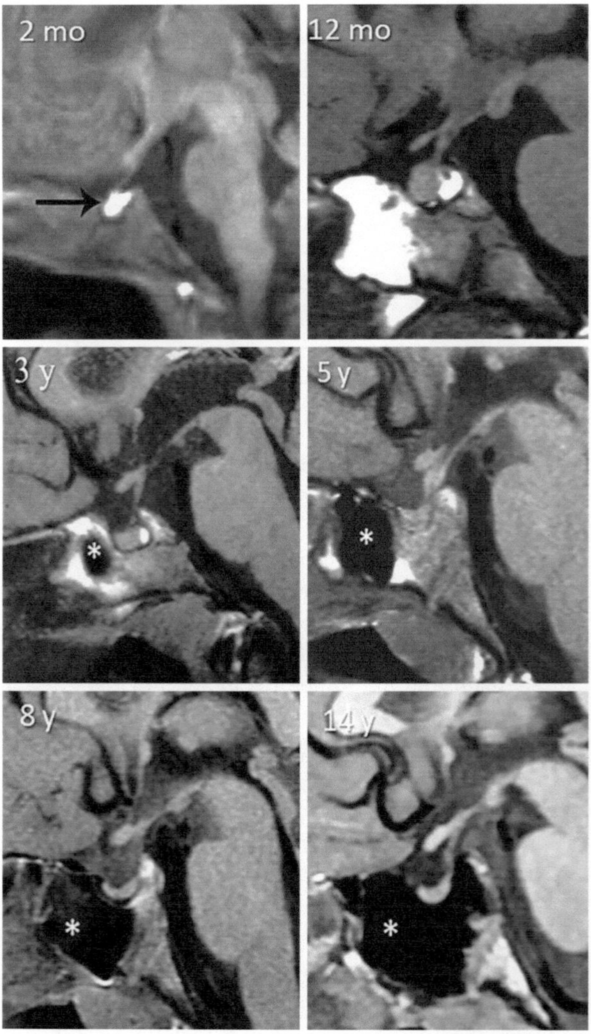

Fig. 4.1 Evolution of sphenoid sinus pneumatization (asterisk) with age. Sagittal T1WIs

sinus concha—may complicate the surgical transsphenoidal approach and necessitate a bone drilling (Fig. 4.2d).

The upper surface of the sphenoid bone which is made of cortical bone—the planum sphenoidale—is undetectable on a sagittal T1W view, its signal being the same as this of the underlying aerated sinus. In the elderly, a fatty transformation occurs and the planum turns to hyperintense on T1W images. Conversely, observation in a young adult of a T1W hyperintense or thick or blistered planum must evoke a meningioma insertion (Fig. 4.3e–h).

A reactional thickening of sphenoidal sinus mucosa is not always related to sinusitis and must draw attention to the overlying sellar content for instance in the case of pituitary apoplexy or hypophysitis (Fig. 20.1).

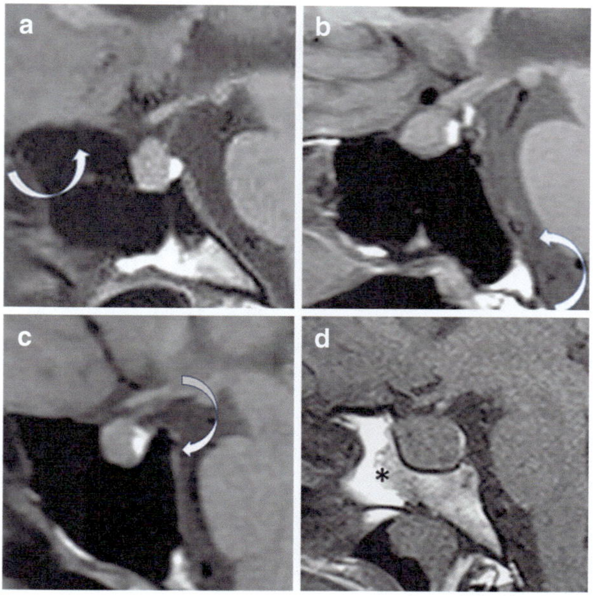

Fig. 4.2 Sphenoid sinus hyperpneumatization responsible of a narrow (**a**), flat (**b**), and short sella (**c**) on sagittal T1WIs. Sinus concha (**d**)

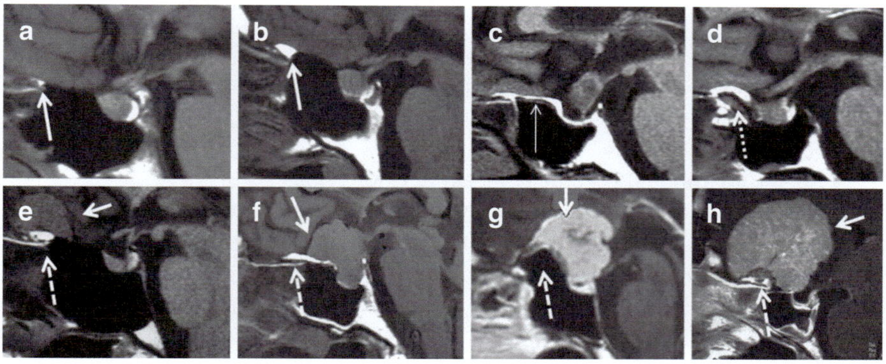

Fig. 4.3 The planum sphenoidale. (**a**, **b**) Normal, in adults. Normal ethmoidal process (thick arrow). (**c**) In the elderly. (**d**) After transsphenoidal surgery and excision of the sphenoid mucosa. (**e–h**) Osteoma and blistering in relation to meningiomas of the planum sphenoidale

The planum may be changed after transsphenoidal surgery: some surgeons resect sphenoid sinus mucosa with consequently a devascularization of the periosteal bone leading to T1 hyperintensity and/or degenerative bony changes mimicking an osteoma (Fig. 4.3d).

If the mucosa is left in place, mucous retention may be observed and possibly lead to a mucoid cyst or even—although rarely—to a mucocele. A tight sphenoid sinus ostium which is best analyzed on axial CT may constitute a contributing factor to this complication. Moreover, fat packing can impede mucus discharge. Mucocele appears as a T1W more or less hyperintense regular mass which may increase slowly in size, distort the sinus walls or even invade the sella (Fig. 4.4).

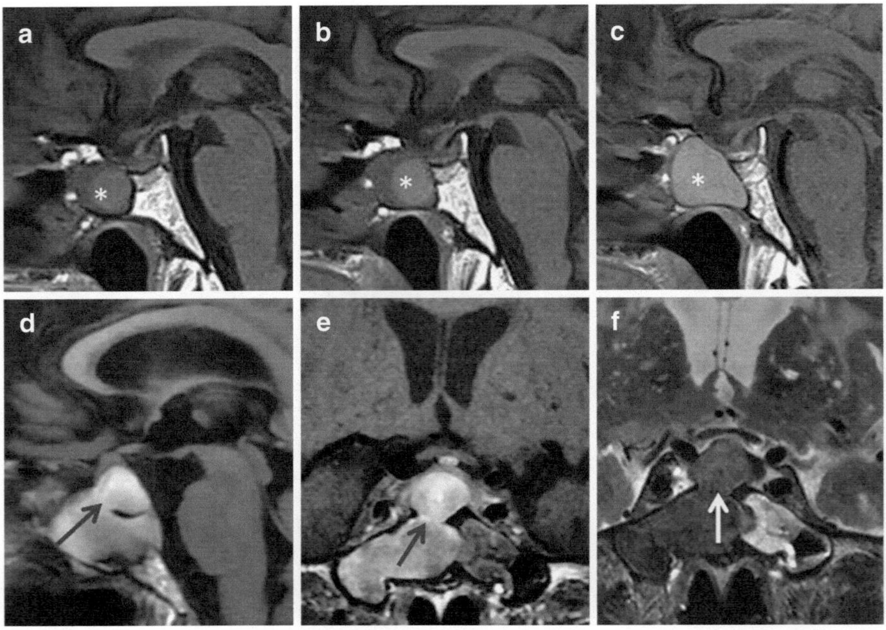

Fig. 4.4 Upper row. Evolution of a common retentional mucoid cyst after sphenoidal surgery. Increased T1W hyperintensity in **c** owing to increased protein concentration. (**a–c**) Sagittal T1WIs. Lower row: Postoperative sphenoid mucocele invading the sella turcica. (**d**, **e**) Sagittal and coronal T1WIs. (**f**) Coronal T2WI

Many different tumors originate in the sphenoid sinus.

The possibility of an ectopic pituitary adenoma has to be kept in mind in front of a pituitary hypersecretion syndrome with inconclusive pituitary MRI.

A sphenoidal tumoral extension is common in prolactinomas in men (Fig. 13.5). A cerebrospinal fluid leak can occur in large prolactinomas after cabergoline: heavily weighted T2W sequences are here useful to precise the site of the leak (Fig. 13.5).

Chordoma is a rare malignant tumor arising at the clivus level, on the midline. It is erosive, invasive, and can be calcified (Fig. 4.5c, d).

The sellar spine is a rare remnant of the notochord (Fig. 4.6a–c) which can be responsible for a troubling magnetic susceptibility artifact.

Ecchordosis physaliphora is a rare benign cystic congenital lesion usually asymptomatic (Fig. 4.6d–f). The absence of enhancement after gadolinium injection is characteristic and permits to eliminate a chondroma (Fig. 4.5a, b).

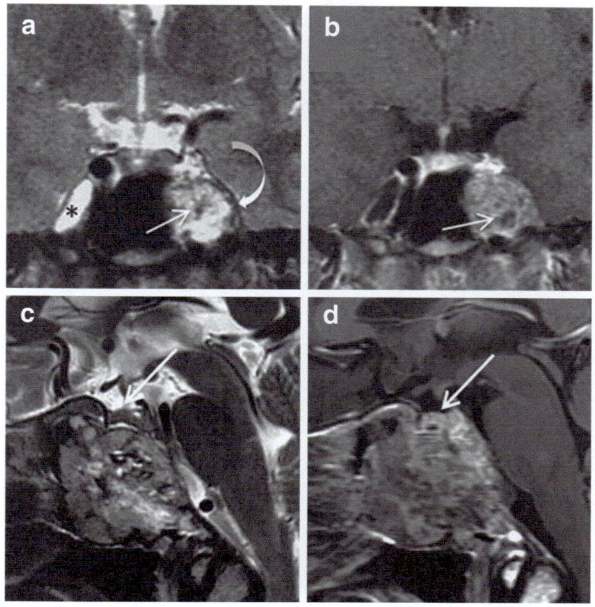

Fig. 4.5 Upper row. Chondroma. Heterogeneously enhanced tumor centered by the left Meckel cave. (**a**, **b**) Coronal T2 and CE T1WIs. Lower row: Chordoma abutting the brain stem. The pituitary gland (arrow) is separated from the tumor. (**c**, **d**) Sagittal T2 and T1 CE WIs

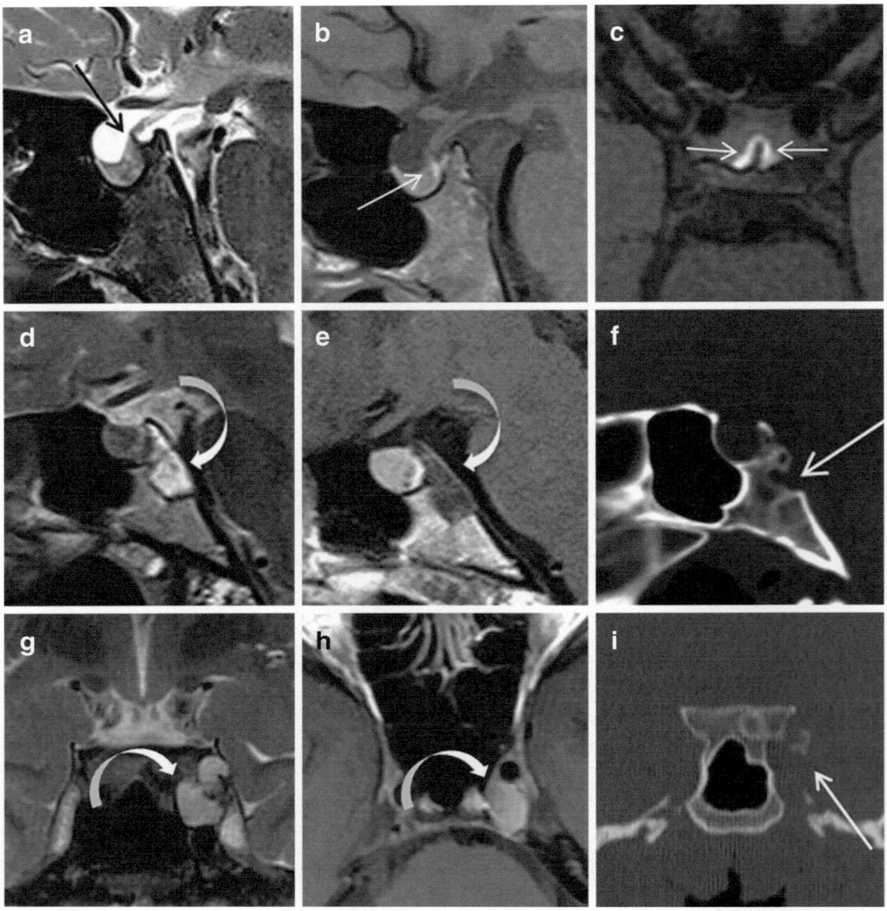

Fig. 4.6 Upper row: Sellar spine, a notochord remnant. (**a**, **b**) Sagittal T2 and T1WIs. (**c**) Axial Fatsat TIWI. Note the induced susceptibility artifact doubling the sella spine image (small arrows). Middle row: Ecchordosis physaliphora, another notochord remnant, in a 36-year-old asymptomatic woman. Unchanged pattern for 10 years. Cystic erosive T2W hyperintense lesion of the clivus, without enhancement. (**d**, **e**) Sagittal T2 and T1CE WIs. (**f**) Sagittal CT. Lower row: Coronal T2WI (**g**), axial CE T1WI (**h**), and coronal CT (**i**)

Further Readings

Kumarasamy S, Kumar A, Singh PK, Suri A, Chandra PS, Kale SS. Non-chordomatous clival bony tumors: a rare experience and systematic literature review. Childs Nerv Syst. 2023; https://doi.org/10.1007/s00381-023-06237-z.

Lee DH, Jang WY, Yoon TM, Lee JK, Jung S, Lim SC. Sphenoid sinus mucocele caused by complications after transsphenoidal pituitary surgery. J Craniofac Surg. 2018;29(7):1859–61. https://doi.org/10.1097/SCS.0000000000004693.

Özgür A, Esen K, Kara E, Yencilek E, Vayisoğlu Y, Kara T, Yıldız A. Ecchordosis physaliphora: evaluation with precontrast and contrast-enhanced fast imaging employing steady-state acquisition MR imaging based on proposed new classification. Clin Neuroradiol. 2016;26(3):347–53. https://doi.org/10.1007/s00062-014-0361-z.

5 The Poorly Known Posterior Lobe

The posterior lobe of the pituitary gland stores vasopressin (or antidiuretic hormone) secreted at the hypothalamic level. This hormone plays a major role in water reabsorption. The recognition of the posterior lobe on MRI is important when reading any examination of the sellar region and more particularly when assessing a polyuro-polydypsia syndrome.

In its normal state, the posterior lobe appears hyperintense on T1WI. Several theories have clashed to explain this signal; the only point of agreement is that this signal is not that of fat, as it does not fade with fat saturation sequence. Importantly, the intensity of the T1 signal varies with plasmatic osmolality. Therefore, when plasma osmolality is increased—as is often the case in the elderly—T1 signal intensity decreases and becomes heterogeneous (Fig. 3.1). The posterior lobe is also found weakly T1 hyperintense in the last trimester of pregnancy (Fig. 5.1) and in different pathological conditions, such as in patients on hemodialysis or with diabetes mellitus. In these different circumstances, the weakly T1W hyperintense signal of vasopressin storage may be unrecognized on sagittal T1WI because it is hidden by the signal of the dorsum sellae but is clearly demonstrated on an axial T1W Fatsat sequence (Fig. 3.2). The normal posterior lobe is more or less hyperintense on T2W images if compared with the anterior pituitary.

The axial T1W sequence, insufficiently used in current practice, has many other advantages. It allows to identify precisely the topography of the posterior lobe which is off midline in half of the cases and strictly adjacent to the anterior surface of the dorsum sellae (Fig. 5.2a, b).

The axial T1W sequence is also the best tool to separate the posterior lobe from an intrasellar mucoid RCC (Figs. 5.2 and 5.3c–e).

It must be remembered that, contrary to what is illustrated in most anatomical textbooks (Fig. 5.3), the normal posterior lobe in adults is much smaller than the anterior lobe, this explaining in part its inconstant demonstration on sagittal T1WIs. A “bright spot” visible on two consecutive sections on a 2–3 mm thick T1W coronal sequence is more likely a Rathke cleft cyst than the posterior lobe. Conversely, the posterior lobe may be proportionally larger in young children.

J.-F. Bonneville, *Tricks and Traps in MRI of the Pituitary Region*,
https://doi.org/10.1007/978-3-031-64710-9_5

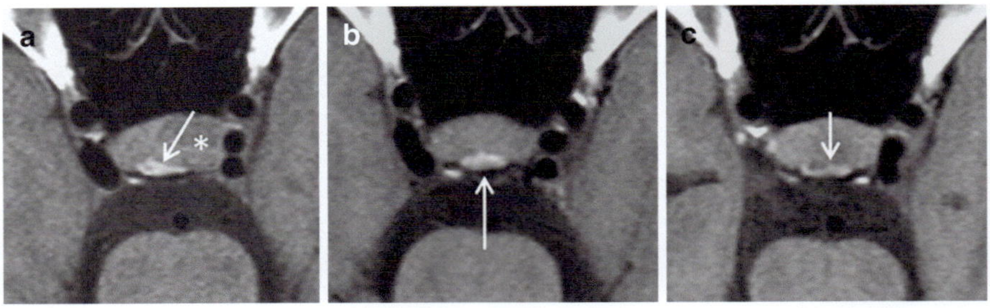

Fig. 5.1 Shape and signal changes of the posterior lobe in a woman harboring a prolactinoma. Axial T1WIs. (**a**) A left-sided prolactinoma (asterisk) encroaches the posterior lobe. (**b**) After cabergoline treatment, shrinkage of the adenoma; the posterior lobe is now symmetrical on midline. (**c**) In the third trimester of pregnancy, decreased T1W signal and flattening of the posterior lobe compressed by the physiological enlargement of the anterior pituitary

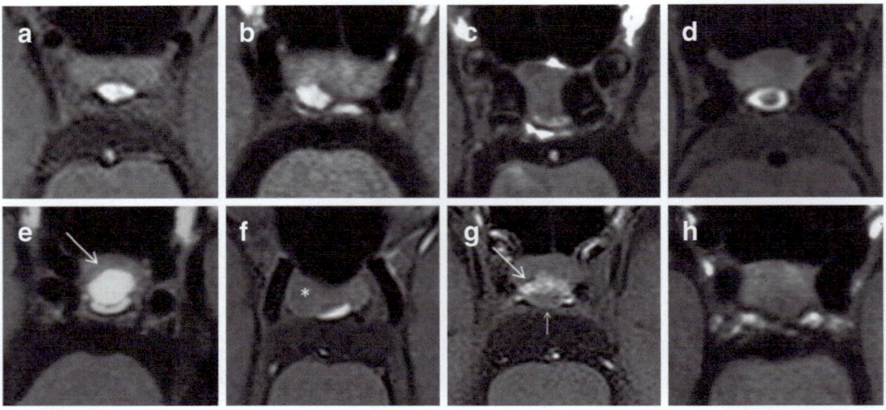

Fig. 5.2 Axial T1WIs of the posterior lobe in various situations. (**a**) Normal posterior lobe stuck to the dorsum sellae. (**b**) Normal off-midline location. (**c**) Poor T1W hypersignal in a 75-year-old man. (**d**) Posterior lobe cyst. (**e**) Perfect delineation of a Rathke cleft cyst (arrow) in front of the posterior lobe. (**f**) Deformation of the posterior lobe by a pituitary microadenoma (asterisk). (**g**) RCC (arrow) in an 80-year-old man. The bright spot is usually weak or absent (small arrow) in an asymptomatic elderly patient. (**h**) Invisibility of the posterior lobe in a patient with vasopressin deficit

If dynamic MR was performed, the posterior pituitary lobe would enhance before the anterior pituitary lobe as a result of its direct arterial blood supply from the internal carotid artery branches.

The posterior lobe is sometimes located in an imprint of the dorsum sellae, the fossula hypophyseos. If it is deep, this dimple may simulate a pituitary adenoma on coronal T2W sequences (Fig. 10.3d–f). Rarely, a sellar spine—a Rathke pouch remnant—can distort the posterior lobe and is easily recognized on axial images (Fig. 10.3a–c).

The presence of a cyst within the posterior lobe is far from infrequent (Fig. 5.2d).

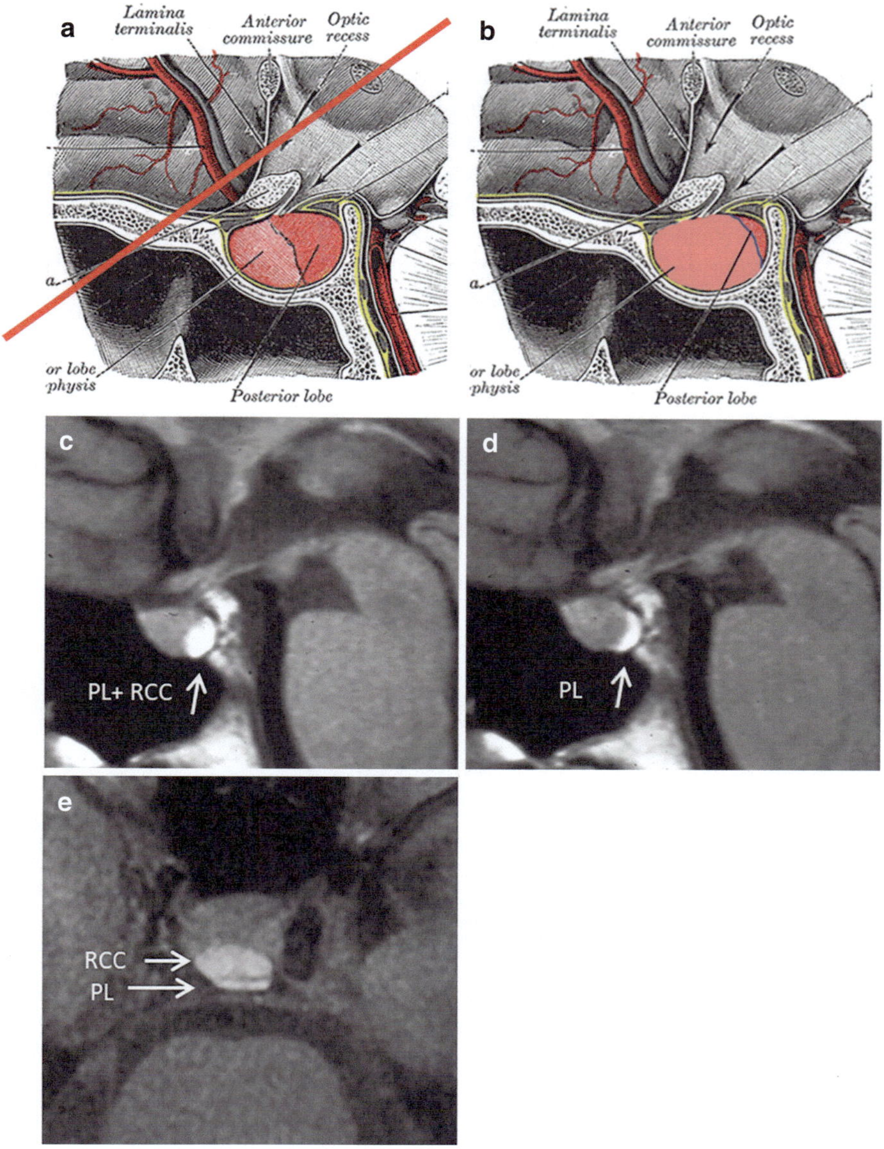

Fig. 5.3 (**a**) Drawing by Henry Vandyke Carter in Gray's Anatomy of the Human Body (1918). (**b**) Our correction: The normal posterior lobe is much smaller than the anterior lobe. (**c**, **e**) Mucoid Rathke cleft cyst mimicking a large posterior lobe on sagittal view and well demonstrated on axial view. (**d**) After spontaneous shrinkage of the Rathke cleft cyst, only the posterior lobe remains visible

Primitive tumors of the posterior lobe are rare. Pituicytomas and spindle cell oncocytomas can be mistaken for nonfunctional pituitary macroadenomas. If they are not recognized, these hypervascularized tumors can be responsible for severe bleeding during surgery. Forward displacement of the pituitary stalk can help. More specifically, T2WIs may demonstrate millimetric hypointense foci corresponding to hemosiderin deposits (Fig. 5.4). Linear or nodular enhancing areas can also be seen.

Metastases of the posterior lobe, particularly from the breast or the lung, are frequent and often tiny and asymptomatic at the end stage of cancer (Fig. 5.5). The erosion of the dorsum sellae is almost the rule when the metastasis is large. A deep acute posterior groove of the mass at the level of the sellar diaphragm is very suggestive of malignancy (Fig. 29.5).

At the end of this chapter, we would remind our assessment that the axial T1W sequence is essential to properly investigate AVP storage. For many years, the standard diagnostic test for the evaluation of polyuria-polydipsia syndrome was the fearsome water deprivation test. Nowadays, infusion of arginine with subsequent copeptin measurement is said a better tolerated test.

In the same time, fiability of MRI in the evaluation of AVP storage has been unfairly denigrated in the endocrinological literature. But it is remarkable that these works have totally ignored the most suitable sequence, i.e., the axial T1W sequence.

If it is true that some overlap may exist in MRI of patients with diabetes insipidus and primary polydipsia, demonstration of an AVP normal storage permits to eliminate a diabetes insipidus of central origin and to spare further unpleasant or expensive tests in daily practice.

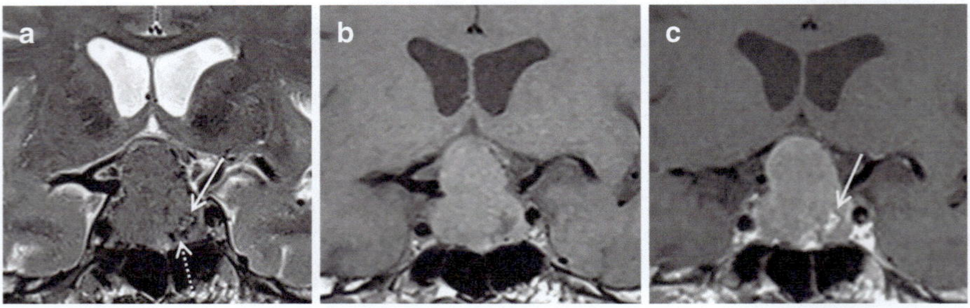

Fig. 5.4 Spindle-cell oncocytoma. (**a–c**) Coronal T2, T1, and CE T1WIS. Enhancing areas (arrows) distinct from hemosiderin deposits (dotted arrow)

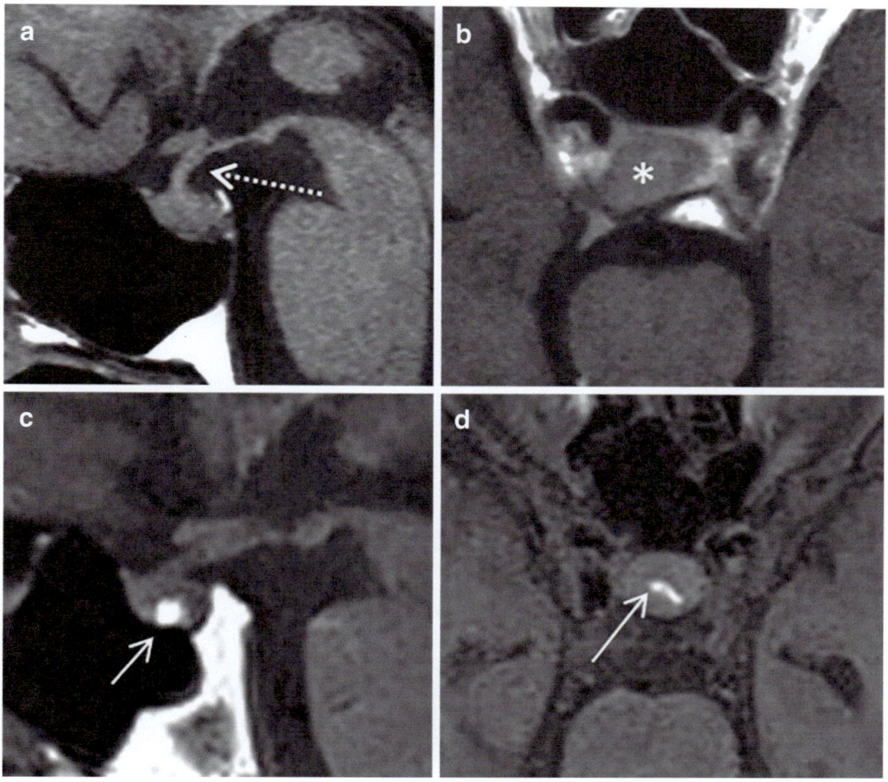

Fig. 5.5 (**a**, **b**) Metastasis of the posterior lobe (asterisk) pushing the pituitary stalk forward (dotted arrow). (**c**, **d**) Metastasis of the posterior lobe and incidental Rathke cleft cyst (arrow) pushed forward by an enlarged tumoral posterior lobe which has lost its T1 hyperintense signal. (**a**, **c**) Sagittal T1WIs. (**b**) Axial CE T1WI. (**d**) Axial T1 Fatsat WI

Further Readings

Christ-Crain M. Diabetes insipidus: new concepts for diagnosis. Neuroendocrinology. 2020;110(9–10):859–67. https://doi.org/10.1159/000505548.

Guerrero-Pérez F, Marengo AP, Vidal N, Iglesias P, Villabona C. Primary tumors of the posterior pituitary: a systematic review. Rev Endocr Metab Disord. 2019;20(2):219–38. https://doi.org/10.1007/s11154-019-09484-1.

Hasiloglu ZI, Ure E, Comunoglu N, Tanriover N, Oz B, Gazioglu N, Mihmanli I. New radiological clues in the diagnosis of spindle cell oncocytoma of the adenohypophysis. Clin Radiol. 2016;71(9):937.e5–937.e11. https://doi.org/10.1016/j.crad.2016.04.022.

6 The Pituitary Stalk and the Infundibular Unidentified Object

The diagnosis of a thickened pituitary stalk (PS) is critical in many diseases of the hypothalamic or hypophyseal regions. Typically, the diagnosis is based on PS measurements. The normal PS size is measured at 3.25 ± 0.56 mm, at the level of the optic chiasm, and at 1.9 ± 0.4 mm at the insertion into the pituitary. In current practice, and despite their apparent precision, these values have little interest because an abnormal PS may be measured inside these limits and conversely a normal PS may be measured beyond these measures. Then, measurements have many limitations.

First, measurements of the pituitary stalk diameter may vary with the MRI sequence:T1, CE T1, or T2W, the slice thickness, 2D or 3D acquisition, and the reformatting technique.

Second, a PS <1.9 mm thick can be abnormal for instance when atrophy occurs as a sequela of an inflammatory process.

Third, an elongated posterior recess of the third ventricle developing inside the infundibulum may mimic an enlarged PS (Fig. 6.1c).

Fourth, in pituitary macroadenoma, the PS is shortened and seems falsely thickened.

In fact, measurements rarely help in questionable cases. Hence, if measurements are not reliable, can morphology be of some help to determine if a PS is abnormal?

- The normal PS displays a flared-up funnel appearance: conversely, a tube-like PS, even in normal limits, constitutes a red flag and enforces a strict follow-up (Fig. 6.1a, b).
- T1 and T2W signals and post gadolinium appearance are essential to recognize pituitary stalk cysts which can mimic stalk thickening (see Chap. 27).
- We have recently described a potential new marker of the normal pituitary stalk. A T2W hypointense flange which is thicker ventrally and can draw an anterior beak circumscribes the lower part of the infundibulum at the level of the distal ending of the posterior recess of the third ventricle. This usually thin flange is undetectable on CE T1WIs (Fig. 6.2) and rarely seen on T1WI as a hyperintense point. Sometimes, only the anterior and posterior sections of this ring are

J.-F. Bonneville, *Tricks and Traps in MRI of the Pituitary Region*,
https://doi.org/10.1007/978-3-031-64710-9_6

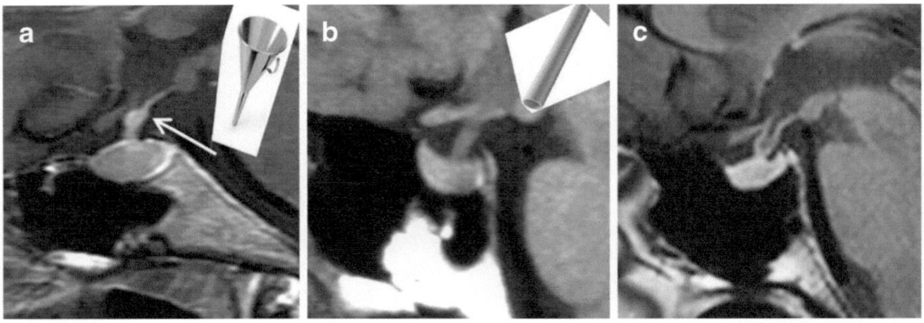

Fig. 6.1 (**a**–**c**) Sagittal T1WIs. (**a**) Funnel-shaped pattern of a normal PS. (**b**) Tube-like appearance of a pathological PS. (**c**) Deep recess of the third ventricle

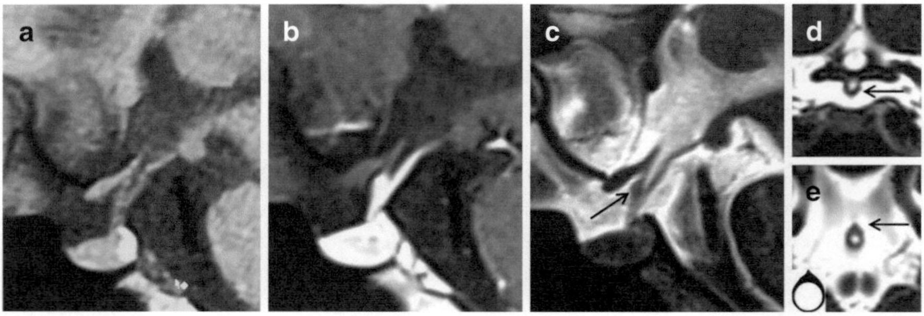

Fig. 6.2 The IUO (Infundibular Unidentified Object) is identified on a sagittal T2WI (**c**, arrow), but not identified on T1 (**a**) nor on CE T1WI (**b**). This peripheral ring is thicker ventrally. (**d**) coronal and (**e**) axial T2WIs

demonstrated on sagittal views (Fig. 6.3b) and axial images confirm its peripheral location (Fig. 6.2e).

- Present in 4 out of 5 normal cases, it is invisible when the PS is elongated or stretched as it is in an empty sella (Fig. 6.3c, d). Rarely, it can be thick enough to mimic a Rathke cleft cyst or even a craniopharyngioma (Fig. 6.4g).
- Its origin is still unclear. We have discussed several potential origins:
  - The arcuate nucleus, a ring surrounding the infundibulum.
  - The pars tuberalis, a tongue of adenohypophysis tissue wrapping partially the pituitary stalk.
  - Squamous cell nests that have been identified at the junction of pars tuberalis with the infundibulum.
  - Embryonic remnants of the Rathke pouch.
  - A focal folding of the median eminence has been evoked since the focal ring here described is blurred when the PS is stretched, for instance in empty sella.
  - A capillary network has been described in the same location: an early enhancement during dynamic MRI finally favors this hypothesis.

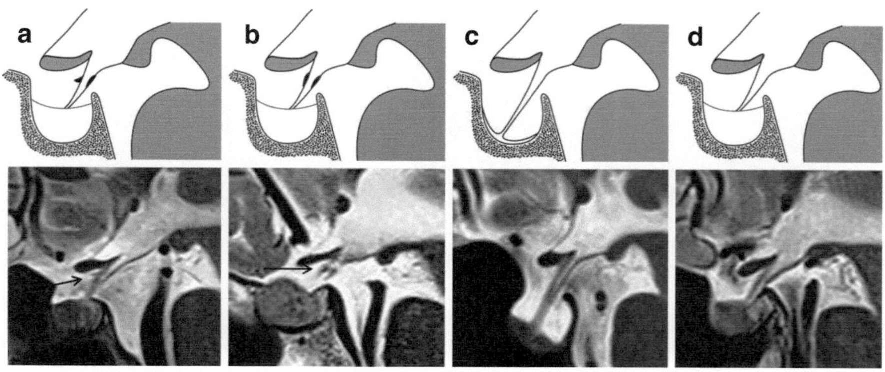

Fig. 6.3 Different patterns of the normal UIO (**a**, **b**) on sagittal T2WIs. The IUO is not demonstrated in case of empty sella (**c**) or deep infundibular recess (**d**)

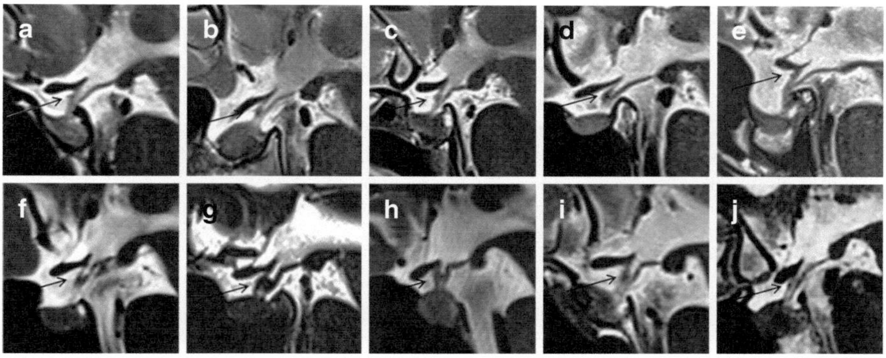

Fig. 6.4 Various appearances of the IUO on sagittal T2WIs (**d–j**, arrows). Note its ventral predominance and specular appearance in (**a–c**)

However, this being only an unproved origin, we proposed the term Infundibular Unidentified Object (IUO) as a denomination for the short T2W hypointense ring circumscribing the inferior part of the infundibulum.

The diagnosis value of this anatomical structure is not fully demonstrated yet, but it is to be recognized as a normal anatomical structure on sagittal T2W MRI. The differential diagnosis is to be made with an ectopic posterior lobe, a pituitary stalk cyst (Fig. 27.3), a craniopharyngioma or fibrous scar after inflammatory disease (Fig. 6.5).

The distortion of the IUO could potentially help for an early diagnosis of pituitary stalk diseases (Fig. 28.1).

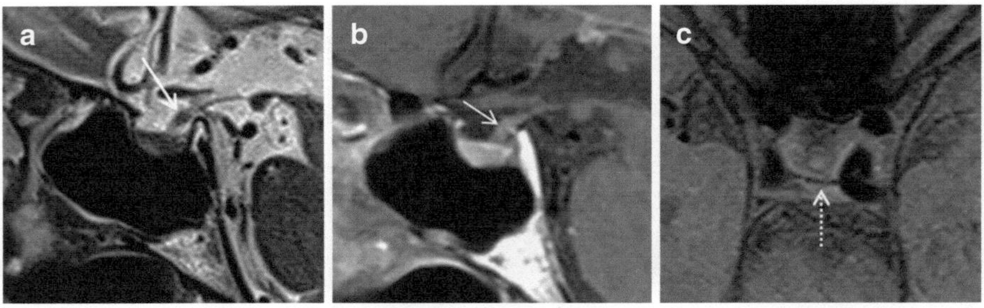

Fig. 6.5 Diabetes insipidus in a 73-year-old woman with a history of Erdheim-Chester disease. Localized T2 hypointensity of the infundibulum (long arrow). Tube-like pituitary stalk (short arrow). The bright spot of the vasopressin storage is missing on (**c**), axial Fatsat T1WI. (**a**, **b**) Sagittal T2 and CE T1WIs

Further Readings

Bonneville JF, Tshibanda L, Beckers A. An infundibular unidentified object (IUO): a new pituitary stalk marker? Pituitary. 2021;24(6):964–9. https://doi.org/10.1007/s11102-021-01169-w.

Satogami N, Miki Y, Koyama T, Kataoka M, Togashi K. Normal pituitary stalk: high-resolution MR imaging at 3T. AJNR Am J Neuroradiol. 2010;31(2):355–9. https://doi.org/10.3174/ajnr.A1836.

Simmons GE, Suchnicki JE, Rak KM, Damiano TR. MR imaging of the pituitary stalk: size, shape, and enhancement pattern. AJR Am J Roentgenol. 1992;159(2):375–7. https://doi.org/10.2214/ajr.159.2.1632360.

7 An Overlooked Venous Sinus

The inferior intercavernous sinus (IICS) is one of the venous connections between both cavernous sinuses. It is located under the sella turcica between the endosteal and the meningeal layers of the dura mater. It is generally considered visible only when it is enlarged by a pathological process: through venous congestion such as with intracranial hypotension (Fig. 7.1), with arteriovenous malformations or fistulas or when a cavernous sinus lesion affects venous outflow (Fig. 7.2).

Occasionally, an IICS can be a source of bleeding complications during the dural opening of transsphenoidal surgery. Bleeding during surgery can hinder proper visualization of normal anatomic structures and pituitary tumors, and can lead to incomplete tumor resection.

Description of the normal IICS is bizarrely quite always absent in radiological textbooks. In anatomical literature, the presence of an IICS is very variously reported, from 100% to 17% of the cases, according to the exploration technique used and whether filiform or plexiform sinuses are taken into account.

The presence or absence of an IICS is quite never mentioned in pre-operative MRI protocols and most of the time, the neurosurgeon is unaware of whether a patent IICS will be found during surgery.

When analyzing a large number of pituitary MRIs, we have noticed that the IICS is almost always visible on coronal T2W sequences when pneumatization of the sphenoid sinus is incomplete, i.e., does not extend beyond the lowest point of the sellar floor, the nadir of the sella turcica (Fig. 7.3).

At the opposite, the IICS is almost never identified when the sphenoid is completely pneumatized (Fig. 7.5e–h), unless in pathological cases, such as with intracranial hypotension (Fig. 7.1)

We hypothesize that a slow extension of sphenoid sinus pneumatization from front to rear and from infancy to adolescence may lead to impaired development of the IICS. An argument is that the IICS is much more frequently identified in children, before sphenoid pneumatization onset, than in adults.

The IICS appears on coronal T2W images as a narrow band-like image visualized between the inferior border of the pituitary gland and the sphenoid, in

J.-F. Bonneville, *Tricks and Traps in MRI of the Pituitary Region*,
https://doi.org/10.1007/978-3-031-64710-9_7

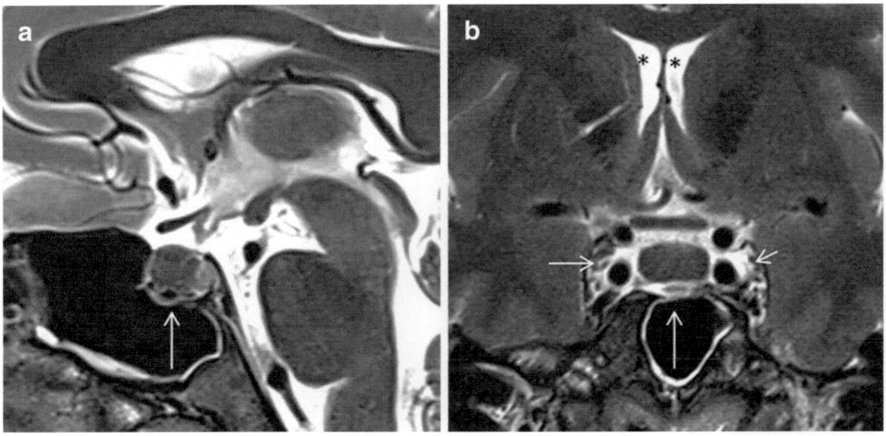

Fig. 7.1 Enlargement of IICS (arrow) and cavernous sinus veins (small arrows) with collapsed frontal horns (*) in a patient with intracranial hypotension. (**a**, **b**) Sagittal and coronal T2WIs

continuity with the parasellar veins, particularly the veins of the carotid sulcus. Its T2 signal is hyperintense in more than 9 out of 10 cases (Fig. 7.3). It is less often visible on CE T1W images. It is harder to identify on a sagittal T1W image where it may appear as a hypo or hyperintense tiny, rounded or target image or as a short band seen just above the sellar floor. On sagittal T2WI, at the difference with Rathke cleft or pars intermedia cyst, the band-like image of ICSS when visible is directed horizontally and not vertically (Fig. 7.4)

When sphenoid pneumatization is asymmetrical, the IICS is detected above the non-pneumatized sphenoid only (Fig. 7.5i–j).

The IICS may be unseen below intrasellar tumors and becomes visible after treatment such as in prolactinomas treated with cabergoline (Fig. 7.6).

The IICS is compressed and then never seen with large sellar tumors such as pituitary macroadenomas. Neurosurgeons know that they do not have trouble with the IICS which is compressed by large tumors but that hemorrhagic bleeding from the IICS may occur with small intrasellar tumors.

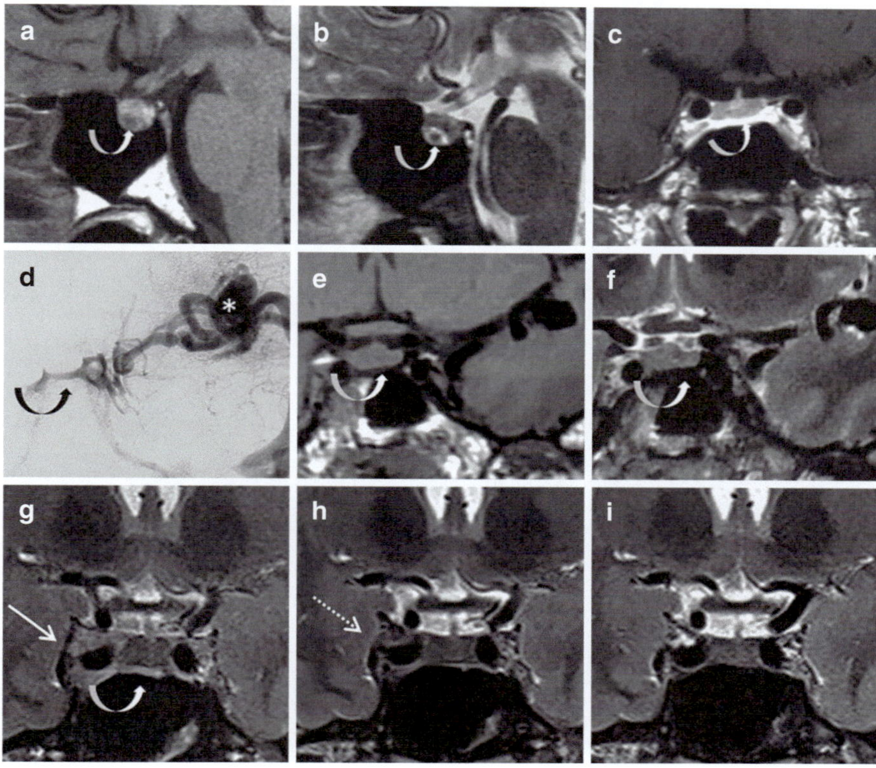

Fig. 7.2 (**a**–**c**) Enlargement of IICS after iterative lumbar punctures and secondary cranial hypotension. (**a**, **b**) Sagittal T1 and T2WIs. (**c**) Coronal CE T1 WI. (**d**–**f**) Enlargement of IICS (black arrow in **d**) with arteriovenous fistula. (**d**) Angiographic demonstration of the vascular shunt *; (**e**, **f**) Coronal T1 and T2WIs. (**g**–**i**) Prolactinoma invading the cavernous sinus in a 23-year-old man. Prolactin level is 1300 μG/L. Enlargement of IICS (curved arrow) which collapsed as well as the intracavernous pituitary adenoma (dotted arrow) after cabergoline treatment at 3 months (**h**) and 1 year (**i**) (**g**–**i**: Coronal T2WI)

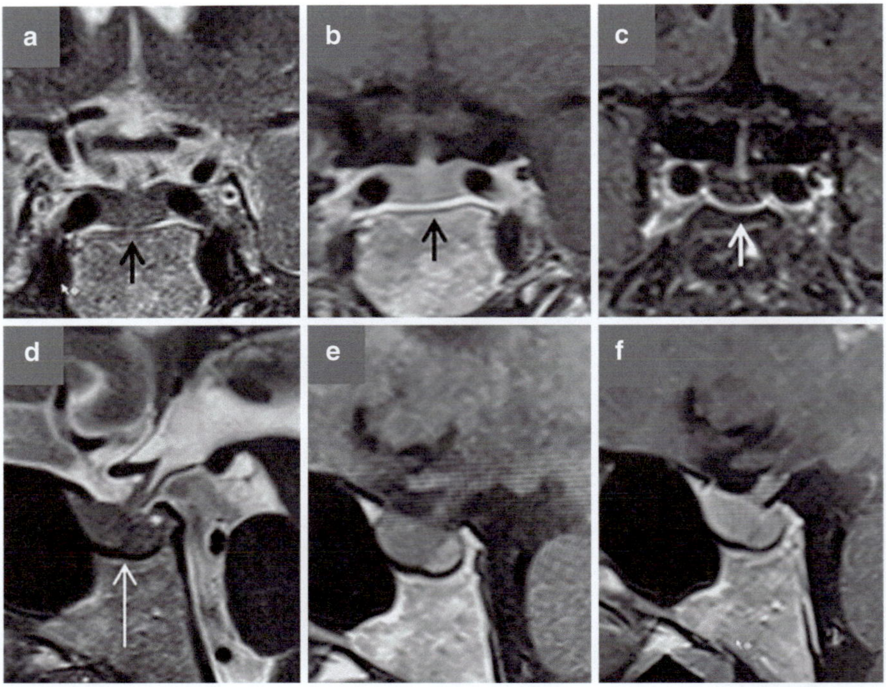

Fig. 7.3 Demonstration of IICS (arrows) above a partially pneumatized sphenoid sinus. The nadir of the sella is marked by a dotted arrow. (**a**–**c**) Coronal T2W, CE T1W and CE 3D FLAIR images. (**d**–**f**) Sagittal T2, T1 and CET1WIs. IICS is usually less visible or invisible on sagittal images unless large

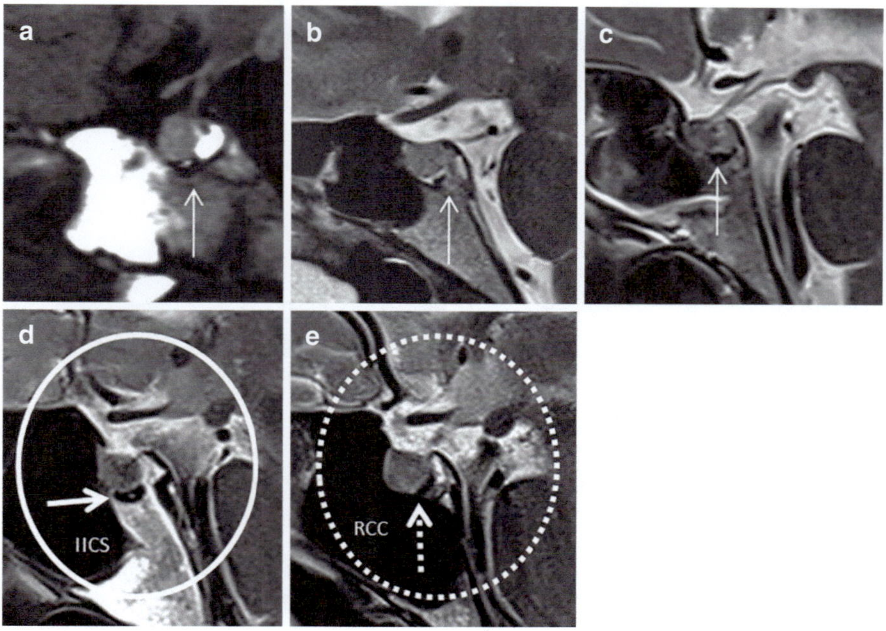

Fig. 7.4 Different aspects of normal IICS on sagittal views (**a–d**, arrows). Note that the sphenoid sinus pneumatization does not extend dorsally beyond the nadir of the sella. IICS is larger in children and then more frequently seen on sagittal images (**a**). At the difference with Rathke cleft cyst (**e**), the band-like image of ICSS is directed horizontally (**d**) and not vertically

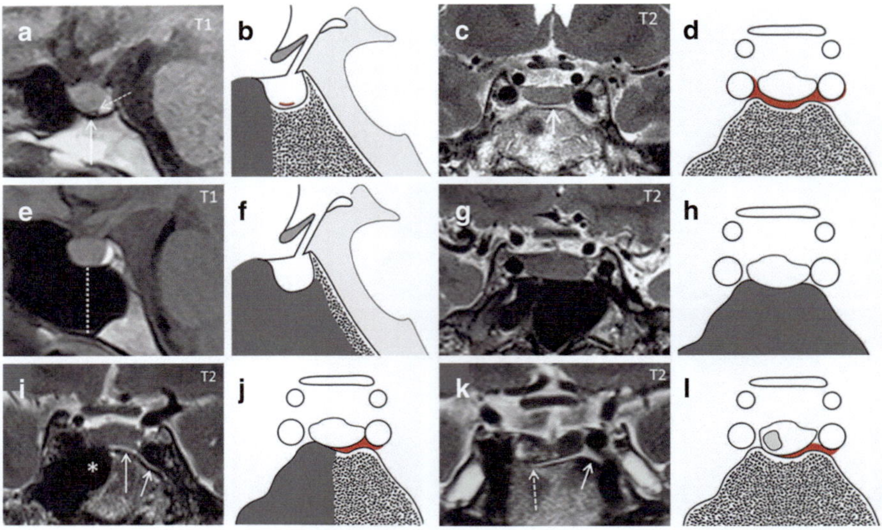

Fig. 7.5 (**a**–**d**) Usual aspect of IICS (arrows and red shapes on drawings) on sagittal T1 and coronal T2WIs. (**e**–**h**) The IICS is not shown when the sphenoid sinus pneumatization extends beyond the nadir of the sella (dotted line). (**i**, **j**) In case of asymmetrical pneumatization of sphenoid sinus, the IICS is demonstrated above the nonaerated sinus only. IICS is in continuity with parasellar veins, particularly the vein of the carotid sulcus (short arrows in **i** and **k**). (**k**, **l**) Compression of IICS by a microadenoma (dotted arrow)

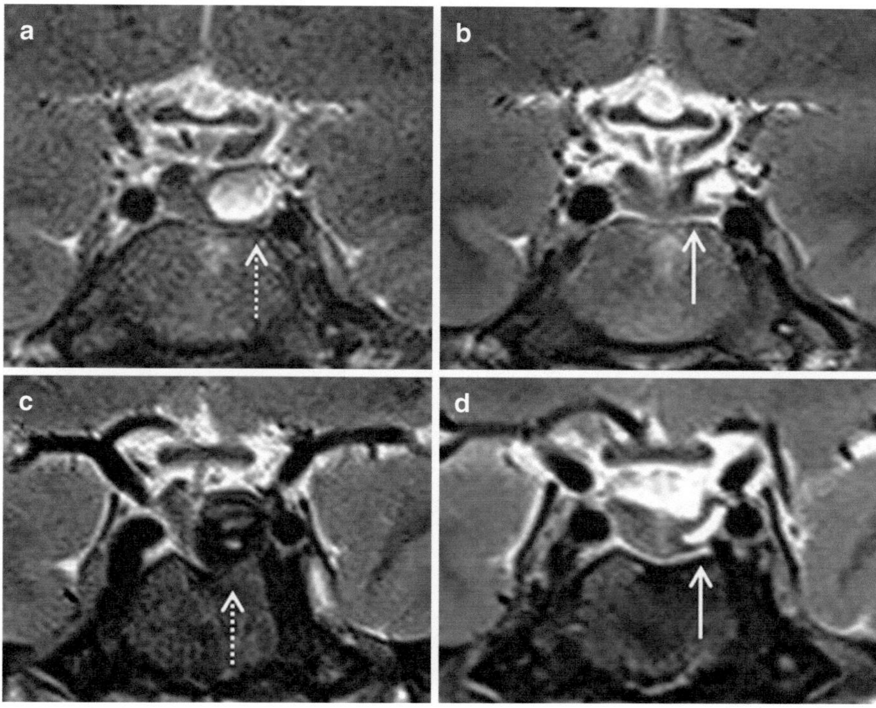

Fig. 7.6 Two examples of IICS compression by pituitary adenomas (**a**, **c**) relieved after treatment and tumor shrinkage (**b**, **d**). Note in both cases that the sphenoid is not pneumatized. (**a–d**) Coronal T2WIs. images

Further Readings

Bonneville JF, Cattin F, Bonneville F. Enlargement of the inferior intercavernous sinus: a new sign for the diagnosis of craniospinal hypotension. Am J Neuroradiol. 2011; https://doi.org/10.3174/ajnr.A2816.

Bonneville JF, Potorac I, Tshibanda L, Martin D, Petrossians P, Beckers A. Demonstration of the inferior intercavernous sinus is closely linked to the extent of pneumatization of the sphenoid sinus: useful information for the pituitary surgeon. Pituitary. 2022;25(6):861–7. https://doi.org/10.1007/s11102-022-01267-3.

Chenin L, Toussaint P, Lefranc M, et al. Microsurgical anatomy of the inferior intercavernous sinus. Surg Radiol Anat. 2021;43:211–8. https://doi.org/10.1007/s00276-020-02581-w.

Deng X, Chen S, Bai Y, et al. Vascular complications of intercavernous sinuses during transsphenoidal surgery: an anatomical analysis based on autopsy and magnetic resonance venography. PLoS ONE. 2015; https://doi.org/10.1371/journal.pone.01447.

8 The Small Sella and the Bulging Pituitary Gland

The upward bulging of the pituitary gland constitutes a frequent cause of concern in daily practice: is it a normal aspect or an indicator of a pituitary disease? Such an upward convexity can lead to unnecessary additional investigations and radiological follow-ups if an anatomical variant is not recognized.

A small sella turcica is a normal anatomical variant responsible for an inadequacy between the sellar volume and its content, with a resultant bulging of the pituitary gland which tends to come out like a brioche out of its mold (Fig. 8.1a, b). If not recognized, a small sella turcica can mimic a pathological enlargement of the pituitary gland and lead to a false diagnosis of pituitary hyperplasia or pituitary tumor. This is particularly true in teenage females who present an additional physiological enlargement of the pituitary gland.

A small sella turcica is frequently related to a hyperpneumatization of the sphenoid sinus defined by aeration extending beyond the spheno-occipital synchondrosis, in the pterygoid processes, in the dorsum sellae, or giving rise to a blistering of the planum sphenoidale. The over-pneumatization of the sphenoid sinus inhibits the complete development of the pituitary fossa and can be associated with a flat or narrow sella and a resultant bulging of the pituitary gland (Fig. 8.1c, d). A thick dorsum sellae, either pneumatized or fatty, can also diminish the anteroposterior diameter of the pituitary fossa.

The sella turcica can also be short transversally: this condition is less clearly perceived because the general image of the sella is much less recognized in coronal than on sagittal views. But there is a good trick: a long time ago, it was noted that only 2 out 100 adults present a sellar floor width of <10 mm. Therefore, an upward convex pituitary gland above a sellar floor <10 mm wide is very likely to be a variant of normal. Such a narrow sellar floor can sometimes be suspected when a short transverse diameter of the head is noted (Fig. 8.2).

In daily practice, in front of an intriguing upward convex pituitary gland with normal T1 and T2 signals and normal enhancement after gadolinium injection, a mismatch between the pituitary volume and the sellar capacity has to be evoked first and a small sella must be looked for. A non-compressed normal posterior pituitary

J.-F. Bonneville, *Tricks and Traps in MRI of the Pituitary Region*,
https://doi.org/10.1007/978-3-031-64710-9_8

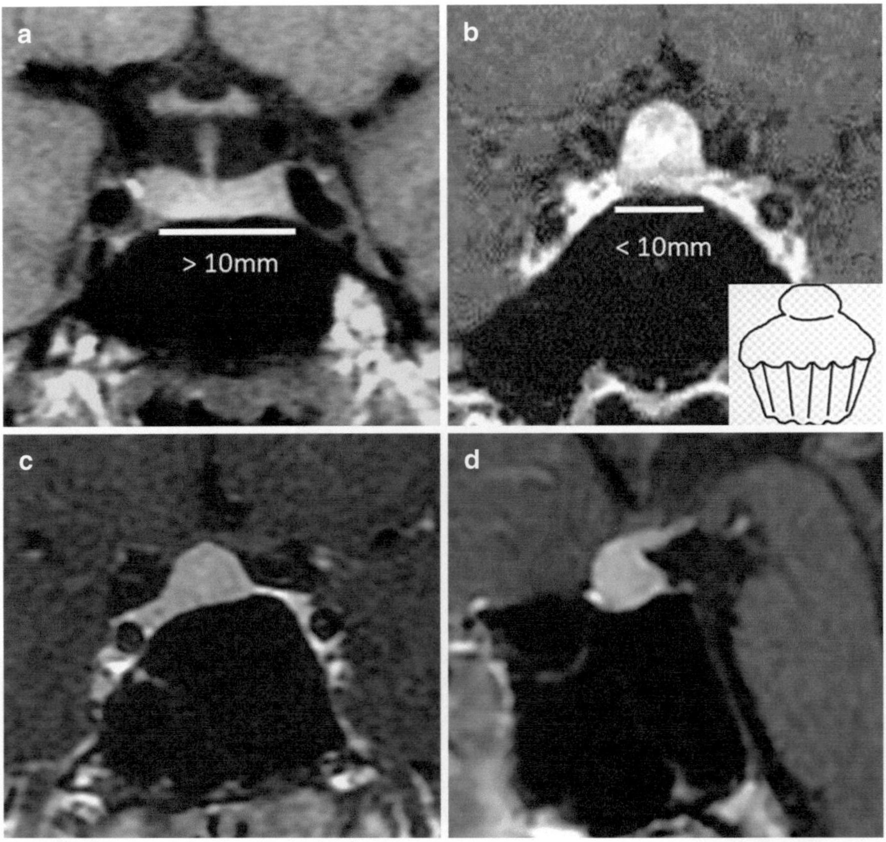

Fig. 8.1 Upper row. Illustration of the relationship between the width of the sellar floor and the shape of the pituitary gland on coronal CE T1WIs. (**a**) Normal sellar floor. (**b**) Narrow sellar floor. Lower row. Bulging pituitary gland in a flat sella above a hyperpneumatized sphenoid sinus. (**a–d**) CE T1WIs

lobe shown on axial view will eliminate a mass effect and confirm a variant of normal (Fig. 3.6).

Other rarer factors can influence the effective volume of the sella turcica, such as tortuous carotid siphons (Fig. 8.3a), a large inferior intercavernous sinus (Fig. 8.3b) or an embryonic remnant emerging from the dorsum sellae called sellar spine (Fig. 8.4 and Chap. 35).

The differential diagnosis of a bulging pituitary gland includes mainly isointense pituitary adenoma or Rathke cleft cyst or pituitary hyperplasia. An ignored or masked pregnancy in a woman of child-bearing age must also be kept in mind.

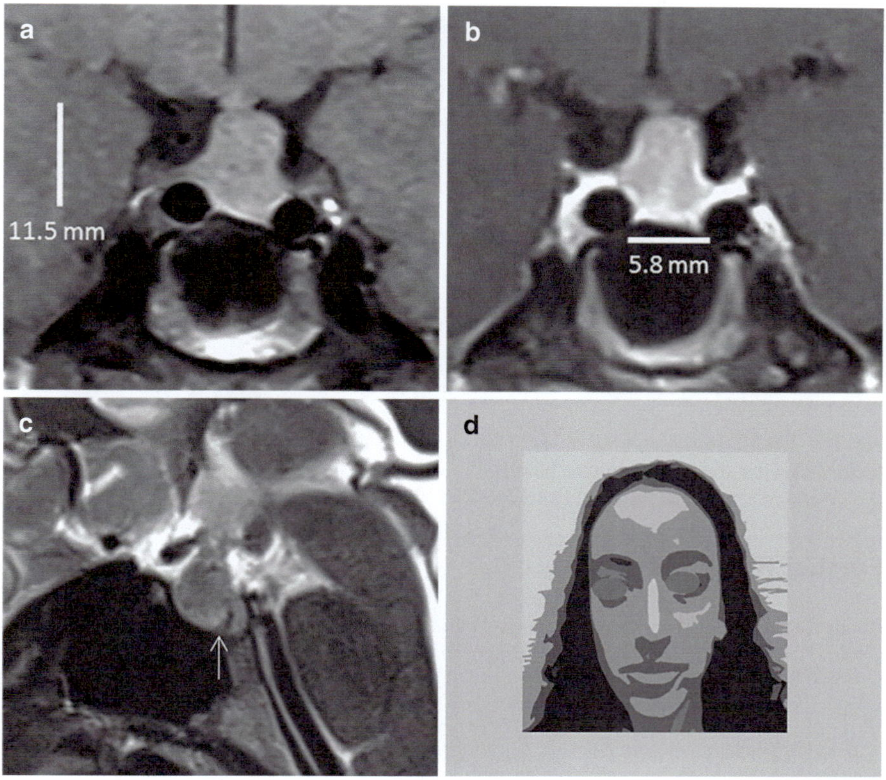

Fig. 8.2 Anatomical variant. Extreme narrowness of the sellar floor and confusing height of the pituitary gland abutting the optic chiasm. Coronal T1 and CE T1WIs (**a**, **b**) and sagittal T2WI (**c**). Note a short transverse diameter of the head (**d**). Incidental common Rathke cleft/pars intermedia cyst (arrow in **c**)

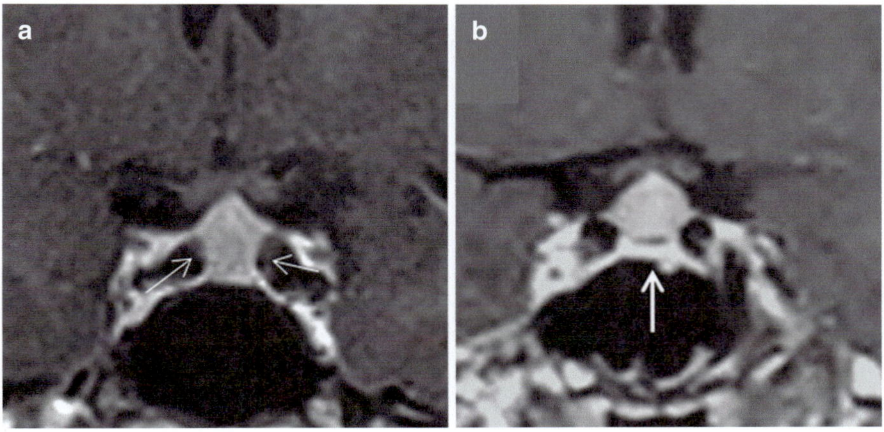

Fig. 8.3 Normal upward convexity of the upper surface of the pituitary gland on coronal CE T1WIs. (**a**) With elongated carotid siphons. (**b**) With a thick inferior intercavernous sinus

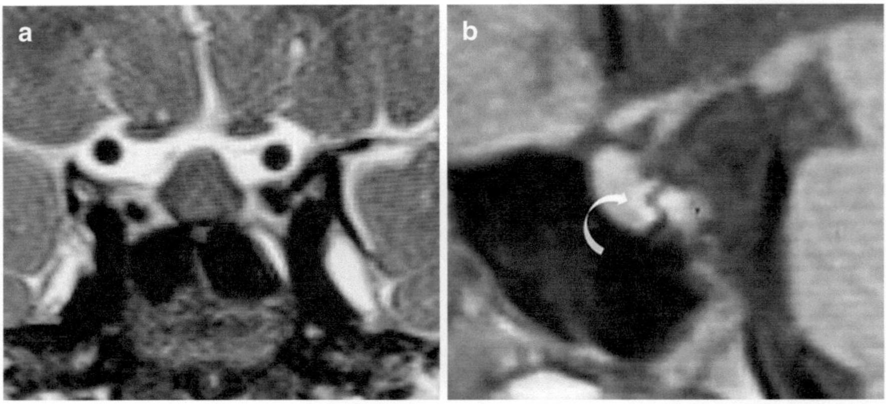

Fig. 8.4 Multifactorial bulging of the pituitary gland. Precocious puberty in a 6-year-old girl. Incidental sellar spine distorting the posterior lobe (arrow). Thick dorsum sellae with short antero-posterior diameter of the sella. (**a**) Coronal T2WI. (**b**) Sagittal TIWI

Further Readings

Bonneville JF. When the pituitary swells up a little. J Radiol. 2002;83(3):319–20.

Cattin F, Bonneville JF, Tang YS. Diagnostic d'une hypophyse convexe. Rev Inst Med. 1990;2:221–8.

9 The Myth of Dynamic MRI

In many radiological centers, dynamic MRI is considered a must and an obligatory part of any MRI of the pituitary region. It is our opinion that this sequence is only really helpful in a very limited number of circumstances and consequently must not be performed routinely. In the specific and very usual situation where a pituitary microadenoma is being looked for, dynamic MRI is no more informative than high-resolution optimized sequences, particularly the T2W sequence. Moreover, dynamic MRI is likely to cause misdiagnoses.

The goal of dynamic imaging is to capture as early as possible the enhancement of the pituitary stalk, the pituitary gland, and the surrounding vascular structures after intravenous injection of gadolinium as well as to follow the washout until about the second minute.

The first application of this principle was dynamic computed tomography in the 1980s: thanks to an ultrafast acquisition time (1–2 s), dynamic CT was able to capture the enhancement of the secondary capillary bed, an unpaired median vascular structure located below the sellar diaphragm, in the prolongation of the pituitary stalk—which we have called the *pituitary tuft*. Its visualization occurred approximately 10 s after the optimal enhancement of the internal carotid arteries. Its displacement was considered the earliest sign of a mass effect in the sella and was a useful adjunct for the diagnosis of isodense microadenomas. Today, the pituitary tuft is inconsistently demonstrated on 3D CE FLAIR (Fig. 9.1e).

Spatial and contrast resolutions of MRI have made dynamic CT quickly obsolete when the tumor was directly demonstrated through its T1 or T2W signal or after gadolinium injection. Dynamic MRI was proposed to try to optimize these results. But, the long acquisition time (20 s) usually required for dynamic MRI, if compared with dynamic CT, is not a favorable factor in catching early enhancement of the pituitary tuft. Recently, a sequence with a reduced acquisition time of a few seconds named GRASP (Golden-Angle Radial Sparse Parallel) has been proposed to overcome this disadvantage, but its spatial resolution is low and its results are not really convincing (Fig. 9.1).

J.-F. Bonneville, *Tricks and Traps in MRI of the Pituitary Region*,
https://doi.org/10.1007/978-3-031-64710-9_9

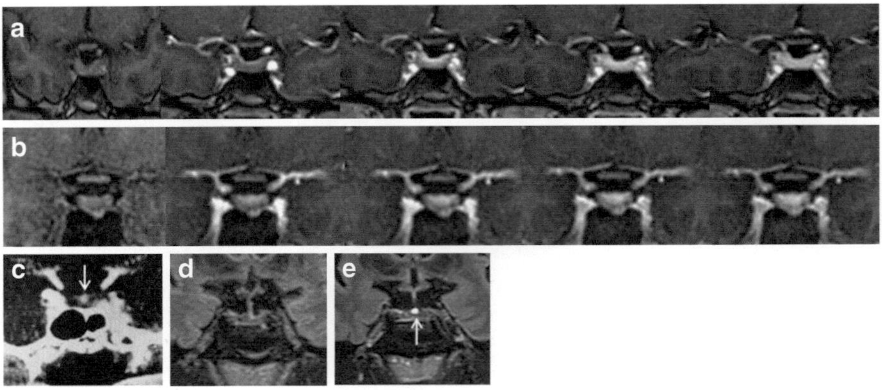

Fig. 9.1 (**a**) Usual dynamic MRI (acquisition time: 20 s) versus; (**b**) GRASP (AT: 4 s). The pituitary tuft on dynamic CT in 1983; (**c**) and 3D CE FLAIR (**d**, **e**)

Dynamic MRI has been proposed to differentiate the different types of secreting pituitary adenomas. For instance, it has been claimed that somatotropinomas present a weaker enhancement pattern in the early and delayed phases. Such an assertion, if confirmed in large series, would have a very poor interest in real life, the diagnosis of acromegaly being made clinically and by hormonal dosage.

In the diagnosis of picoadenomas of Cushing disease, dynamic MRI has not proved its superiority over 3D Gradient Echo contrast-enhanced MRI with inframillimetric acquisitions.

It has been said that defects in enhancement during dynamic MRI could favor the diagnosis of cysts versus pituitary adenomas, but this statement is invalid with cystic or hemorrhagic pituitary adenomas.

Generally speaking, dynamic MRI is not useful for the diagnosis of pituitary microadenomas and must not be systematically performed. Moreover, dynamic MRI may be the source of a misdiagnosis: an off-midline posterior lobe, a frequent anatomical variant, may be mistaken for a displaced secondary capillary bed (Fig. 9.2). Asymmetry of the pituitary gland is another common trap.

We consider that dynamic MRI should be reserved for research purpose or for specific rare cases such as to differentiate a meningioma extending to the sella from a pituitary adenoma extending outside the sella although T2WI usually makes the diagnosis (Fig. 9.3).

Hypophysitis is another potential indication: the inflammatory process could be better shown in the early phase of dynamic MRI (Fig. 9.4).

Dynamic MRI could help for differentiating symptomatic and non-symptomatic RCCs in difficult cases (Fig. 25.3) but 3D CE FLAIR is more reliable (Fig. 25.4).

Cavernous sinus hemangioma is a rare example of the real usefulness of dynamic MRI. This vascular malformation lies in the cavernous sinus and can extend into the sella turcica. Its T2W hypointense signal is not specific at all. Dynamic MRI demonstrates the characteristic pattern of a slow centripetal enhancement of the mass (Fig. 9.5).

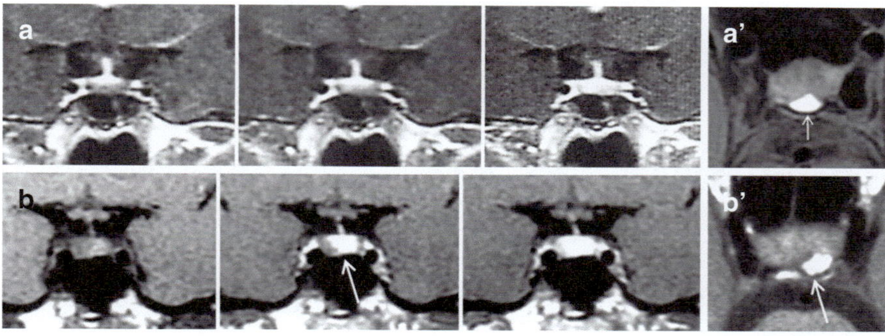

Fig 9.2 (**a**) Normal dynamic MRI with a posterior lobe on midline (short arrow). (**b**) Normal dynamic MRI with a posterior lobe off midline (long arrow): asymmetrical early enhancement and pituitary stalk tilting mimicking a pituitary adenoma at the early phase of dynamic MR. (**a′**) and (**b′**) are axial T1WIs

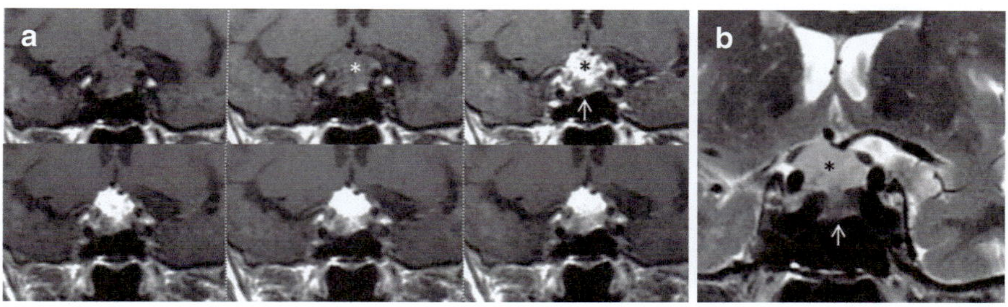

Fig. 9.3 Suprasellar meningioma. (**a**) Dynamic MRI. Strong enhancement of the meningioma (*) well before that of the pituitary gland (arrow). (**b**) Coronal T2WI

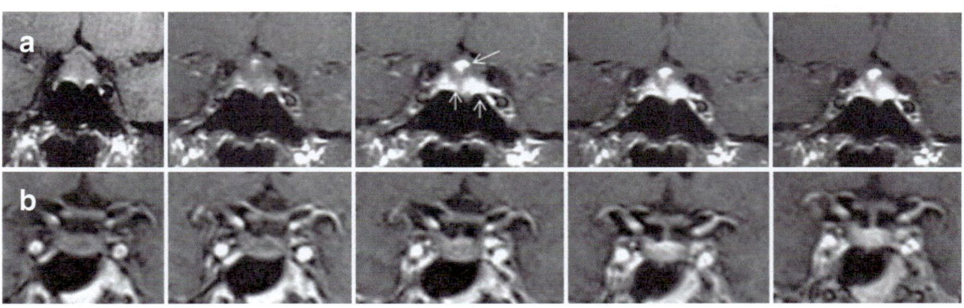

Fig. 9.4 Upper row. Lymphocytic hypophysitis at its early phase (**a**). Rapid and intense enhancement of patchy areas (arrows). Lower row. Post immunotherapy hypophysitis (**b**). Delayed pituitary enhancement at the phase of hypophysitis sequellae

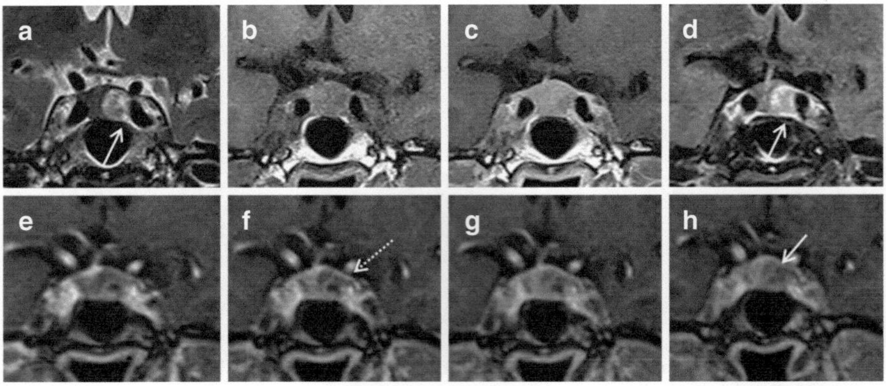

Fig. 9.5 Cavernous sinus hemangioma. (**a**) T2W hyperintense intracavernous and intrasellar mass. The lesion is poorly demonstrated on T1 and CE T1WIs (**b**, **c**), but well shown on a delayed CE T1WI (**d**). On dynamic MRI (**e–h**), slow centripetal enhancement from the peripheral (dotted arrow) to the central zone of the mass (arrow)

In conclusion, we would like to remind that dynamic MRI has no place as a first choice in the diagnosis of sellar masses, nor in the assessment of hyperprolactinemia and must be reserved for rare and specific cases or for research purpose.

Further Readings

Amano T, Masumoto T, Akutsu H, Sakamoto N, Hoshiai S, Mori K, Nakajima T. The utility of dynamic MRI in differentiating the hormone-producing ability of pituitary adenomas. Jpn J Radiol. 2021;39(8):741–8. https://doi.org/10.1007/s11604-021-01121-9.

Bonneville JF, Cattin F, Gorczyca W, Hardy J. Pituitary microadenomas: early enhancement with dynamic CT--implications of arterial blood supply and potential importance. Radiology. 1993;187(3):857–61. https://doi.org/10.1148/radiology.187.3.8497646.

Hainc N, Stippich C, Reinhardt J, et al. Golden-angle radial sparse parallel (GRASP) MRI in clinical routine detection of pituitary microadenomas: first experience and feasibility. Magn Reson Imaging. 2019;60:38–43. https://doi.org/10.1016/j.mri.2019.03.015.

Pitfalls and Traps

10

A high number of artifacts mimicking or masking a pituitary lesion have to be clarified when reading a pituitary MRI. Many can be solved by technical means or by changing MR parameters. The most frequent artifacts and several common anatomical variants are shown here only.

Partial volume effects from the carotid artery or the sphenoid sinus (Fig. 10.1) are cleared by millimetric slices, multiplanar acquisition, or better by volume acquisition. In their absence, Flair can help (Fig. 10.1g–i).

Magnetic susceptibility artifacts occur at air and bone or soft tissue interfaces and are more pronounced with curved surfaces. They result in localized geometric distortion and signal intensity changes. At the sellar floor level, they can mask a pituitary abnormality and at the planum level mimic a blistering announcing a meningioma (Fig. 10.2c, d). More prominent at 3.0 Tesla, they can be eliminated by changing the bandwidth or by using a FLAIR sequence.

The sellar spine, a notochordal bony remnant arising from the dorsum sellae, can induce a disturbing target-like picture (Fig. 10.3a–c).

Chemical shift artifacts are related to the T1W high signal of some tissues, for instance fat in the dorsum sellae; they are eliminated by a fat saturation sequence which must be systematically used for assessment of vasopressin storage on axial T1W sequence (Fig. 3.2).

A small sella, a flat sella, or a narrow sella with a sellar floor width of less than 10mm can be responsible for an upward bulging of the pituitary simulating a sellar mass (Fig. 10.4a–c).

A deep imprint of the posterior lobe thinning the dorsum sellae could also be tricky on coronal T2W images (Fig. 10.3d–f).

Flow artifacts can be troublesome, such as those from the CSF in the suprasellar or peduncular cistern on coronal T2W images (Fig. 10.2a, b) which can mask the pituitary stalk or from the intracavernous internal carotid artery (Fig. 10.1d–f). Application of saturation bands is a way to reduce them. Flow artifacts are also reduced on the 3D FLAIR sequence.

J.-F. Bonneville, *Tricks and Traps in MRI of the Pituitary Region*,
https://doi.org/10.1007/978-3-031-64710-9_10

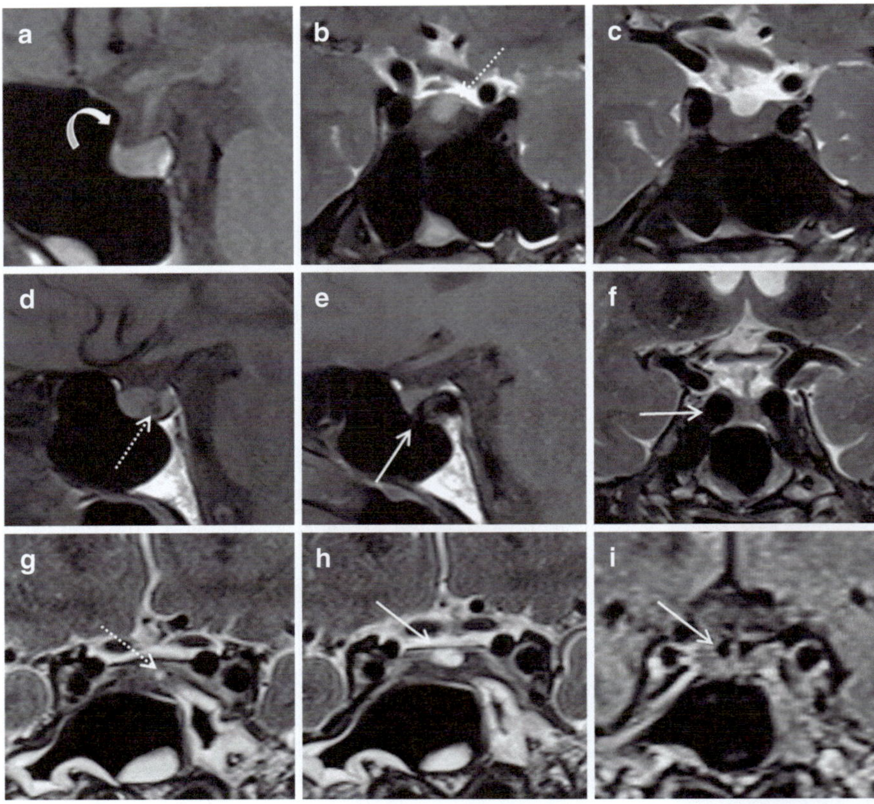

Fig. 10.1 Partial volume artifacts (dotted arrows). Upper row. Resulting from a cornice-like tuberculum sellae (curved arrow) overhanging the pituitary fossa. (**a**–**c**) Sagittal T1 and coronal T2WIs. Middle row. Resulting from kissing carotid arteries (arrows). (**d**, **e**) Sagittal T1WIs; (**f**) Coronal T2WI. Lower row. Partial empty sella simulating a microincidentaloma. (**g**, **h**) Coronal T2WIs. (**i**) Coronal FLAIR favors intrasellar CSF extension

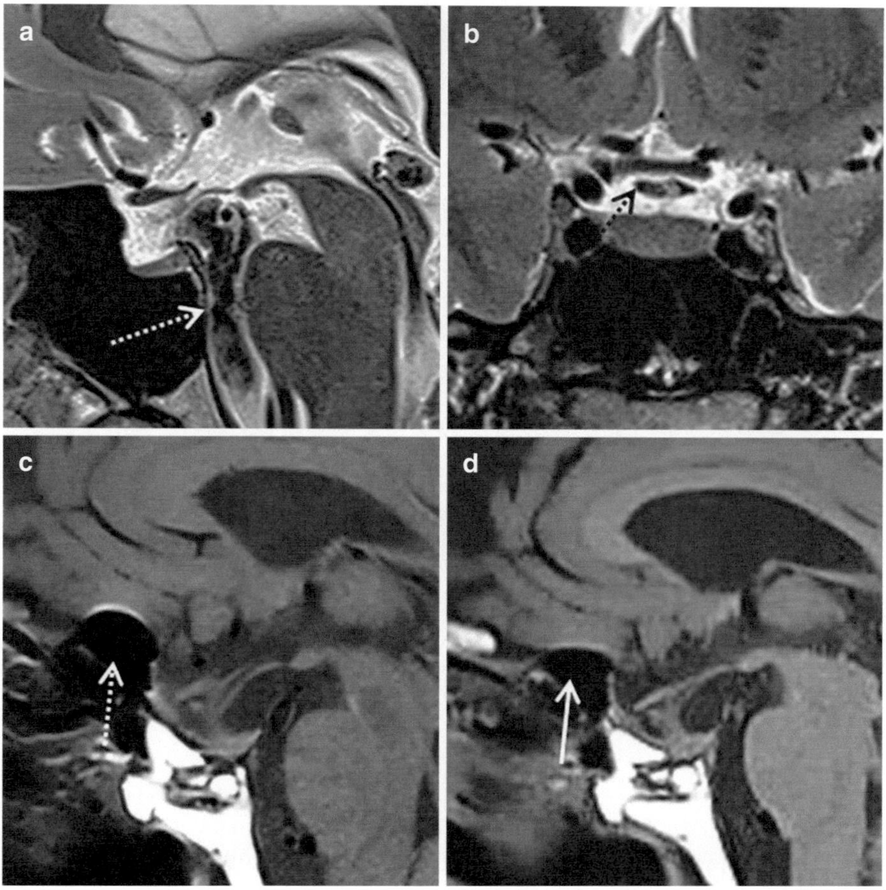

Fig. 10.2 Upper row. Flow artifacts. (**a**) From the CSF and the basilar artery in the pre-pontine cistern. (**b**) False double optic chiasm image resulting from flow artifacts from CSF in the suprasellar cistern. Lower row. Magnetic susceptibility artifact responsible of a false blistering of the jugum sphenoidale (dotted arrow in **c**). Correction of the artifact after changing the bandwidth (**d**). (**a**, **b**) Sagittal and coronal T2WIs. (**c**, **d**) Sagittal T1WIs

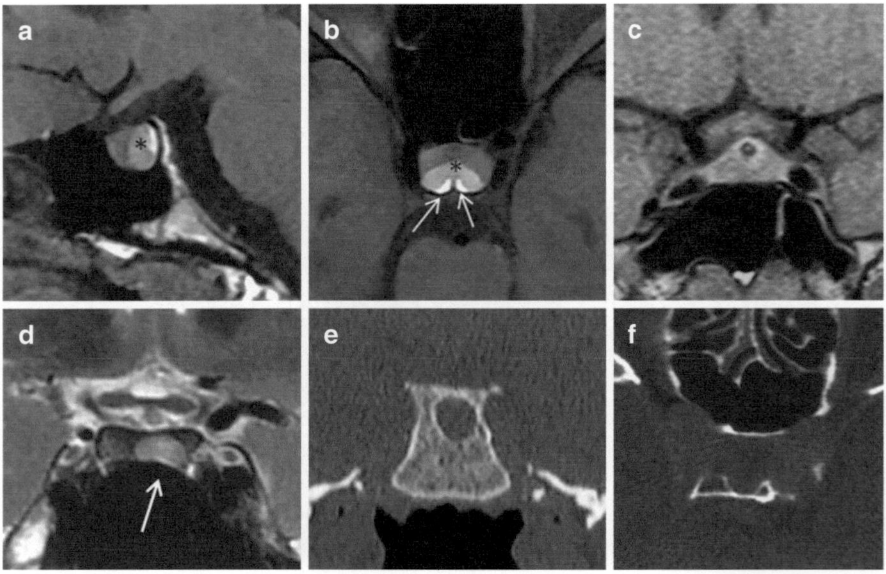

Fig. 10.3 Upper row. Sellar spine piercing the posterior lobe (arrows) and a Rathke cleft cyst (*). (**a**, **b**) Sagittal T1 and axial T1 Fatsat WIs. (**c**) Sellar spine surrounded by the distorted posterior lobe on coronal T1WI in another patient. Lower row. Imprint of the posterior lobe on the dorsum sellae simulating a pituitary adenoma (arrow). (**d**) Coronal T2WI. (**e**, **f**) Coronal and axial CT

A large inferior intercavernous sinus can simulate a microadenoma on a sagittal view (Fig. 10.4g–i). The concomitant presence of an incomplete sphenoid sinus pneumatization can draw attention (see Chap. 7). *Anterior and posterior intercavernous sinuses* also are sometimes visible (Fig. 10.4d–f).

Differential diagnosis of a thickened pituitary stalk is discussed in Chap. 6. We will mention here the most usual, such as the lengthening of the infundibular recess of the third ventricle, the Rathke cleft cyst localized at the stalk level, and what we have named an Infundibular Unidentified Object (IUO).

Artifacts caused by *dynamic imaging* are related to the asymmetry of the pituitary gland wings or an off-midline position of the posterior lobe. Dynamic imaging should not be used routinely but reserved for rare specific situations (see Chap. 9).

The misjudgment of a pituitary tumor or remnant growth is unfortunately common in everyday practice and can lead to erroneous management. This mistake will not occur when coronal views are always rigorously obtained in the same projection, as recommended in several places in this book (Fig. 10.5)

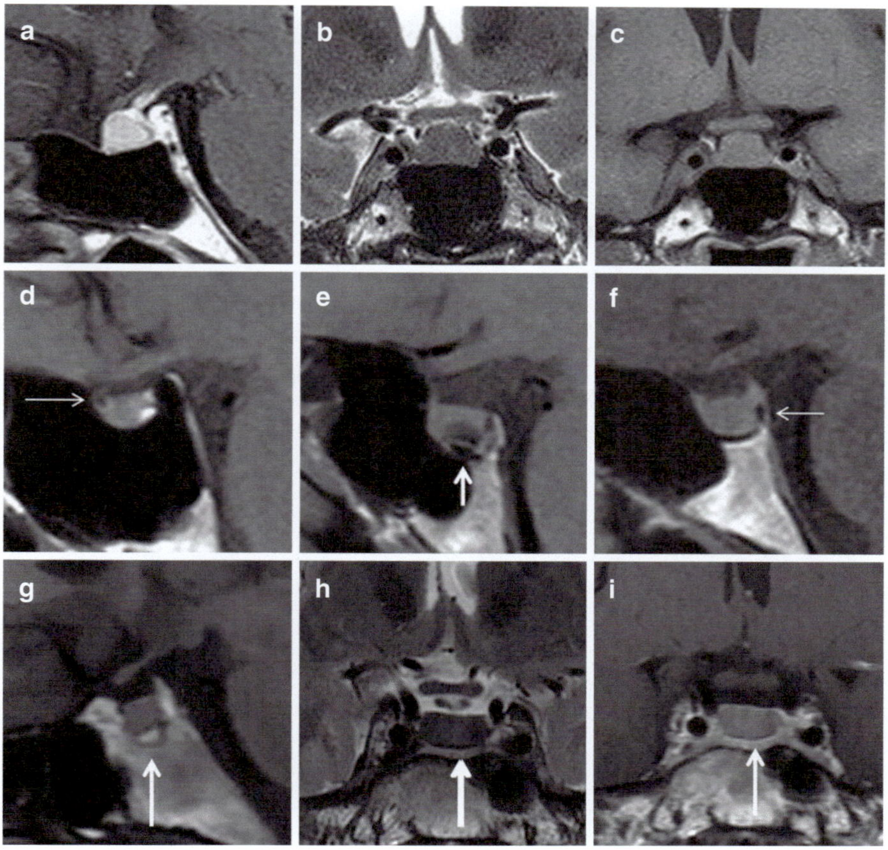

Fig. 10.4 Upper row. Flat sella. Normal pituitary gland abutting the optic chiasm mimicking a sellar mass. (**a**) Sagittal CE T1WI. (**b**, **c**) Coronal T2 and T1WIs. Middle row. Intercavernous venous connections. (**d**) Anterior, (**e**) Inferior, (**f**) Posterior intercavernous sinuses. (**d–f**) Sagittal T1WIs. Lower row (**g–i**) Inferior intercavernous sinus (thick arrows). (**g**) Sagittal T1WI. (**h**, **i**) Coronal T2 and CE T1 WIs

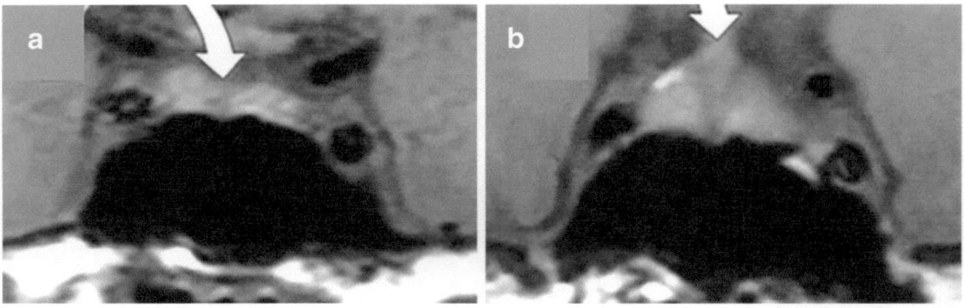

Fig. 10.5 During follow-up of pituitary lesions, coronal sections must be always oriented according to the same landmark. The subcallosal line is very convenient to draw and remains unchanged whatever the evolution or the treatment. Changing the orientation of the sequences between two examinations may lead to an erroneous measure of the pituitary content. (**a**, **b**) Coronal T1WIs performed with different projections on the same day

11 In Young Children, Made Quick and Simple

We will only consider here the most common indications of MRI of the hypothalamic-pituitary region in children, that is, growth retardation or puberty troubles. MRI of pituitary hypersecretion syndromes such as Cushing's disease or hyperprolactinemia is presented in dedicated chapters as well as polyuro-polydipsic syndrome which, in a child, must lead to fear the presence of a germinoma. Pilocytic astrocytoma of the suprasellar region is evoked in Chap. 29.

Many young children dread MRI and may be restless, making the examination of poor quality or even impossible, but it is often possible to avoid general anesthesia or even premedication. A few simple rules are to be followed by the radiologist:

- Give the child a short explanation of the examination.
- Tell him/her that there will be no injection.
- The presence of a parent, usually the mother, within the MRI room can help.
- Of course, the presence of the radiologist is mandatory to choose if necessary the MR sequences in real time.
- The localizer can bring useful information (it is not a joke) and must not be neglected in a restless child. For instance in a girl with advanced puberty who cannot stand still, the localizer image obtained in seconds may give an acceptable image of the stalk, the pituitary gland, and the bright spot of the posterior lobe and can help to decide if it worth to schedule a MRI with sedation or general anesthesia.
- A brain axial FLAIR sequence eliminates a tumor or a malformation at distance from the pituitary region.
- Select a limited number of MR sequences, the sagittal T1 and T2W sequences being essential and could be enough in some cases, if the child does not accept one more.
- Of course if a tumor is revealed, an additional MRI will be scheduled and under general anesthesia if necessary.

J.-F. Bonneville, *Tricks and Traps in MRI of the Pituitary Region*,
https://doi.org/10.1007/978-3-031-64710-9_11

In a child with precocious puberty, pay particularly close attention to boys where advanced puberty is rare and more frequently caused by tumors than in girls. Indeed, precocious puberty appears idiopathic in 90% of girls affected versus only 30% of boys. Therefore, it can be recommended that MRI be performed in all boys with precocious puberty and only in girls with pubertal symptoms starting before age of six years and with hormone levels higher than expected for pubertal stage. Tumors of the pineal gland which are exceptionally responsible of precocious puberty have to be differentiated from common pineal cysts.

In idiopathic precocious puberty, the pituitary gland may be enlarged with bulging of the sellar diaphragm. A tongue-like upward extension of the anterior pituitary is sometimes observed (Figs. 11.1 and 21.1).

Hypothalamic hamartomas can induce precocious puberty. They are made of normal gray matter located in an ectopic position at the tuber cinereum level (Fig. 11.2). The tuber cinereum belongs to the hypothalamus and is part of the floor of the third ventricle (Fig. 1.1). It is recognized on a T2W sagittal view as a thin hypointense short band extending from the infundibulum to the mammillary bodies which enhances after gadolinium injection. Hamartomas must not be mistaken with the mammillary bodies which are located just behind. The size of hamartomas can vary from a few millimeters to a few centimeters (Fig. 11.2d–f). Rarely, a tiny hamartoma can develop within the hypothalamus and be barely visible on sagittal view. Hamartomas are usually pedunculated but can be sessile and these may cause gelastic seizures. The signal of hamartomas is usually similar to this of the gray matter in all sequences and they usually do not enhance after gadolinium injection. In case of abnormal signal or enhancement, a hypothalamic glioma may be suspected.

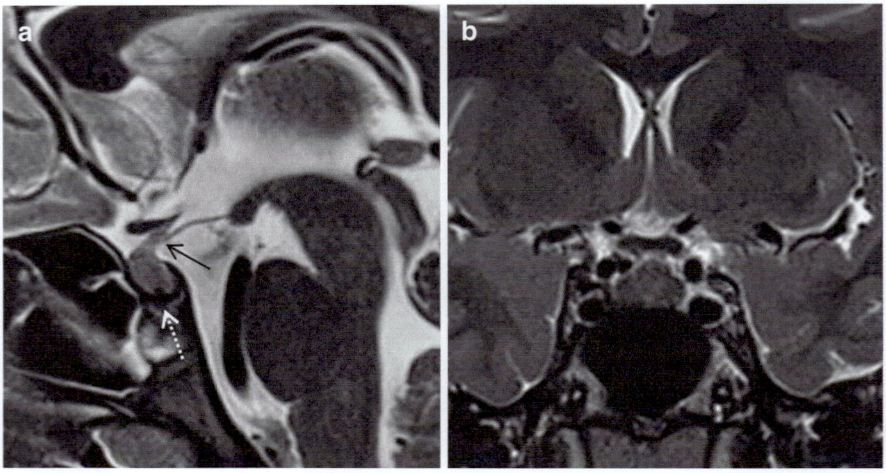

Fig. 11.1 Physiologic advanced puberty in a 7-year-old girl. Sagittal T2WI (**a**) shows a convex sellar diaphragm with an upward tongue-like extension of the anterior pituitary gland (black arrow). Normal well-developed inferior intercavernous sinus (dotted arrow). (**b**) Physiological pituitary hyperplasia in a 13-year-old pubescent girl on coronal T2WI

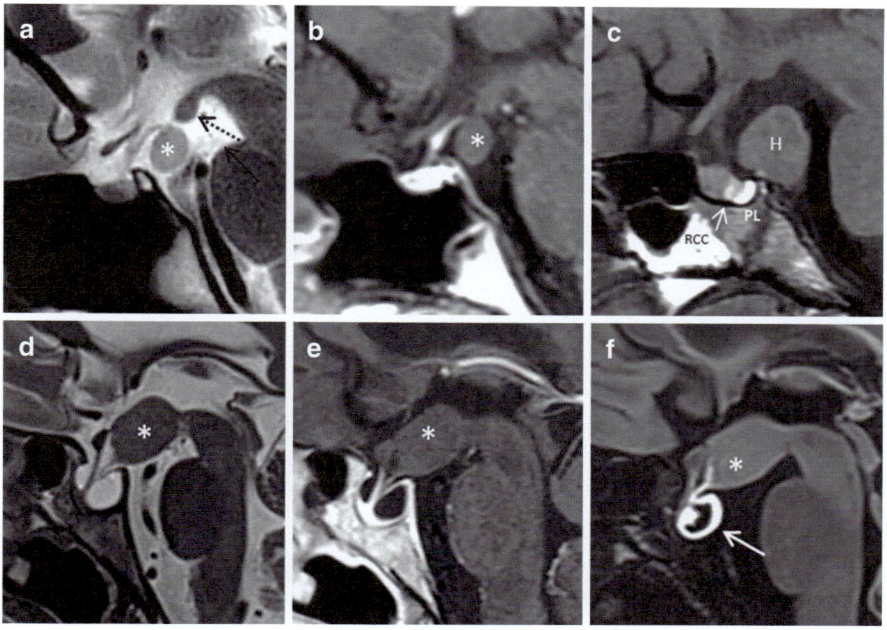

Fig. 11.2 Upper row. Pedunculated hamartomas*. Normal mamillary bodies (black dotted arrow). (**a**, **b**) Sagittal T2 and CE T1WIs. (**c**) Sagittal T1WI. Large hamartoma (h) seeming free in the prepontine cistern. Incidental Rathke cleft cyst (arrow)Lower row. Large sessile hamartoma (*) in a patient with Pallister-Hall syndrome and polydactyly. 3D CE T2 FLAIR (f) reveals an intrasellar cystic lesion inconspicuous on T2 (**d**) and CE T1WI (**e**)

In a child with growth retardation and growth hormone deficiency, a craniopharyngioma must be first eliminated (Chap. 28). Afterward MRI must look for an abnormality of the pituitary stalk and/or the posterior pituitary and evaluate the anterior pituitary volume. Anomaly of these three anatomical structures constitute the classical triade. Sagittal T1 and T2W sequences are here clearly complementary. In accordance with recent recommendations, a gadolinium injection is spared in the first intention, the CE T1W sagittal sequence being advantageously replaced by a T2W sequence.

– *The posterior lobe* must be sharply shown, normally in front of the dorsum sellae and strictly adjacent to its anterior surface as best appreciated on an axial T1W view and distinguished from a possible mucinous Rathke cyst which is not rare in children (Figs. 11.2c and 3.3). The posterior lobe can be ectopic either at the infundibulum or at different levels along the pituitary stalk (Fig. 11.3a–d). Vasopressin storage can be also seen together in eutopic position and along the pituitary stalk (Fig. 11.4c and d). An ectopic posterior lobe located at the infundibulum can mimic a lipoma attached to the tuber cinereum (Fig. 11.3 e and f).

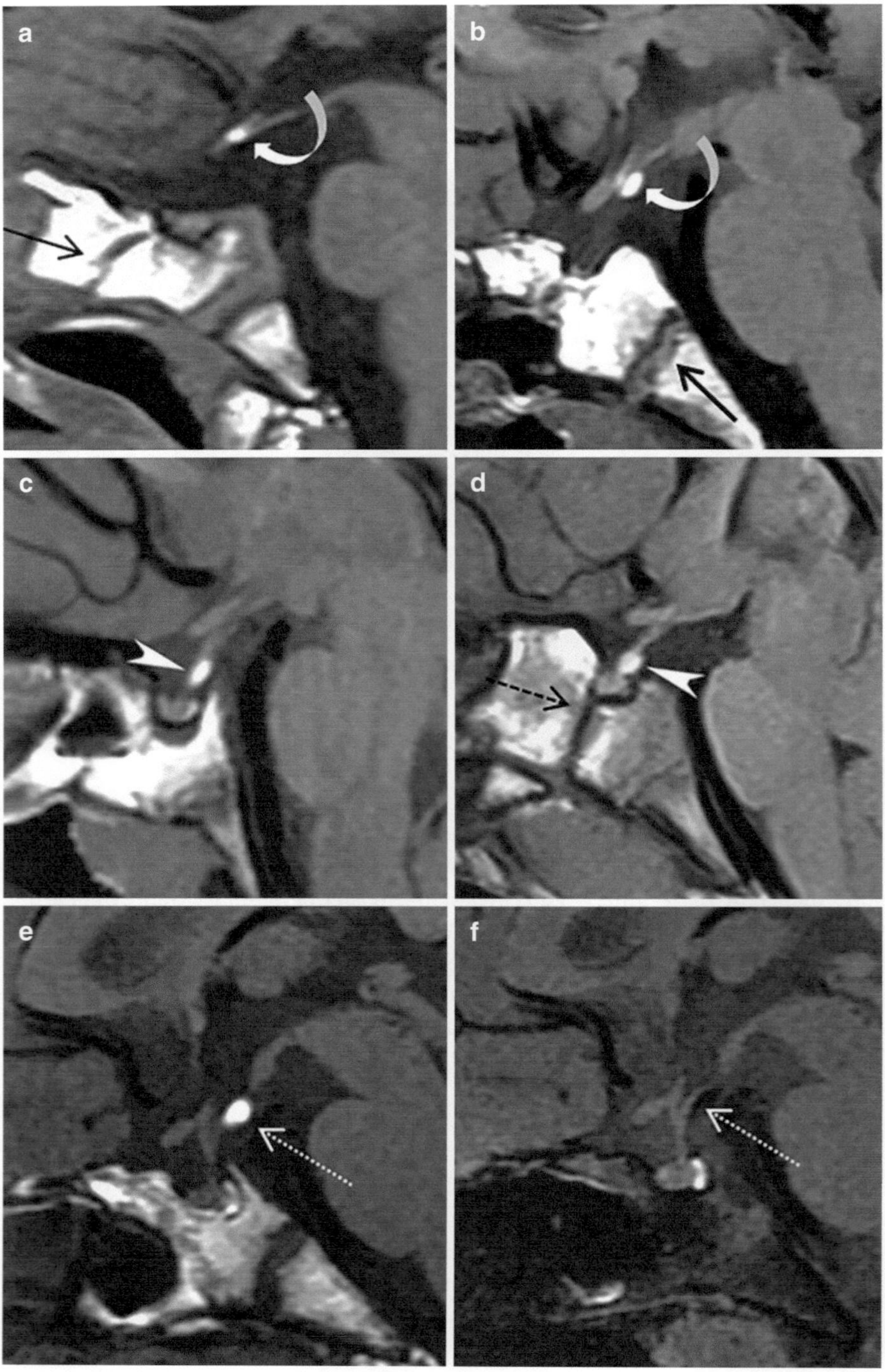

Fig. 11.3 Interrupted Pituitary Stalk Syndrome (IPSS) in four children. Ectopic posterior lobe at the infundibulum and along the pituitary stalk on sagittal T1WIs (**a–d**). (**a**) Septo-optic dysplasia. Intersphenoid suture (arrow). Large spheno-occipital synchondrosis in (**b**) Persistent craniopharyngeal canal in d. (**e** and **f**) Differential diagnosis. Lipoma of the tuber cinereum on sagittal T1WI (**e**), erased on Fatsat T1WI (**f**)

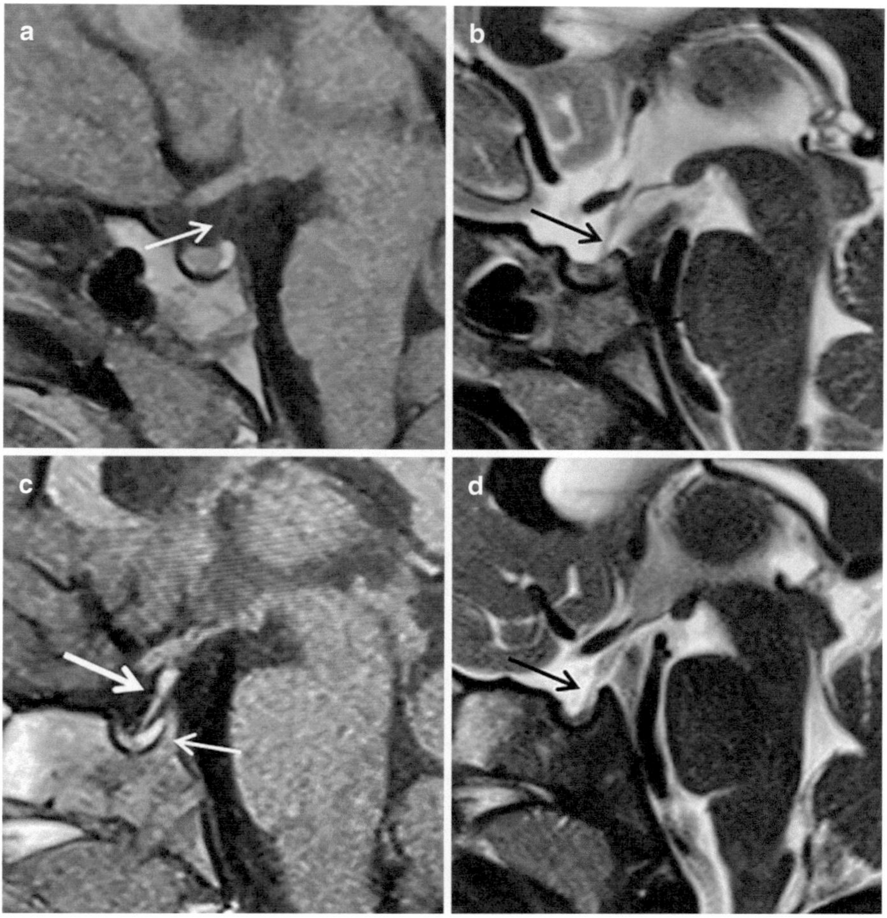

Fig. 11.4 IPSS in two 7-year-old children. (**a** and **b**) With partial GH deficit. Anterior pituitary gland and posterior lobe are normal. The only abnormality is a hypoplastic pituitary stalk (arrow). Delayed sphenoid pneumatization. (**c** and **d**) With multihormonal deficit. Complete triade: hypoplastic pituitary stalk + hypoplastic anterior pituitary + ectopic vasopressin storage at the infundibulum and along the pituitary stalk (large arrow). Note in this particular case an ectopic plus eutopic AVP storage in front of the dorsum sellae (small arrow). (**a** and **c**) Sagittal T1WIs. (**b** and **d**) Sagittal T2WIs

A relation has been established between the level of the so-called ectopic posterior pituitary and the severity of the malformation: if the vasopressin storage is located at the infundibulum and the pituitary stalk completely missing, the deficit is usually multihormonal, growth hormone deficit will persist in adult and associated brain malformations are frequently observed.

If the ectopic posterior lobe is attached to a thin but present pituitary stalk, growth hormone deficit is usually isolated and can be reversible.

- *The pituitary stalk* is ideally demonstrated on a sagittal T2W or a heavy T2W sequence. It can be normal, thin, incomplete, or completely missing. An incomplete triade is frequently observed in children with growth retardation and partial growth hormone deficit, the only abnormality being a thin pituitary stalk, best appreciated on T2WI (Fig. 11.4).
- *A small anterior pituitary lobe* is the last component of the classical radiological triade seen with growth hormone deficiency. If this diagnosis is clear when the anterior pituitary height is less than 2 mm (Fig. 11.4c and d) or in case of empty sella, the diagnosis of a so-called small pituitary is difficult to affirm in the other cases since normal variations are numerous. In practice, precise pituitary size measurement is rarely of help in the diagnosis of growth retardation.

Delayed pneumatization of the sphenoid bone, delayed closure of sutures, synchondroses, or persistence of the craniopharyngeal canal can come with hormonal deficiency (Fig. 11.3).

Numerous gene defects can cause abnormal pituitary development.

Among these, PROP-1 gene mutation is a rare but exciting cause of multiple hormone deficiencies. A lack of pituitary gland development leads to its replacement by a T1W hyperintense mass which has characteristics similar to those of Rathke cysts and can shrink spontaneously as do Rathke cleft cysts (Fig. 11.5). It is very likely that intrasellar lesions described in PROP-1 are RCC.

Kallmann syndrome is an intriguing disease with an association of hypogonadotropic hypogonadism and anosmia or hyposmia. In face of this condition, a T2W coronal section through the olfactory bulbs is essential to support the diagnosis.

Lastly, a reminder of several specificities of pituitary MRI in children can be useful:

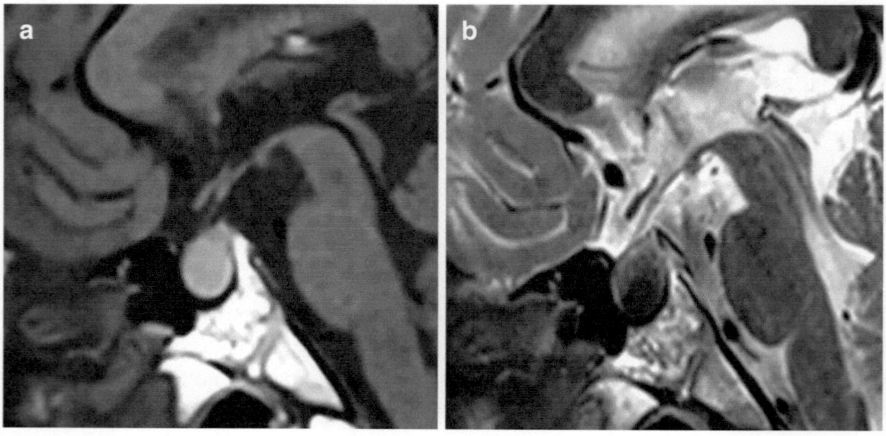

Fig. 11.5 PROP-1 gene mutation in an 18-year-old man. Multiple hormonal deficiencies. (**a** and **b**) Sagittal T1 and T2WIs. Spontaneously T1 hyperintense, T2 hypointense sellar mass pushing the pituitary stalk forward and presenting the characteristics of a Rathke

- The normal anterior pituitary gland is hyperintense on T1W images during the first two months of life (Fig. 4.1) as is the posterior pituitary, except in the case of neonatal hypoglycemia which can be revealing of growth hormone deficiency.
- The normal posterior lobe is proportionally larger than in adults and can mimic a Rathke cleft cyst on sagittal T1WI.
- The inferior intercavernous sinus (Chap. 7) is frequently well developed in young children above a still incompletely pneumatized sphenoid bone and can mimic a pituitary microadenoma or a Ratke cleft cyst on a sagittal view (Figs. 11.1 and 7.3).

Further Readings

Almaghraby A, Jaju A, Ryan ME, Rychlik K, Habiby RL, Brickman WJ. Is gadolinium contrast necessary for pituitary mri in the evaluation of pediatric short stature and growth hormone deficiency? Horm Res Paediatr. 2021;94(5–6):201–10. https://doi.org/10.1159/000519031. Epub 2021 Aug 23. PMID: 34425574

Fava D, Calandrino A, Calevo MG, Allegri AEM, Napoli F, Gastaldi R, Patti G, Casalini E, Bassi M, Accogli A, Alyasin ARAA, Ramaglia A, Rossi A, Maghnie M, Morana G, Di Iorgi N. Clinical, endocrine and neuroimaging findings in girls with central precocious puberty. J Clin Endocrinol Metab. 2022;107(10):e4132–43. https://doi.org/10.1210/clinem/dgac422. Erratum in: J Clin Endocrinol Metab. 2023 Feb 15;108(3):e45

Vuralli D, Gonc EN, Alikasifoglu A, Kandemir N, Ozon ZA. Central nervous system imaging in girls with central precocious puberty: when is necessary? Arch Endocrinol Metab. 2020;64(5):591–6. https://doi.org/10.20945/2359-3997000000259: 34033300; PMCID: PMC10118962

12 Hyperprolactinemia in Women

Hyperprolactinemia represents one of the most common indications of pituitary MRI in women. A radiological diagnosis of prolactinoma is not always easy due to the high frequency of incidentalomas and possible artifacts. Thereby, clinical and biological contexts are essential to achieve the diagnosis. The classical presentation of prolactinoma associates secondary amenorrhea and galactorrhea in a young woman, but amenorrhea is frequently masked by oral contraceptives, and galactorrhea may be absent or unrecognized. A recent weight gain is often noticed. Different presentations may be misleading, such as primary amenorrhea or galactorrhea in women after menopause. Combined prolactinoma and polycystic ovary syndrome are not unusual. Isolated infertility with normal menses is rarely related to prolactinoma. Headaches and visual symptoms are observed with large macroadenomas only. Asking for a visual field examination in a woman harboring a microprolactinoma is a non-sense and a waste of time and money.

Hyperprolactinemia has multiple causes: non-tumoral etiologies, for instance polycystic ovary syndrome, have to be eliminated, as well as macroprolactinemia or drug intake, such as neuroleptics, anxiolytics, antiemetics, etc. Such information is rarely included in the prescription, therefore making questioning by the radiologist himself and medical history essential.

Microprolactinomas are lateralized in the sella and in the large majority of cases more or less T2W hyperintense. When such an image is in accordance with medical history and prolactin levels, it is our practice to spare a post-gadolinium sequence. An optimal T2W signal resolution is essential (Fig. 12.1). T1W hypointensity of the adenoma is common but less obvious. Conversely, gadolinium injection is mandatory when MRI is negative in the same situation. T2W hypointense microadenomas are rare.

The macroprolactinoma pattern is not different from that of non-secreting PitNETs with a similar frequency of cavernous sinus invasion.

It is very important to consider the level of hyperprolactinemia—but this is unfortunately usually not transmitted to the radiologist. Two types of prolactin assays are still in used: if the result is given in international milliunits per liter

J.-F. Bonneville, *Tricks and Traps in MRI of the Pituitary Region*,
https://doi.org/10.1007/978-3-031-64710-9_12

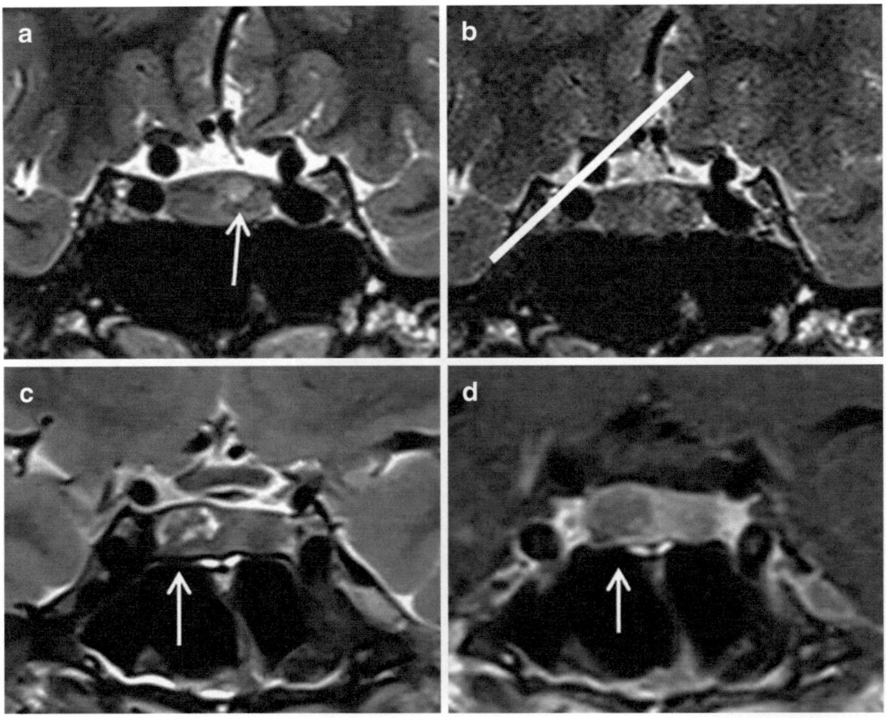

Fig. 12.1 Upper row. Microprolactinoma in an 18-year-old amenorrheic woman. Prolactin is 42 µg/L. T2WI optimal quality is indispensable (**a**). Poor quality image must be rejected (**b**). Lower row. Microprolactinoma in a 36-year-old woman with amenorrhea-galactorrhea. Prolactin is 80 µg/L. The microadenoma is heterogeneous but sufficiently well demonstrated on coronal T2WI (**c**). Gadolinium injection (**d**) could have been spared

(mIU/L), divide by 20 to get the value in micrograms per liter (µg/L) or nanograms per millimeter (ng/mL). In our experience, it is exceptional to demonstrate a pituitary microadenoma if the prolactin level is below 35 µg/L, i.e., 700 mIU/L. Drug-induced hyperprolactinemia is common and can reach and exceed 200 µg/L, this is more than what is commonly observed in microprolactinomas. A positive correlation between prolactin level and pituitary adenoma volume is usual and very useful for the diagnosis: a microadenoma—less than 10 mm in diameter—usually corresponds to a prolactin level between about 35 and 120 µg/L but a small lateralized prolactinoma invading the cavernous sinus may correspond to a much higher prolactinemia as does a macroprolactinoma. Demonstration of a non-cystic pituitary macroadenoma with mild hyperprolactinemia more likely indicates a nonfunctioning adenoma than a prolactinoma. Correlation between adenoma volume and prolactin levels is in default with hemorrhagic and T2 hyperintense tumors and with the rare T2W hypointense microprolactinomas. The latter corresponds either to a tumoral subtype with high prolactin levels, to a calcified prolactinoma or to a hemorrhagic transformation, spontaneous (Figs. 12.2 and 12.3) or after cabergoline

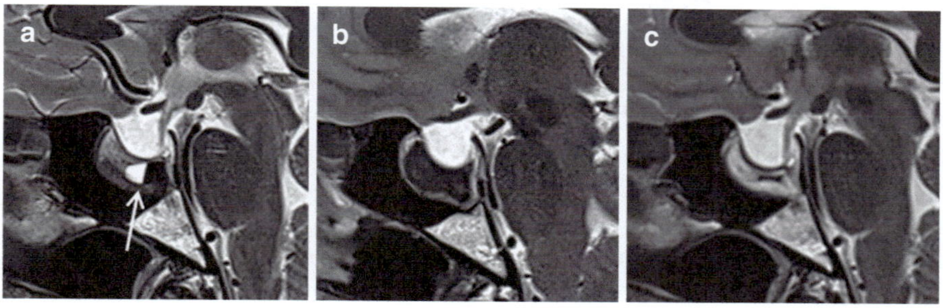

Fig. 12.2 Spontaneous hemorrhage of a macroprolactinoma in an 18-year-old amenorrheic woman (**a**). Prolactin is 52 µg/L. Enlarged sella with depressed sellar diaphragm indicating a macroadenoma spontaneous partial shrinkage. A fluid level (arrow) indicates a previous hemorrhage. (**b**) After 6 months of cabergoline treatment. T2 hypointensity of the sellar content indicates extension of the hemorrhagic component without adenoma size change. (**c**) At 12 months, T2W hyperintensity and decreased size of the residual prolactinoma. (**a–c**) Sagittal T2WIs

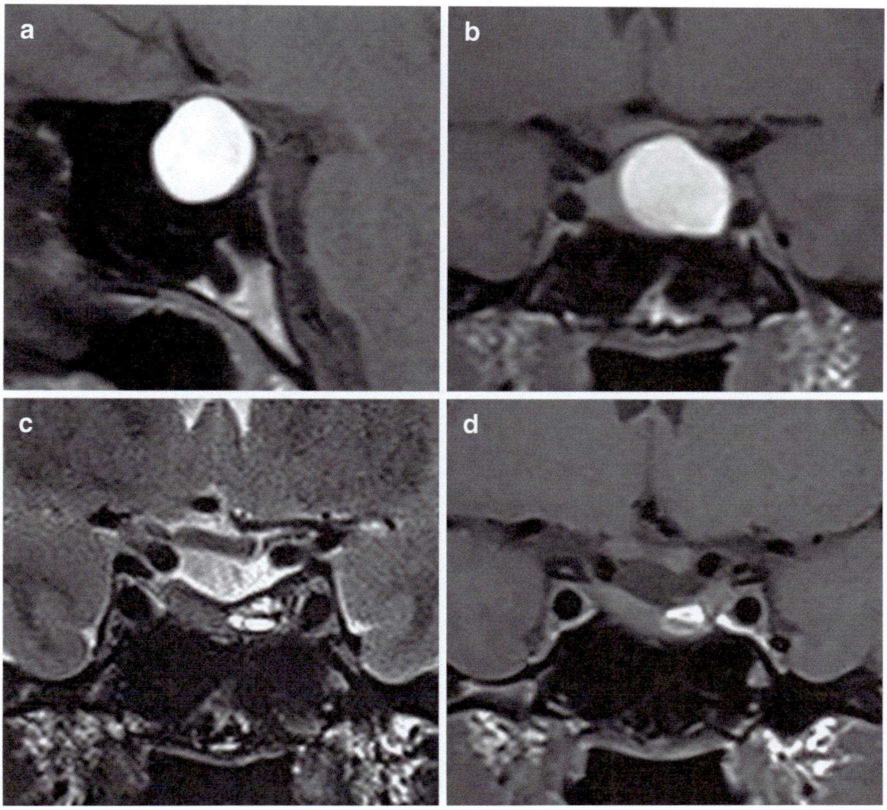

Fig. 12.3 Post pill amenorrhea in an 18-year-old woman. No headache. Almost complete hemorrhagic transformation of a large macroprolactinoma (**a**, **b**). Prolactin is 75 µg/L only. Impressive shrinkage after 8 months of medical treatment (**c**, **d**). (**a**, **b**) Sagittal and coronal T1WIs. (**c**, **d**) Coronal T2 and T1WIs

treatment. Collision lesions, that is microprolactinoma and Rathke cleft cyst for instance, may complicate the diagnosis (Fig. 34.2).

Indications for pituitary MRI during pregnancy are exceptional, for instance when a visual field defect or a severe acute headache occurs. In these circumstances, MRI would visualize an optic chiasm compression or a hemorrhage which can mimic the T1 hyperintensity of the normal pituitary tissue (Chap. 22). Apoplexy is rarely observed.

When treated with dopaminagonists, prolactinoma shrinks quickly, sometimes in a few days and demonstrates an increased T2W hyperintensity. The cavernous sinus compartment shrinks as well.

A T2W hypointense peripheral ring encircling a T1W hyperintense lesion indicates a benign hemorrhagic transformation observed as well before than after medical treatment (Fig. 12.4).

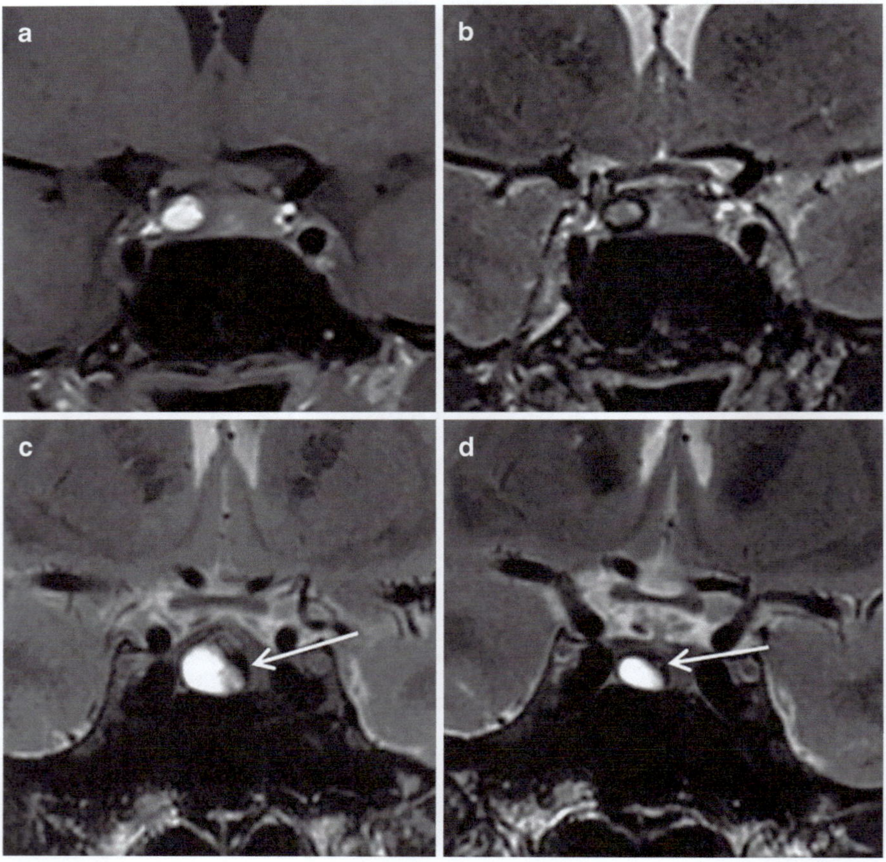

Fig. 12.4 Hemorrhagic microprolactinomas. Upper row. Prolactin level is 51 µg/L. Rounded T1W hyperintense right-sided lesion (**a**) with T2W hypointense ring (**b**). Lower row. T2W hyperintense hemorrhagic prolactinoma with incomplete hypointense ring (arrow). Prolactin is 80 µg/L. Slight shrinkage after 6 months of cabergoline treatment (**d**). (**c**, **d**) T2WIs

The stabilization of the size and of the signal of the adenoma is variable, usually around after 1 year of treatment with dopamine agonists. Nevertheless, shrinkage of the adenoma is delayed in case of hemorrhage, even if the prolactin level is normalized.

Persistence of a focal T2 hyperintensity after years is the rule even in cured microprolactinomas (Fig. 12.5). Unfortunately, MRI is unable to differentiate strictly a persistent active prolactinoma from a scar. This information must be given in the radiological report to avoid unnecessary prolonged medical treatment. After several years of treatment and/or after one or two pregnancies, dopaminagonists may be withdrawn for a therapeutic window of 6–12 months; if the T2W hyperintense signal remains unchanged, prolactinoma can be considered cured after confirmation by normalization of prolactin levels. The MRI follow-up may then be stopped.

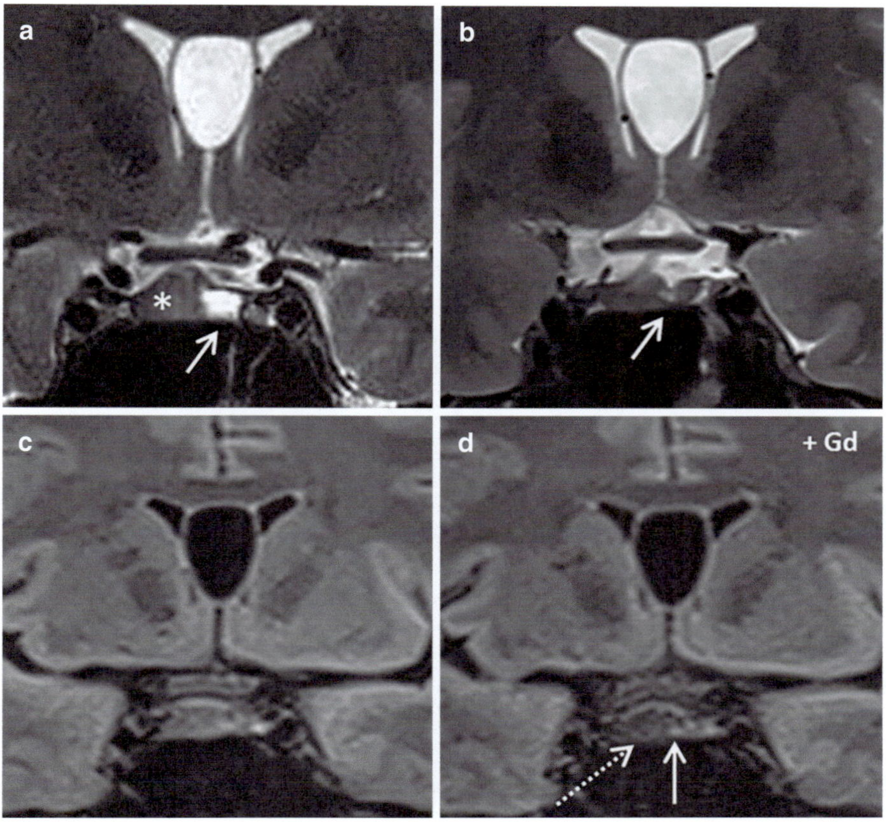

Fig. 12.5 Microprolactinoma (small arrows) in a flat sella before (**c**) and after withdraw of cabergoline given for 2 years (**d**). Initial prolactin level was 45 μg/L, then normalized without treatment. The normal pituitary gland (*) is displaced by the adenoma and is bulging upward due to a reduced sellar volume through a sphenoid sinus hyperpneumatization (not shown). Note that the signal of the normal pituitary (dotted arrow) is deleted after gadolinium injection in FLAIR (**d**). Incidental cyst of the septum lucidum. (**a**, **b**) Coronal T2 WIs. (**c**, **d**) 3D FLAIR before and after 0.03 mmol/kilo Gadolinium

Further Readings

Auriemma RS, Pirchio R, Pivonello C, Garifalos F, Colao A, Pivonello R. Approach to the patient with prolactinoma. J Clin Endocrinol Metab. 2023;108(9):2400–23. https://doi.org/10.1210/clinem/dgad174. Epub ahead of print

Kim SI, Yoon JH, Park DC, Yang SH, Kim YI. What is the optimal prolactin cutoff for predicting the presence of a pituitary adenoma in patients with polycystic ovary syndrome? Int J Med Sci. 2023;20(4):463–7. https://doi.org/10.7150/ijms.80891. PMID: 37057215; PMCID: PMC10087626

Tritos NA, Miller KK. Diagnosis and management of pituitary adenomas: a review. JAMA. 2023;329(16):1386–98. https://doi.org/10.1001/jama.2023.5444.

13 Prolactinoma in Man

When microadenomas represent 80% of prolactinomas in women, macroadenomas are by far the most frequent in men as they represent up to 80% of these tumors. Even if the clinical symptoms—altered libido, erectile dysfunction—are recognized quite late, thus delaying the diagnosis, this does not explain the usual difference in prolactinoma size in women and in men. In addition, a very high prolactin level, up to thousands of micrograms per liter, rarely seen in women, is not unusual in men. In microadenomas too, the prolactin level is considerably higher in men than in women (Fig. 7.2).

A greater trend in the invasiveness of men's tumors is probably related to specific markers of cellular proliferation.

Massive sphenoid sinus invasion, mimicking a sphenoid tumor, is a characteristic pattern of prolactinomas in men: a wise rule is to systematically check the prolactin level in front of every "sphenoid sinus tumor" (Fig. 13.1). Similarly, the diagnosis of prolactinoma must be evoked first in front of any giant tumor of the sellar region in men (Fig. 13.2). The frequency of cavernous sinus invasion is similar to what is observed in macroprolactinomas in women.

If the MRI signal of prolactinomas is usually similar in women and men, a T2 hypointensity is more frequently noted in men (Fig. 13.3a and b). In addition, the presence of hypointense T2W intra-tumoral nodules could reflect calcifications (Fig. 13.3c and d) rarely seen in other types of pituitary adenomas, except in thyrotroph adenomas. A very low intensity on T2WI can also correspond to characteristic amyloid deposits better shown on CT (Fig. 13.4a and b). Areas of T1W hyperintensity giving evidence of hemorrhage, or T2W marked hyperintensity representing focal necrosis or old hemorrhage may be seen.

Treatment with dopamine agonist is as a rule quickly efficient clinically and with a spectacular fall in prolactin level together with tumor shrinkage and change in signal toward T2 hyperintensity or rarely asymptomatic hemorrhage. A too quick shrinkage of the sphenoid compartment tumor may lead to a CSF fistula or exceptionally to a pneumatocyst (Fig. 13.5d and e). The risk of CSF fistula is not always reduced through a progressive increase in cabergoline dosage (Fig. 13.5a–c).

J.-F. Bonneville, *Tricks and Traps in MRI of the Pituitary Region*,
https://doi.org/10.1007/978-3-031-64710-9_13

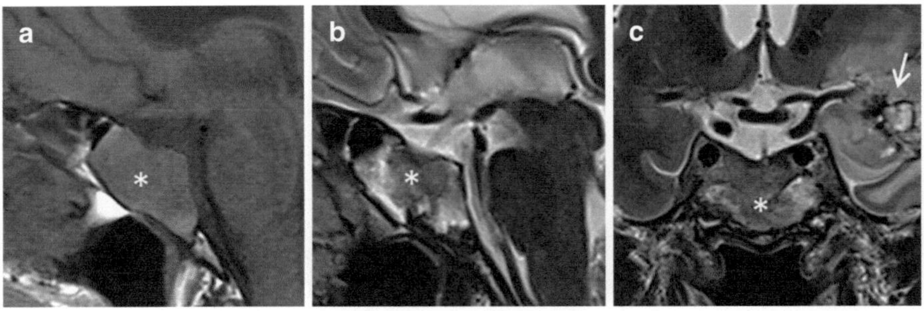

Fig. 13.1 Usual pattern of a macroprolactinoma (*) invading massively the sphenoid sinus in a 57-year-old man. Prolactin is 6000 ng/mL. (**a**, **b**) Sagittal T1 and T2WIs. (**c**) Coronal T2WI. Incidental temporal vascular malformation (arrow)

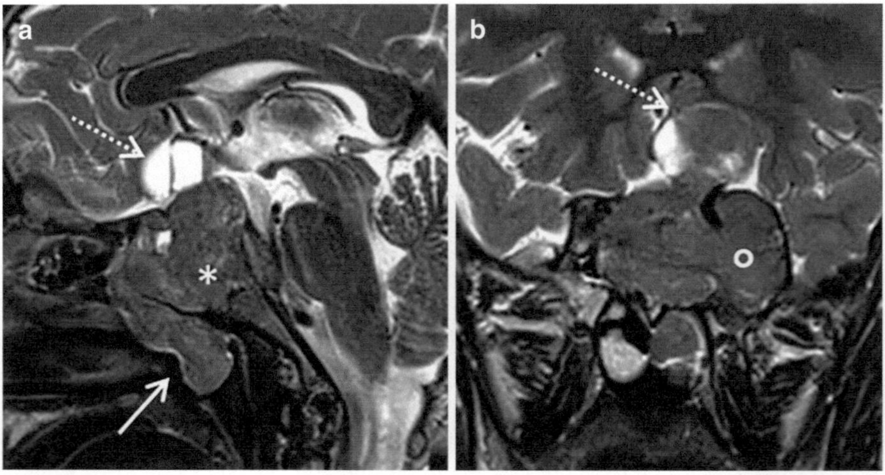

Fig. 13.2 Giant prolactinoma in a 19-year-old man. Suprasellar necrotic extension (dotted arrow). Sphenoid sinus and cavernous sinus invasion (circle). Cavum extension (arrow). (**a** and **b**) Sagittal and coronal T2WIs

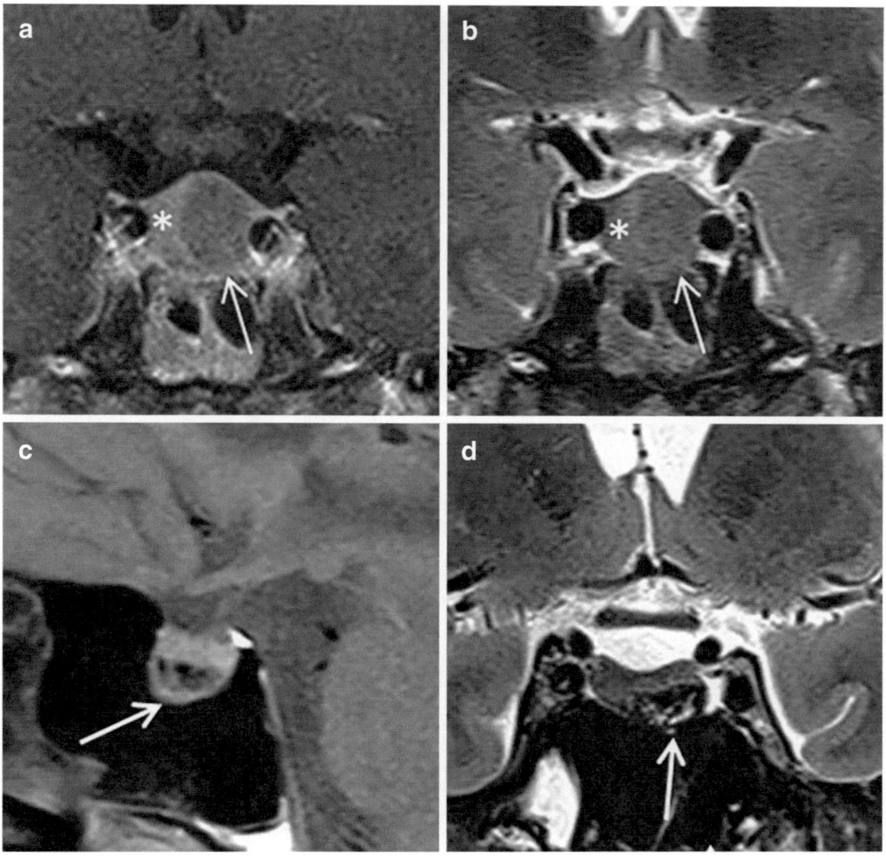

Fig. 13.3 Upper row. Intrasellar prolactinoma in a 20-year-old man. Prolactin is 400 ng/mL. The adenoma (arrow) is hypointense if compared with the normal pituitary (*). (**a**) Coronal CE T1WI. (**b**) Coronal T2WI. Lower row. Calcified prolactinoma in a 46-year-old man. Prolactin is 72 ng/mL. (**c**) Sagittal T1WI. (**d**) Coronal T2WI

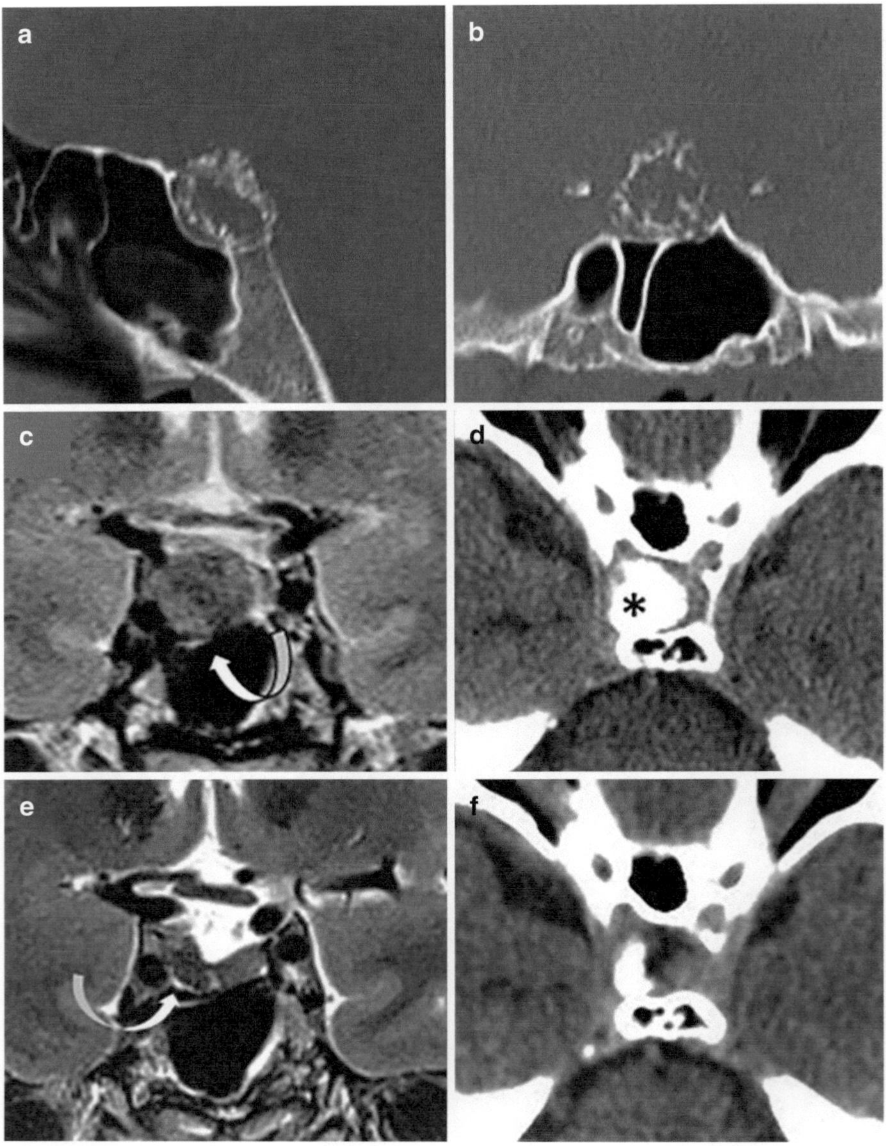

Fig. 13.4 Upper row. Prolactinoma in a 49-year-old man with presumed amyloid deposits. The adenoma is hypointense on T1 and T2WIs (not shown). On CT (**a**, **b**), punctiform peripheral hyperdensities evoking amyloid deposits. Middle and lower row. Calcified prolactinoma before (**c**, **d**) and after 2 years of cabergoline treatment (**e**, **f**). Shrinkage of the adenoma on coronal T2WI (**e**) and of the corresponding hyperdense mass on CT (**f**)

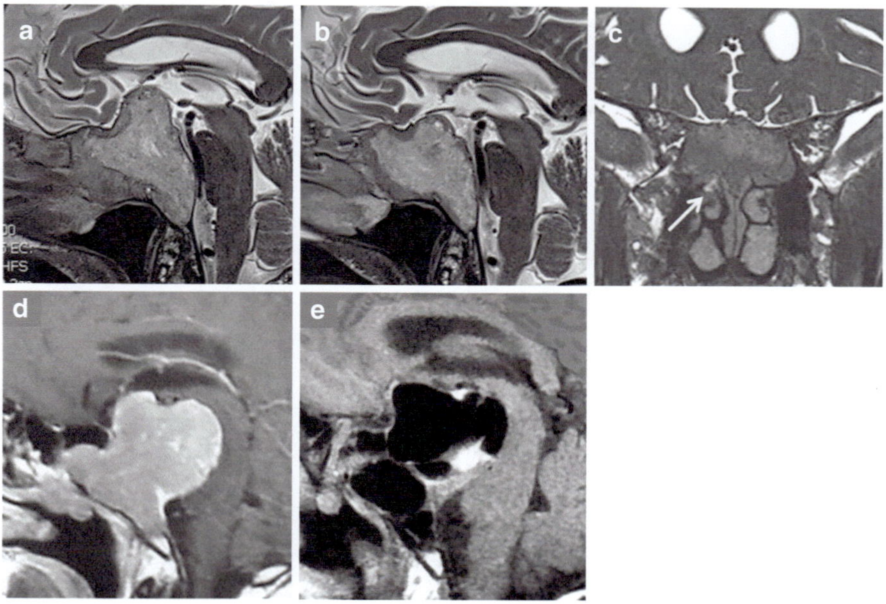

Fig. 13.5 Rare complications of medical treatment. Upper row. Rhinorrhea in a 78-year-old man treated for 3 months with a low cabergoline dosage. Baseline prolactin was 12,000 ng/mL. (**a**, **b**) Sagittal T2WIs before and after treatment. Partial tumoral shrinkage in **b**. CSF fistula demonstrated in coronal heavy T2 WI (arrow in **c**). Lower row: Pneumatocyst after 6 months of cabergoline treatment of a giant prolactinoma in a 60-year-old man suffering from hemiparesis and headache. (**d**, **e**) Sagittal T1WIs before and after treatment

Further Readings

Colao A, Sarno AD, Cappabianca P, et al. Gender differences in the prevalence, clinical features and response to cabergoline in hyperprolactinemia. Eur J Endocrinol. 2003;148(3):325–31.

Iglesias P, Bernal C, Villabona C, et al. Prolactinomas in men: a multicentre and retrospective analysis of treatment outcome. Clin Endocrinol. 2012;77(2):281–7.

Kreutz J, Vroonen L, Cattin F, et al. Intensity of prolactinoma on T2-weighted magnetic resonance imaging: towards another gender difference. Neuroradiology. 2015;57(7):679–84.

Acromegales and Giants

14

Acromegaly is a rare but fascinating disease. Radiologic features of the responsible pituitary somatotroph adenoma are frequently specific and may orient the management of the patient. Despite the obvious character of clinical features, the diagnosis is most of the time delayed by an average of 4 years. Changes in morphotype, particularly of extremities, sleep apnea, and canal tunnel syndrome draw attention late and the diagnosis is frequently evoked by persons far from the patient for years. When the diagnosis has been confirmed by hormonal status—mainly GH, oral glucose suppression test, and IGF1—the role of MRI is to demonstrate the responsible pituitary adenoma, identify a subset, and indicate whether it is invasive.

Pituitary macroadenomas count for more than 70% of cases. A unique feature is their predominantly downwards extent, within the sphenoid sinus. Therefore, distortion of the optic chiasm by a suprasellar tumoral extension is observed in less than 20% of the cases—that explaining the rarity of visual field defects in acromegaly if compared with their occurrence in non-secreting adenomas (Fig. 14.1). Therefore, the downward extension of the pituitary adenoma constitutes an adjunct factor explaining the usually delayed diagnosis. In some situations, the inferior extension is so marked that the pituitary gland seems healthy, the adenoma mimicking a sphenoidal polyp (Fig. 14.2). Many theories have been proposed to explain this pattern of extension, the most likely being that growth-hormone-induced sphenoid sinus hyperpneumatization makes the sellar floor frail.

There are two different pathological subtypes of the somatotropic adenomas: the densely granulated tumors, the most frequent, and the sparsely granulated ones. The first ones express the somatostatin receptors STTR 2 and respond frequently well to medical treatment with first-generation somatostatin analogs. The latter respond poorly or not at all and invade the cavernous sinus in more than half of the cases. Their treatment is then more complicated and the prognosis less favorable.

MRI is able to recognize these two entities by providing a rigorous technical approach, mainly an optimal signal resolution. Densely granulated adenomas are T2 hypointense while densely granulated ones are hyperintense if compared with the normal pituitary gland (Fig. 14.3).

J.-F. Bonneville, *Tricks and Traps in MRI of the Pituitary Region*,
https://doi.org/10.1007/978-3-031-64710-9_14

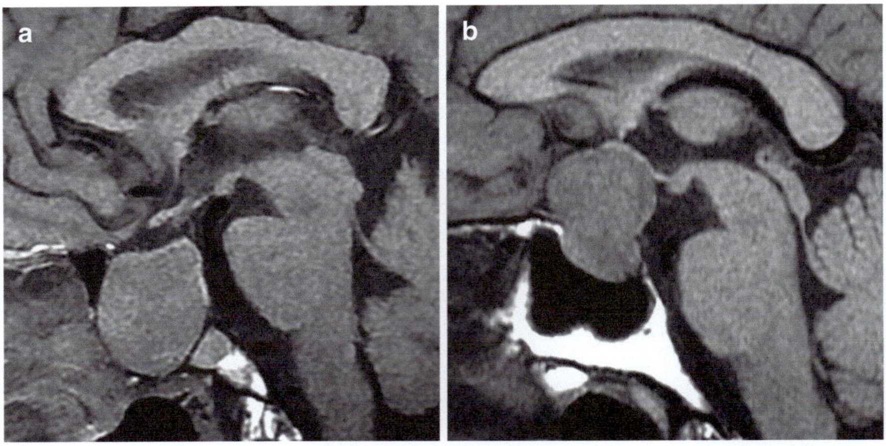

Fig. 14.1 Typical downward extension of a somatotroph macroadenoma (**a**) versus suprasellar usual extension of a nonsecreting PitNET (**b**). Sagittal T1WIs

But the referential tissue is debated: in the literature, the selected referential tissue is most commonly white and grey cerebral matters together, which, in our experience, is uneasy to apply. For us, the most logical reference is the normal anterior pituitary gland. In the cases where the normal pituitary tissue is invisible, masked by a large adenoma, we have shown that in the adult the pituitary gland has a T2W signal very similar to this of the adjacent cortex, i.e., the grey matter of the temporal lobe. The proximity of the brain cortex to the sellar content makes the comparison of both signals very easy to the eye.

Another important issue concerns isodense pituitary adenomas (Fig. 14.3c). It is clear that their demonstration depends on signal resolution, therefore on MR parameters. In our experience, isointense adenomas account for about 15% of the tumors and have a behavior close to that of T2W hyperintense somatotroph adenomas regarding cavernous sinus invasion and response to medical treatment. But the proportion of isointense adenomas will be found much higher if the spatial resolution of the T2W sequence is not optimized. Similarly, distinction between densely and sparsely granulated tumor is impossible without a high-resolution T2W sequence (Figs. 2.2 and 14.4).

When most GH-secreting adenomas are macroadenomas, microadenomas as well as giant adenomas do exist. The diagnosis of microadenomas may be difficult in the case of associated aneurysmal enlargement of intracavernous internal carotid arteries responsible for flow artifacts or in case of empty sella secondary to a spontaneous shrinkage of the adenoma.

The thickening of the soft palate, tongue, and pharynx walls is responsible for sleep apnea (Fig. 14.5a and b). It regresses inconsistently after treatment (Fig. 14.5c and d).

Enlargement of the sheath of the third cranial nerve is another little-known marker of acromegaly (Fig. 14.6).

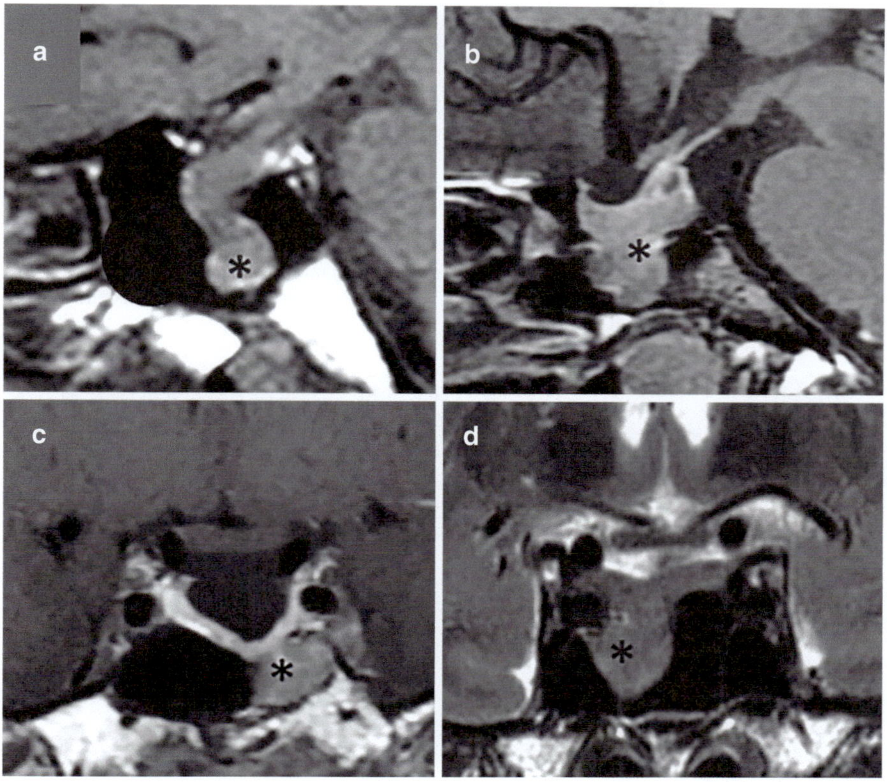

Fig. 14.2 GH-secreting adenomas (*) mimicking sphenoid sinus polyps; (**a**, **b**) Sagittal T1WIs. (**c**, **d**) Coronal CE T1 and T2WIs

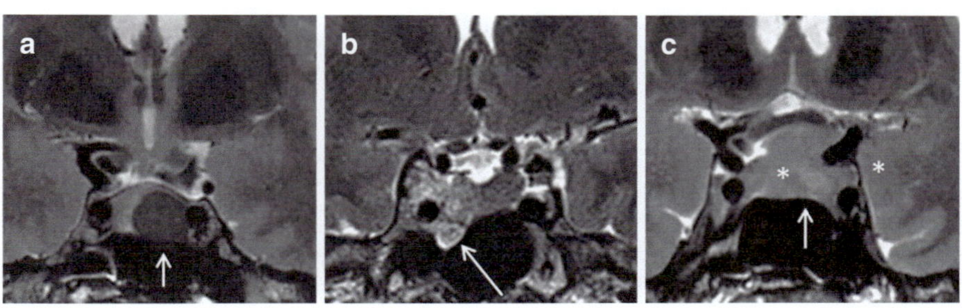

Fig. 14.3 T2W hypointense well-limited pituitary adenoma suggestive of a densely granulated tumor (**a**). T2W hyperintense tumor invading cavernous sinus and sphenoid sinus suggestive of a sparsely granulated adenoma (**b**). (**c**) T2W isointense adenoma whose signal is very similar to that of the temporal cortex (*). The normal pituitary gland is not demonstrated. (**a–c**) Coronal T2WIs

Surgical removal of the adenoma which is the first line of treatment is frequently incomplete, particularly with cavernous sinus invasion. Medical treatment lies on first-generation somatostatin analogs, then on GH receptor antagonists. After

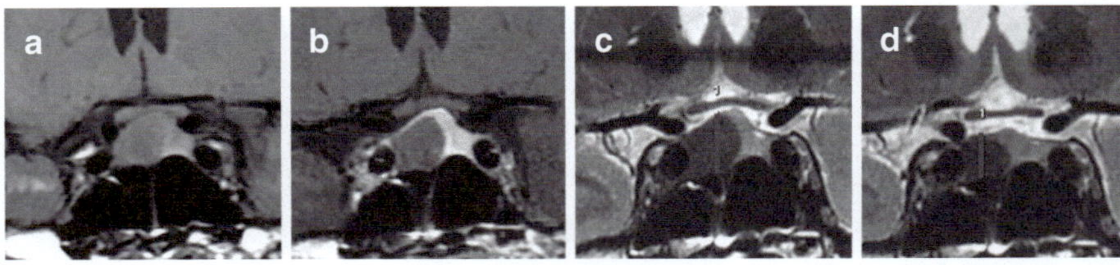

Fig. 14.4 Densely granulated pituitary adenoma. Well-limited, homogeneous T2 hypointense lesion without cavernous sinus invasion which shrinks after 3 months of somatostatin analogs (**d**). (**a**, **b**) Coronal T1 and CE T1WIs. (**c**, **d**) Coronal T2WIs. Note that the somatotroph adenoma subtype is given by the T2W sequence only

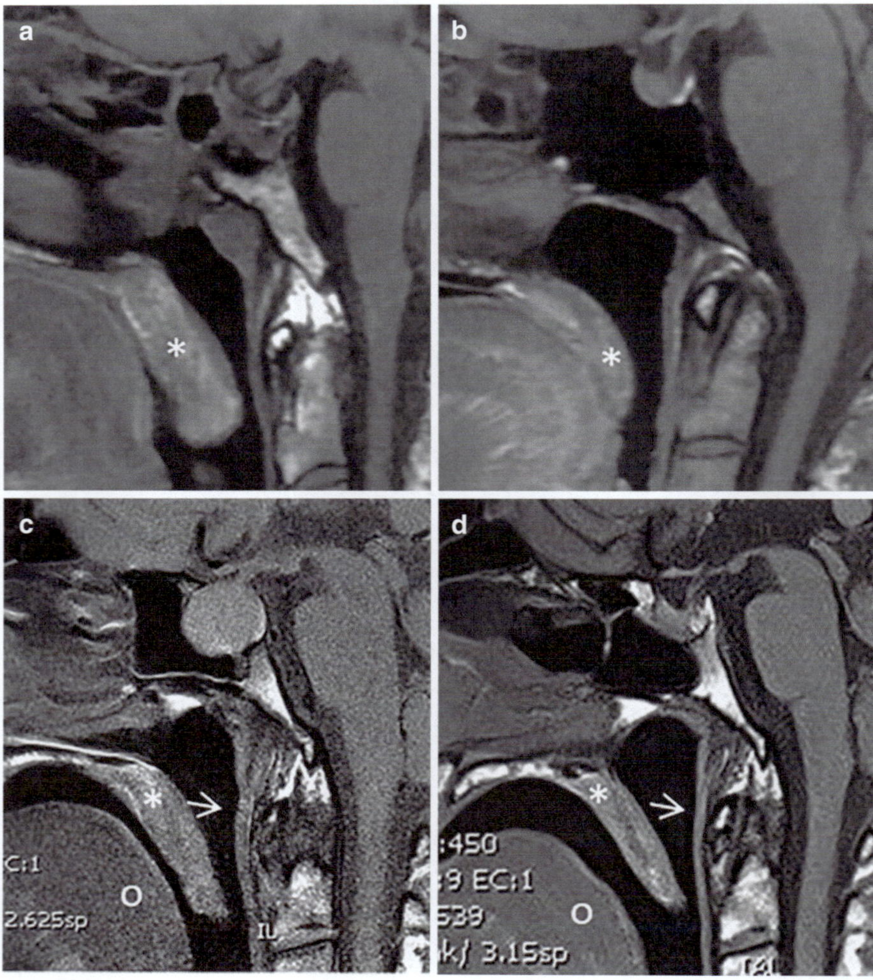

Fig. 14.5 ENT manifestations of acromegaly. Upper row. Thickening of the soft palate (*) in an acromegalic patient (**a**) versus a normal individual (**b**). Lower row. Decreased size of the soft palate (*), tongue (°), and pharyngeal wall (arrow) after surgery in another patient (**c**, **d**): (**a–d**) Sagittal T1WIs

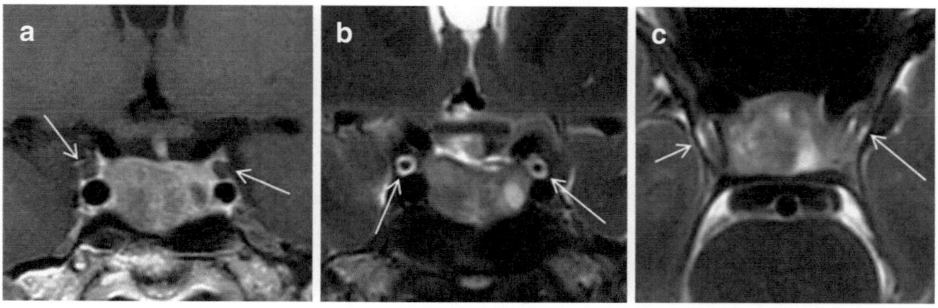

Fig. 14.6 Enlarged meningeal sheaths of the third cranial nerves (arrows) in a patient with a heterogeneous T2W hyperintense somatotroph adenoma. (**a** and **b**) Coronal CE T1 and T2WIs. (**c**): Axial T2WI

treatment, tumor shrinkage and T2W hyperintensity are more frequently observed in T2W hypointense tumors (Fig. 14.7). The role of medical treatment in the preoperative period is controversial.

Acromegaly occurring early in childhood or adolescence gives rise to gigantism; the responsible pituitary adenoma may be giant but it is not the rule.

Neuroendocrine tumors may produce growth hormone-releasing hormone (GHRH) and lead to increased levels of GH and IGF 1 and therefore to acromegaly (see Chap. 15).

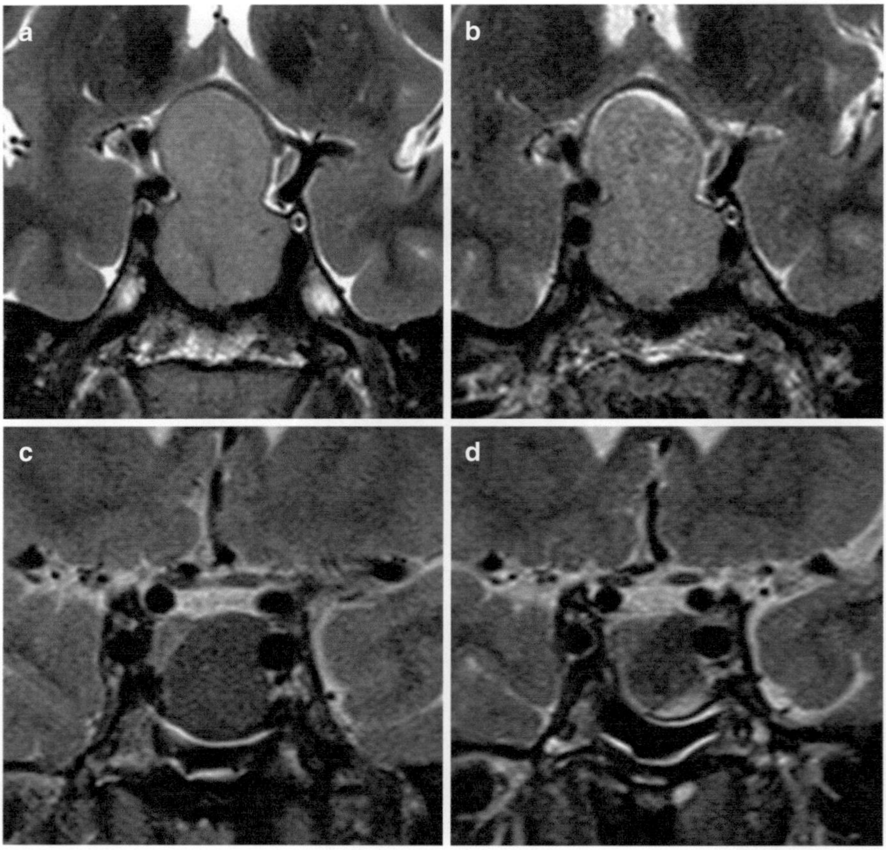

Fig. 14.7 Different efficacy of medical treatment in a T2W hyperintense sparsely granulated adenoma (**a** and **b**) and in a T2W hypointense densely granulated adenoma (**c** and **d**) after 6 months of somatostatin analogs. (**a–d**) Coronal T2WIs

Further Readings

Ilie MD, Tabarin A, Vasiljevic A, Bonneville JF, Moreau-Grangé L, Schillo F, Delemer B, Barlier A, Figarella-Branger D, Bisot-Locard S, Santos A, Chanson P, Raverot G. Predictive factors of somatostatin receptor ligand response in acromegaly-A prospective study. J Clin Endocrinol Metab. 2022;107(11):2982–91. https://doi.org/10.1210/clinem/dgac512.

Potorac I, Beckers A, Bonneville JF. T2-weighted MRI signal intensity as a predictor of hormonal and tumoral responses to somatostatin receptor ligands in acromegaly: a perspective. Pituitary. 2017;20(1):116–20. https://doi.org/10.1007/s11102-017-0788-8.

Potorac I, Petrossians P, Daly AF, Schillo F, Ben Slama C, Nagi S, Sahnoun M, Brue T, Girard N, Chanson P, Nasser G, Caron P, Bonneville F, Raverot G, Lapras V, Cotton F, Delemer B, Higel B, Boulin A, Gaillard S, Luca F, Goichot B, Dietemann JL, Beckers A, Bonneville JF. Pituitary MRI characteristics in 297 acromegaly patients based on T2-weighted sequences. Endocr Relat Cancer. 2015;22(2):169–77. https://doi.org/10.1530/ERC-14-0305. Epub 2015 Jan 2

15 Syndromic and Familial Acromegaly

If acromegaly is usually a sporadic disease, it can also be a manifestation of a syndromic or familial disease. These rare diseases are fascinating and can be discovered when elucidating a gigantism in a child for instance.

The McCune-Albright syndrome reunites the triad polyostotic osteodysplasia, café-au-lait skin spots, and endocrinopathies, particularly peripheral precocious puberty. Acromegaly or gigantism are present in one-third of the cases and pituitary MRI reveals a pituitary hyperplasia or a pituitary adenoma which can be multiple. A T2W hypointense signal of the sellar content similar to that observed in densely granulated adenomas has been observed (Fig. 15.1).

Carney complex is a rare multiple endocrine and non-endocrine neoplasia. The main manifestations are skin-pigmented peri-orificial spots, cardiac myxoma, and primary pigmented nodular adrenal disease. Growth hormone pituitary adenoma and acromegaly can be present.

Acromegaly can also be part of *multiple endocrine neoplasia-type 1 (MEN1)* with a frequent association with endocrine tumors of the parathyroids and pancreas principally.Isolated pituitary gigantism or acromegaly may occur in a familial pattern. The disease is defined as the development of pituitary adenomas in at least two members of a family in the absence of genetic abnormality *(familial isolated pituitary adenomas, FIPA)*.

A genomic duplication has been identified in what is called *X-linked acrogigantism (X-LAG)*. This rare disease involves preferentially boys and is responsible for strikingly early gigantism with a median age of onset of 12 months. MRI reveals a homogeneous pituitary mass. At the difference with what is observed in acromegalic adult patients, tumoral extension is strictly upwards, perhaps because the sphenoid bone is not yet pneumatized (Fig. 15.2). Surgery is mandatory since medical treatment is ineffective. Pathology reveals pituitary hyperplasia or pituitary adenoma.

Ectopic growth hormone -releasing hormone (GHRH) secretion from a neuroendocrine tumor is another extraordinary etiology of acromegaly. This condition has long been ignored and up to 30% of patients with this disease have

J.-F. Bonneville, *Tricks and Traps in MRI of the Pituitary Region*,
https://doi.org/10.1007/978-3-031-64710-9_15

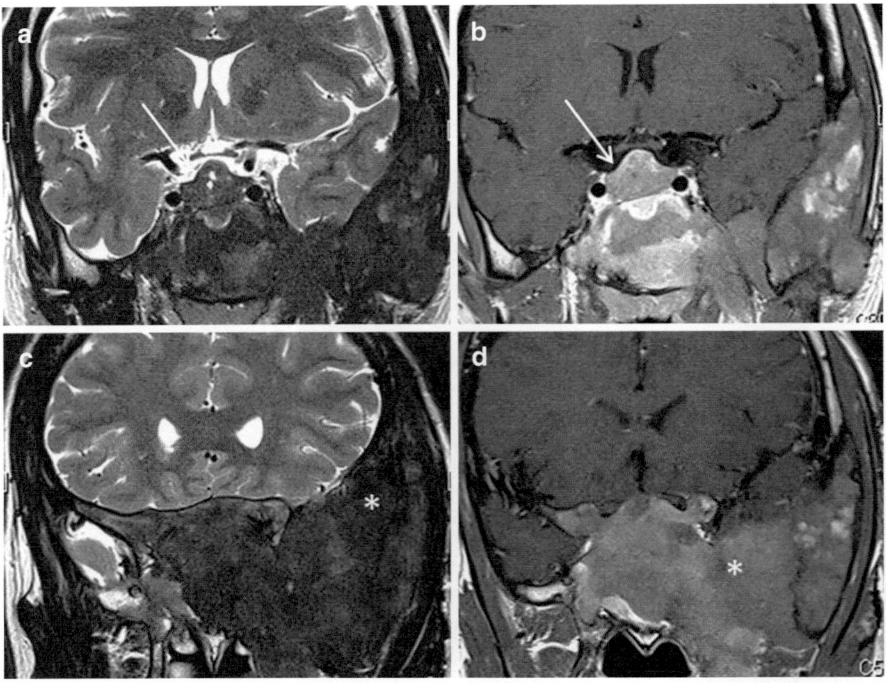

Fig. 15.1 GH-secreting pituitary adenoma and McCune–Albright syndrome. (**a**, **c**) Coronal T2WIs. (**b**, **d**) Coronal CE T1WIs. Characteristic pattern of polyostotic fibrous dysplasia (*asterisks*) and T2W hypointense PitNET (*arrow*). (Courtesy of G. Raverot)

unfortunately been inefficiently operated at the sellar level. The diagnosis was frequently missed because GHRH dosage is usually not made in acromegaly. The result of this hypersecretion of GHRH from a pancreatic or a bronchial tumor is an elevated value of GH and IGF1 as it is observed in GH-PitNETs but the radiological pattern is different: a symmetrical enlargement of the sellar content without or with minimal sellar floor changes and without visualization of the normal pituitary gland sign pituitary hyperplasia but a more or less T2W hypointense signal of the mass is fundamental for the diagnosis of ectopic GHRH secretion (Fig. 15.3). The diagnosis is particularly difficult in the elderly or in patients with empty sella where the normal pituitary is smaller than in adults and where hyperplasia can mimic a normal-sized gland. Observation of the T2W signal as well as the symmetrical, homogeneous signal of the sellar content are fundamental to establishing the diagnosis. After successful retrieval of the neuroendocrine tumor, the pituitary gland returns to normal size and tends frequently to recover a normal T2W signal (Fig. 15.4). Differential diagnosis is pituitary metastasis from the neuroendocrine tumor: metastases are not T2 hypointense and tend to grow quickly (Fig. 15.5).

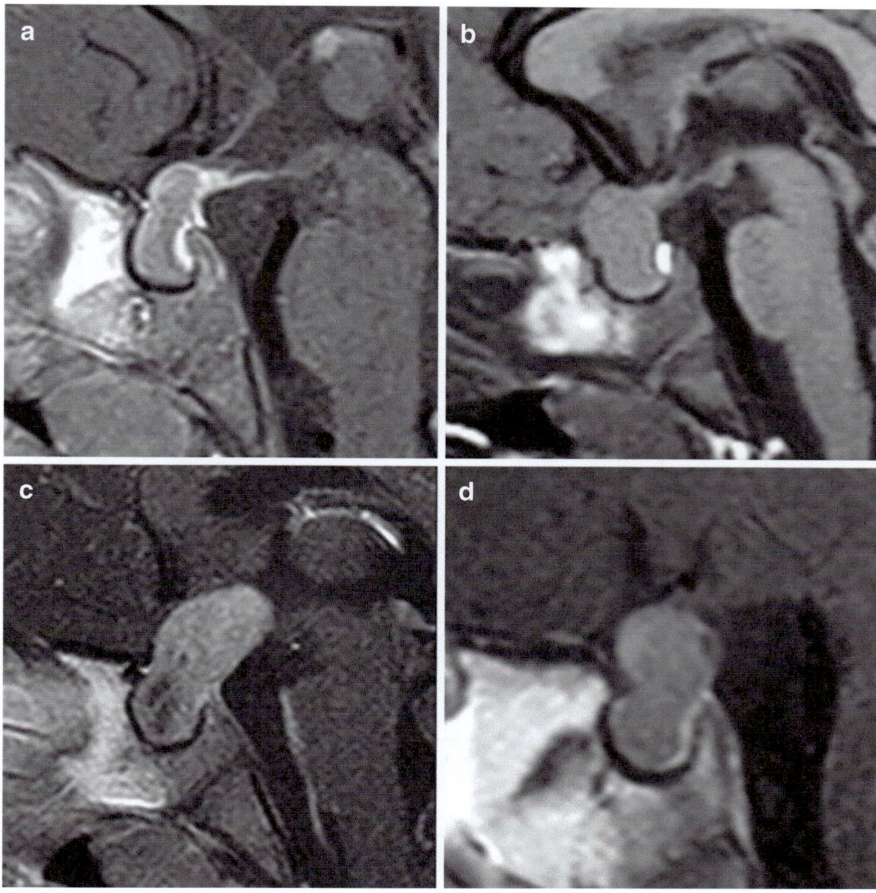

Fig. 15.2 Characteristic pattern of pituitary macroadenomas simulating hyperplasia in four very young children with X-linked acrogigantism (X-LAG). Note the upward extension of the mass, at the difference with what is observed in sporadic acromegaly in adults. (**a–d**) Sagittal T1WIs

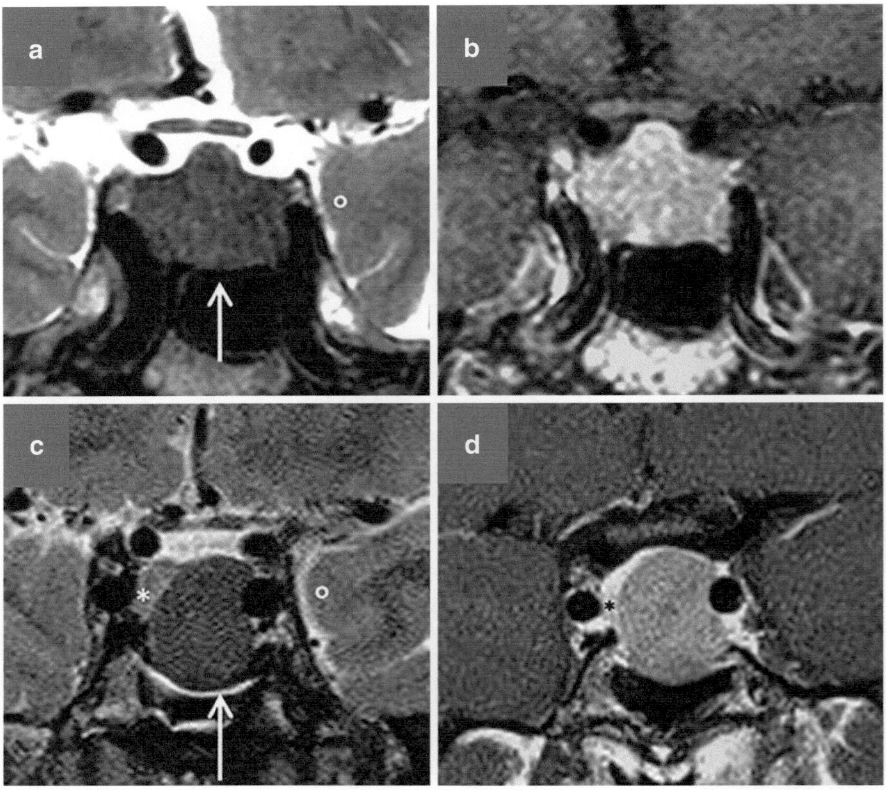

Fig. 15.3 Pituitary hyperplasia (**a**, **b**) versus densely granulated somatotroph adenoma (**c**, **d**). Both lesions (arrows) demonstrate a T2W hypointense signal—if compared with the temporal cortex (°). In hyperplasia (**a**), the normal pituitary gland is not visible while it is in pituitary adenoma (*). Moreover, the sellar floor (arrow) is nearly unchanged in hyperplasia while it is deformed with PitNET. (**a**, **c**) Coronal T2WIs. (**b**, **d**) Coronal CE T1WIs

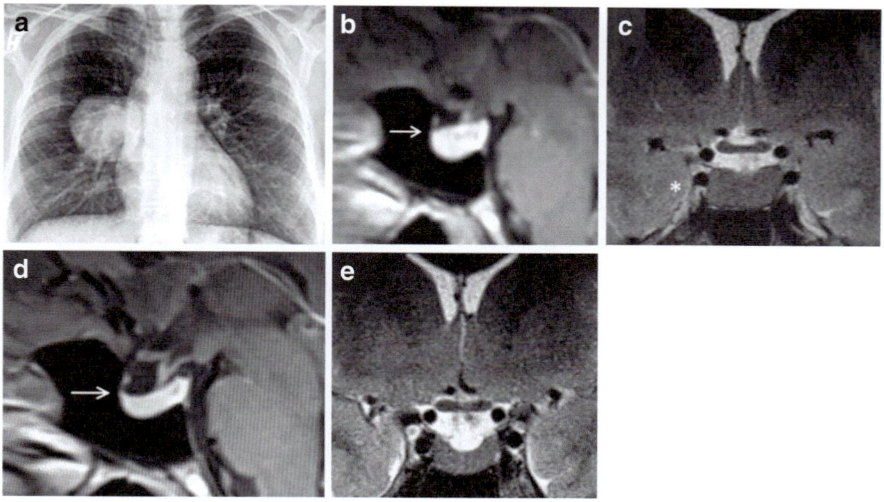

Fig. 15.4 Pituitary hyperplasia in a 35-year-old acromegalic female with a GHRH-producing bronchial carcinoma (**a**). Homogeneous T2W hypointense sellar content (**c**) which shrinks after surgery of the bronchial tumor and becomes almost T2W isointense. The T2W signal of the pituitary is compared with that of the temporal cortex (*). (**b**, **d**) Sagittal CE T1WIs. (**c**, **e**) Coronal T2WIs

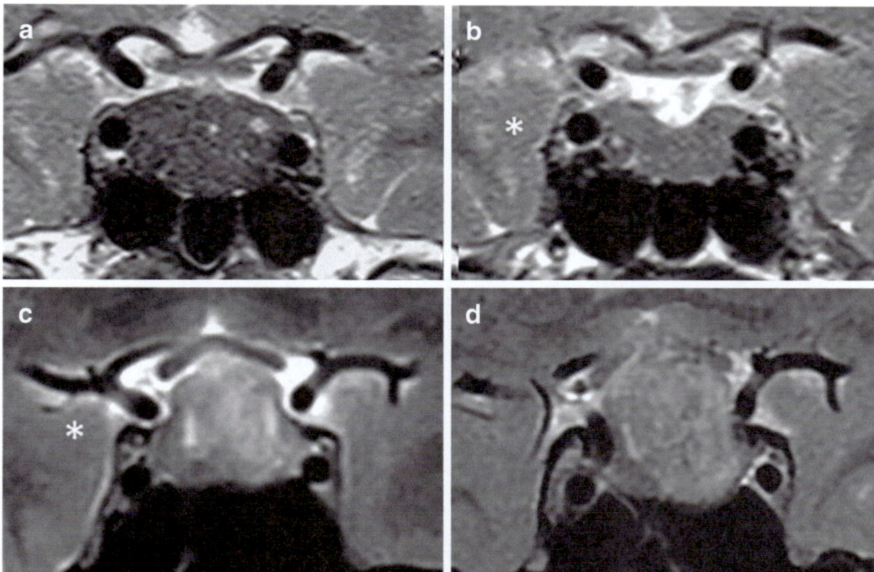

Fig. 15.5 Upper row. Pituitary hyperplasia from a GHRH-producing pancreatic tumor before and after surgery (**a**, **b**). T2 signal and volume changes are obvious. Lower row. Pituitary metastasis from a GHRH bronchial tumor (**c**, **d**). The sellar mass displays a T2W hyperintense signal and increases in size despite surgery of the bronchial tumor. (**a–d**) Coronal T2WIs. The referential tissue is the temporal cortex (*)

Further Readings

Beckers A, Rostomyan L, Potorac I, Beckers P, Daly AF. X-LAG: how did they grow so tall? Ann Endocrinol (Paris). 2017;78(2):131–6. https://doi.org/10.1016/j.ando.2017.04.013. Epub 2017 Apr 27

Potorac I, Bonneville JF, Daly AF, et al. Pituitary MRI features in acromegaly resulting from ectopic GHRH secretion from a neuroendocrine tumor: analysis of 30 cases. J Clin Endocrinol Metab. 2022;107(8):e3313–20. https://doi.org/10.1210/clinem/dgac274.

Salenave S, Boyce AM, Collins MT, Chanson P. Acromegaly and McCune-Albright syndrome. J Clin Endocrinol Metab. 2014;99(6):1955–69. https://doi.org/10.1210/jc.2013-3826. Epub 2014 Feb 11. PMID: 24517150; PMCID: PMC4037730

Cushing's Disease: The Grail of the Radiologist

16

A pituitary picocorticotropinoma responsible for Cushing's disease is frequently hard to find but its demonstration is so rewarding that it may be named "the Grail of the neuroradiologist". Indeed, the cure for this severe disease is closely dependent on the MRI localization of the responsible pituitary adenoma. In a patient with an ACTH-dependent Cushing syndrome, a negative MRI embarrasses the endocrinologist and can force the surgeon to make multiple incisions in the pituitary in search of tumoral tissue, or to perform partial hypophysectomy, both giving lower results and possibly complications. Inferior petrosal sinus sampling can also be proposed: this invasive procedure can localize the tumor in 2 out of 3 cases but is ineffective with a midline located tumor.

Thus, MRI remains crucial for the localization of the pituitary adenoma.

In about 50% of the cases, the corticotropinoma is a macroadenoma or a microadenoma more than 5 mm in diameter and its demonstration is nowadays relatively easy whatever the MRI protocol. It should be noted that, unlike what is observed in prolactinomas, there is no correlation between the tumor size and the severity of hypercortisolism.

MR signal of corticotropinoma is usually slightly T1 hypointense and T2 hyperintense as most PitNETs, but may be isointense on both sequences and then difficult to show if the tumor is tiny. Even after half-dose of gadolinium, a microadenoma can be masked by the enhancement of the normal surrounding pituitary tissue. Partial volume artifacts can be misleading (Fig. 16.1a, b). A coexisting empty sella, not infrequent in Cushing disease, further makes the demonstration of the lesion harder (Fig. 16.1c, d). Demonstration of cavernous sinus invasion is of uppermost importance for the prognosis (see Chap. 18).

We will focus on the particular research of the tiniest adenomas—3 mm in diameter or less we named picoadenomas—for which a first MRI is frequently negative. We must confess at once that detection of the responsible tumor remains negative in a significant percentage of cases, even in the most expert hands and there is reason to believe that technical improvements such as hybrid imaging combining PET and MRI will solve the diagnosis of corticotropic picoadenomas in the future.

J.-F. Bonneville, *Tricks and Traps in MRI of the Pituitary Region*,
https://doi.org/10.1007/978-3-031-64710-9_16

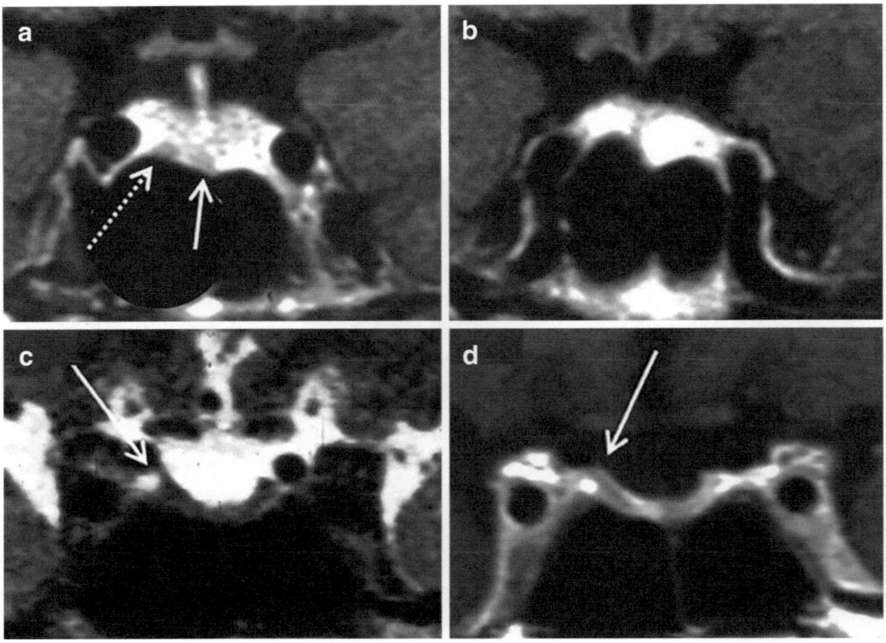

Fig 16.1 Upper row. Asymmetrical hyperpneumatized sphenoid sinus responsible of a partial volume artifact (dotted arrow). An ACTH-producing adenoma lies on the midline (arrow). (**a**, **b**) Coronal CE T1WIs. Lower row: Corticotropinoma and empty sella. (**c**, **d**) Coronal T2W and late CE T1WIs

Optimal MRI technique and skilled interpretation are pivotal to demonstrating these adenomas and avoiding false attributions to artifacts or incidentalomas.

- A 3.0 T scanner is to be preferred. The advantage of 7.0 T has not been really proven yet.
- A long examination time must be scheduled. Let us recall once again the crucial importance of a high-resolution T2 sequence.
- Gadolinium half dosage at maximum (0.05 mmol/kg) must be used for CE T1 W sequences.
- Specifically for picoadenomas, 3D imaging is superior to 2D imaging (Fig. 16.2). Indeed, volumetric acquisitions provide infra-millimetric slices, minimize partial volume effects, and permit multiplanar reformats.
- 3D Gradient-Echo (3D GE) is generally considered more informative than 3D Spin-Echo (3D SE), but we use to perform both sequences after a first negative MRI (Fig. 16.3) each bringing specific advantages. Indeed, 3D SE sequences reduce motion and susceptibility artifacts if compared with the 3D GE sequence. 3D SE is also beneficial for the demonstration of pituitary adenomas located within the cavernous sinus or in contact with it (Fig. 16.5b).

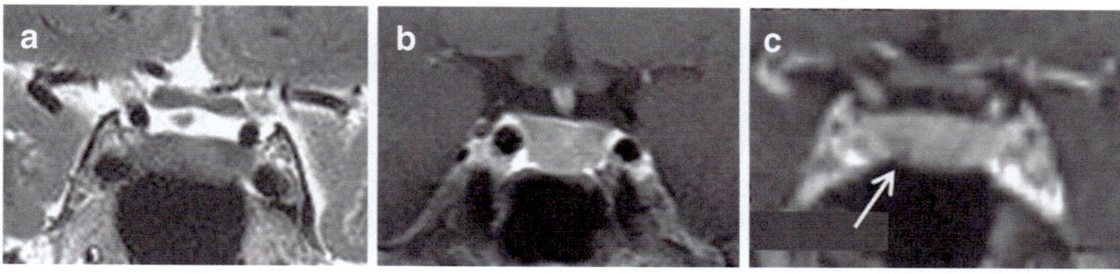

Fig 16.2 ACTH-secreting PitNET. A right-sided non-enhanced area is demonstrated only on a 3D GE-enhanced sequence. (**a–c**) Coronal T2, 2D CE T1 and 3D GE CE T1WIs

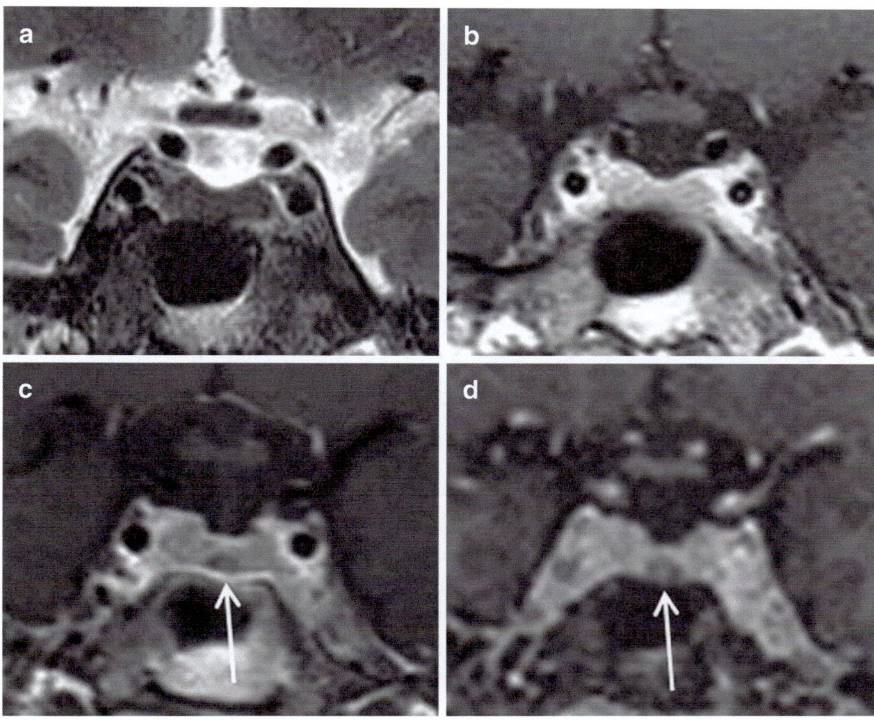

Fig 16.3 ACTH-secreting PitNET. (**a–d**) Coronal T2, 2D CE T1, 3D SE CE T1, and 3D GE CE T1WIs. 3D images only demonstrate the picoadenoma

- Dynamic imaging has pros and cons. Even though we were pioneers of dynamic CT in another millennium, we consider today dynamic MRI mostly as lost time and a potential source of errors (see Chap. 9). To try to overcome the disadvantage of a long acquisition time, a more rapid dynamic MRI technique combined with 3D submillimeter isotropic acquisitions (GRASP) has been proposed but has not proven its utility for the diagnosis of picoadenomas due to its relatively poor spatial resolution.

- Immediate or late post-gadolinium 2D or 3D T2 FLAIR (fluid-attenuated inversion recovery) sequences may be interesting. By injecting a large dosage of contrast—two or three times the usual dosage—the pituitary gland appears as nonenhanced at the difference of the adenoma, probably because of T2 shortening due to high gadolinium blood concentration (Fig. 16.4). It has been also suggested that delayed T2 FLAIR MRI could make the diagnosis between solid microadenomas which demonstrate late wash-out and cystic or necrotic lesions which did not. Unfortunately, cysts and cystic microadenomas have a similar dynamic profile.
- Lastly, if a pituitary MRI managed by a skilled neuroradiologist remains negative, inferior petrosal sinus sampling (IIPS) could affirm ACTH pituitary hypersecretion but not the adenoma lateralization.
- We must also remember the possibility of ectopic adenomas, such as in the sphenoid sinus or the cavernous sinus (Fig. 16.5).
- Furthermore, Cushing's disease could be in relation with an ectopic ACTH secretion by a neuroendocrine tumor which can be large as bronchial carcinomas or small such as bronchial carcinoids. Other responsible tumors can be carcinomas of the thyroid or the pancreas, pheochromocytomas, or thymic carcinoids. Ectopic or paraneoplastic Cushing is frequently more severe and associated with a worse prognosis than Cushing related to a corticotroph pituitary adenoma. High-resolution thoraco-abdominal CT/MRI is then essential if pituitary MRI is negative. A marked hyperplasia of the adrenal glands could point to an ectopic source of ACTH secretion.

Visualizing an abnormal image within the pituitary does not make the diagnosis of the responsible ACTH-producing pituitary adenoma. If the diagnosis of intrasellar Rathke cleft cyst is easy that of a nonfunctioning adenoma is not because most PitNETs present similar characteristics. Characterization remains a major issue. It has been suggested that late wash-out of the lesion on CE T2 3D FLAIR could occur later in corticotropinomas if compared with non-secreting ones, but this interesting observation has to be confirmed. We have shown a long time ago that such a late wash-out can be demonstrated not only on FLAIR but also on enhanced SET1 W sequences in pituitary adenomas regardless of the adenoma secretion.

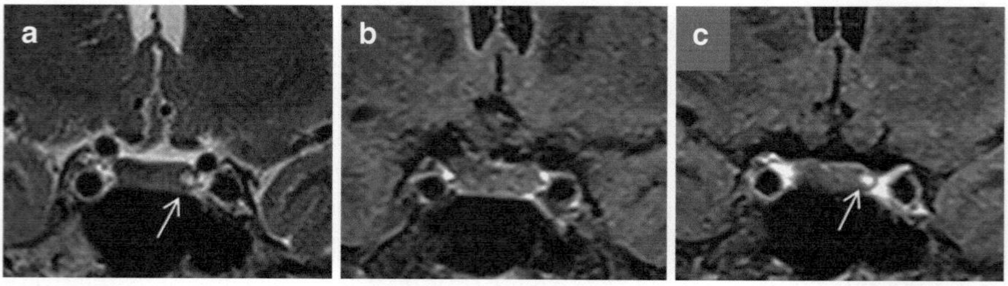

Fig 16.4 Potential usefulness of CE FLAIR with high dose of gadolinium. (**a**) Coronal T2WI. (**b**, **c**) Coronal 2D 3 mm FLAIR without (**b**) and after high dose of contrast (**c**). The pituitary gland is non-enhanced in (**c**), rendering the adenoma image more accurate

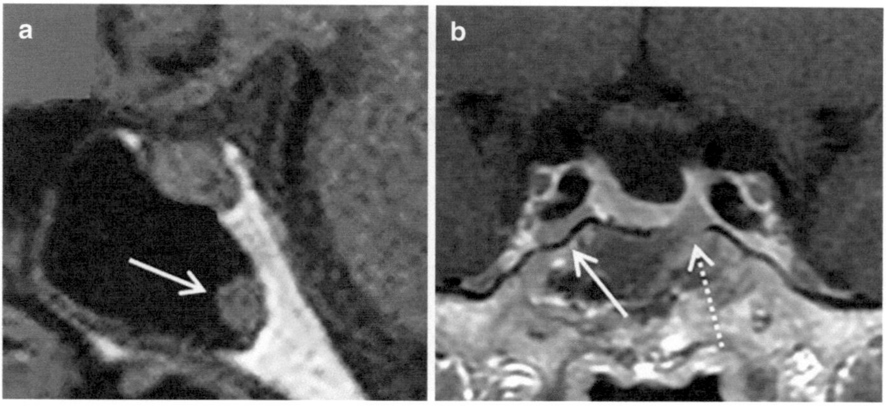

Fig 16.5 Ectopic corticotropic PitNETs in the sphenoid sinus (**a**, sagittal T1WI) and in the cavernous sinus (arrow in **b**, 3D SE CE T1WI). The adenoma has taken the place of the vein of the carotid sulcus. The dotted arrow points to the trace of a previous negative surgical approach

In summary, it is very likely that PET imaging will in a near future overcome the shortcomings of MRI for the diagnosis of ACTH-producing picodenomas.

For now, there is no doubt that a Cushing's patient will have a greater chance of being cured if its MRI is performed and read by an expert neuroradiologist, as well as if pituitary surgery is realized by an expert pituitary neurosurgeon.

Lastly, if machine learning is a hot research topic today to differentiate clinically Cushing disease from ectopic ACTH secretion, it seems a poor help for the MRI diagnosis of picocorticotropinomas.

Further Readings

Bashari WA, Gillett D, MacFarlane J, Powlson AS, Kolias AG, Mannion R, Scoffings DJ, Mendichovszky IA, Jones J, Cheow HK, Koulouri O, Gurnell M. Modern imaging in Cushing's disease. Pituitary. 2022;25(5):709–12. https://doi.org/10.1007/s11102-022-01236-w. Epub 2022 Jun 6.

Bonneville J-F, Potorac I, Petrossians P, Tshibanda L, Beckers A. Pituitary MRI in Cushing's disease—an update. J Neuroendocrinol. 2022:e13123. https://doi.org/10.1111/jne.13123.

Chatain GP, Patronas N, Smirniotopoulos JG, et al. Potential utility of FLAIR in MRI-negative Cushing's disease. J Neurosurg. 2018;129:620–8. https://doi.org/10.3171/2017.4.JNS17234.

17 Silent and Unusual Pituitary Adenomas

Silent pituitary adenomas are tumors of the anterior pituitary gland with hormone synthesis but without any sign of hypersecretion. A few are partially silent and are called "whispering "adenomas. Silent PitNETs are usually discovered when they are large, and they are responsible for the same symptoms as non-secreting adenomas. Otherwise, they are discovered incidentally when neuroimaging is performed for another reason.

Silent corticotroph pituitary adenomas are considered to be more aggressive than non-secreting adenomas which they look like: they frequently invade the cavernous sinus, may have a more rapid growth, and can recur. In addition, they have a tendency to bleed and can present with pituitary apoplexy. Rarely, a silent corticotroph PitNET may transform into an active adenoma responsible for Cushing disease. For all these reasons, it would be essential to evoke this diagnosis in front of a seemingly banal history evoking a non-secreting PitNET.

Fortunately, the diagnosis of silent ACTH-producing adenoma can be considered—not formally made—in many circumstances. In fact, a particular microcystic pattern—well seen on T2W images—must draw attention (Fig. 17.1), particularly if the cysts diameter is less than 3 mm and if these cysts cover at least 25% of the solid part of the tumor. However, this feature is not absolutely specific and can be observed—albeit more rarely—in true corticotropic adenomas and in non-secreting PitNETs. However, in our experience, microcystic non-secreting PitNETs may present a more aggressive evolution (Fig. 17.2). A macrocystic pattern is less suggestive of silent adenomas. Recently, dynamic MRI has been proposed to differentiate silent corticotroph adenomas from non-functioning pituitary adenomas through their time-intensity curves but this research has to be confirmed in a large series of patients.

Silent somatotroph pituitary adenomas are frequently identified immunohistochemically. They are more frequently sparsely granulated than densely granulated. IGF-1 is normal or barely elevated. Some are mixed GH-prolactin-secreting adenomas. A female predominance is noted. The T2W signal of silent somatotroph PitNETs has not been reported in the literature yet. Sparsely granulated ones are reputed as more invasive and presenting higher recurrence rates than their

J.-F. Bonneville, *Tricks and Traps in MRI of the Pituitary Region*,
https://doi.org/10.1007/978-3-031-64710-9_17

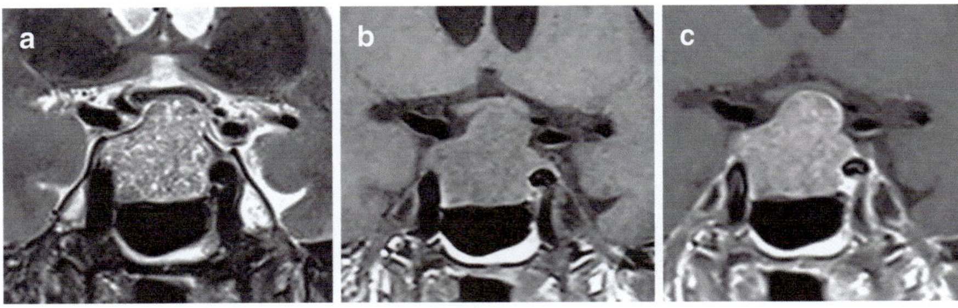

Fig. 17.1 Silent corticotroph PitNET. Characteristic microcystic pattern best demonstrated on (**a**) Coronal T2WI. (**b**, **c**) Coronal T1 and CE T1 WIs

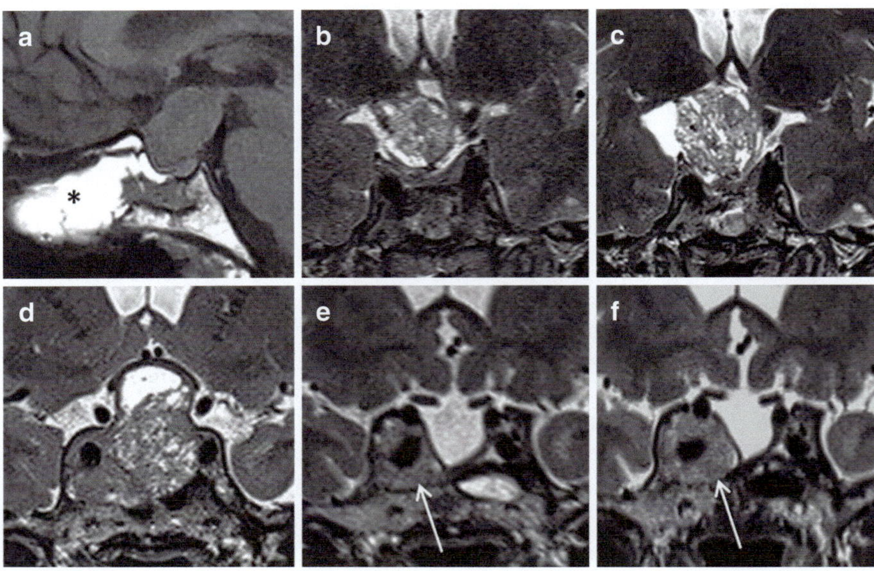

Fig. 17.2 Upper row. Evolution of a microcystic non-secreting PitNET remnant. Large unusual fat packing in the surgical approach (*). (**a**) Sagittal T1WI. (**b**, **c**) Coronal T2WIs 15 years apart. Lower row. Micro-macrocystic non-secreting PitNET invading the cavernous sinus. Rapid evolution of a post-surgical remnant (arrow). Nine months only separate the images presented in (**e**) and (**f**). (**d**–**f**) Coronal T2WIs

symptomatic counterparts. For these reasons, it has been proposed to perform a complete hormonal staining panel for all PitNETs.

Calcified pituitary adenomas are rarely seen and could sometimes signal a previous hemorrhage. They are described mainly in prolactinomas and particularly in men. They are better seen on CT where they are observed in two forms: eggshell-like capsular calcifications and intratumoral nodular calcifications or "pituitary stones". Calcifications in pituitary adenoma raise special diagnostics and therapeutic challenges, even if soft calcifications do not always make surgery riskier (Fig. 13.4). The diagnosis of craniopharyngioma must always be cleared in front of a calcified sellar mass.

Thyrotropin-secreting pituitary adenomas represent a very rare cause of hyperthyroidism, with symptoms being less severe than in peripheral hyperthyroidism. They are characterized by elevated serum levels of free thyroid hormones with measurable TSH levels. These tumors may present a fibrous compartment and/or calcifications (Fig. 17.3). TSH microadenomas are also described. If surgery is refused by the patient or inefficient, medical treatment with somatostatin analogs is another option. Shrinkage of the pituitary adenoma can occur quickly (Fig. 17.4). The main differential diagnosis of TSH-PitNET is thyroid hormone resistance syndrome.

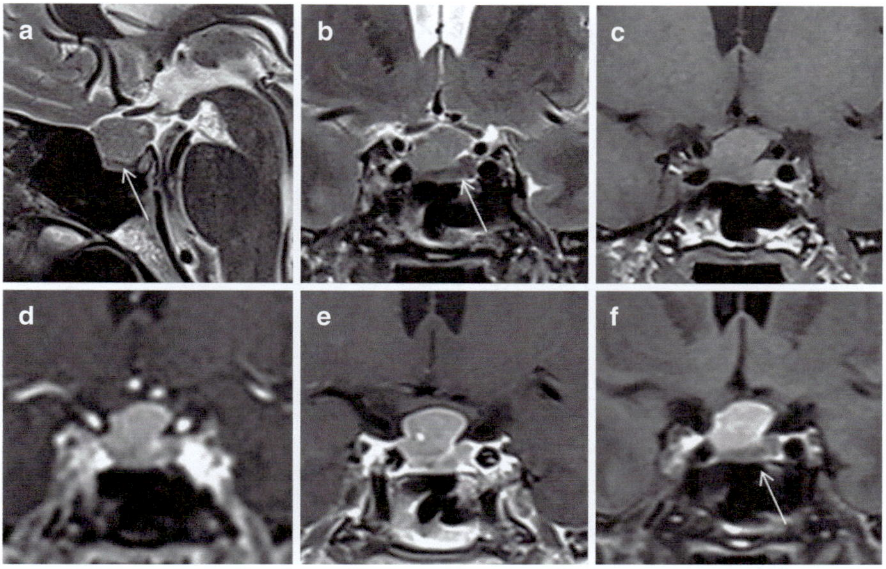

Fig. 17.3 TSH-secreting PitNET. The lower T2W hypointense compartment of the tumor (arrow) is fibrous and enhances differently if compared with the upper part. (**a**) Sagittal T2WI. (**b**–**f**) Coronal T2, T1, early phase of dynamic sequence, late post-contrast, and CE FLAIR WIs

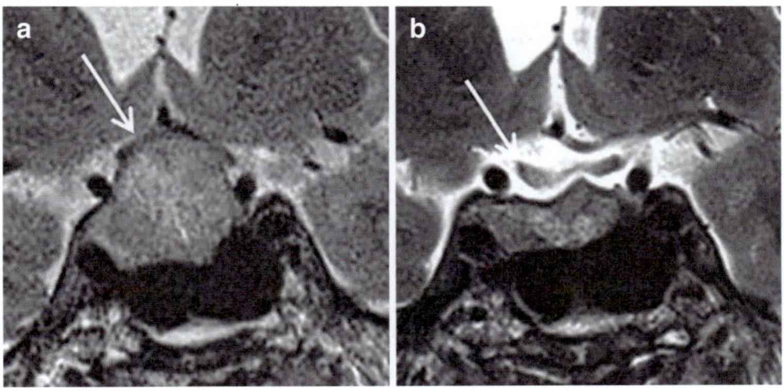

Fig. 17.4 TSH-secreting PitNET with optic chiasm compression (arrow) before (**a**) and after 3 months of somatostatin analog treatment (**b**). Very quick tumoral shrinkage. (**a**, **b**) Coronal T2WIs

T2W hypointense pituitary adenomas are much rarer than hyperintense ones. Prolactinomas, particularly in men may exhibit a T2W hypointense signal. Some of the latter can contain calcifications or amyloid deposits better shown on CT (Fig. 13.4). In women, T2W hypointense prolactinomas represent a subtype with a higher prolactin level and sometimes a different response to dopamine agonists. A T2W hypointense signal is characteristic of densely granulated GH-secreting PitNETs.

Ectopic pituitary adenomas are defined as located outside the sella and are distinctly separate from the pituitary gland. The most common sites are the sphenoid sinus and the cavernous sinus. All types of PitNETs can be ectopic. In Cushing disease, an ectopic corticotropic adenoma may mimic a sphenoid polyp (Fig. 16.5).

Hypervascular sellar tumors displaying serpiginous flow-void images are rarely pituitary adenomas (Fig. 17.5) and should suggest a meningioma (Fig. 32.1), a rare oncocytoma (Fig. 5.4) or a metastasis from a hypervascular tumor, such as a kidney carcinoma.

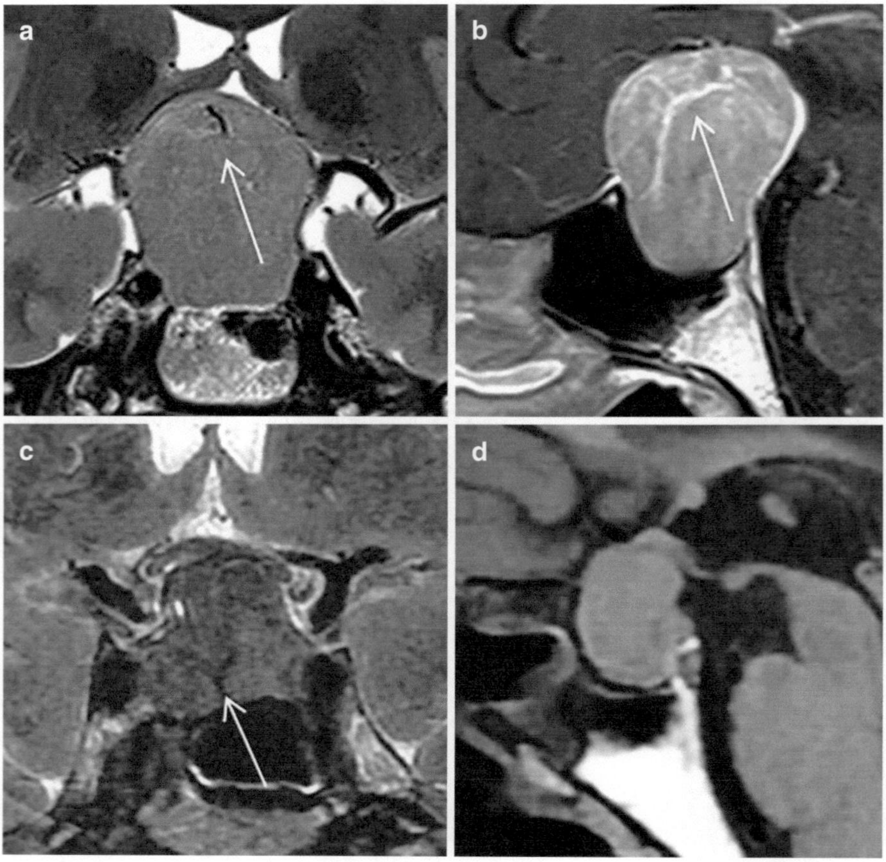

Fig. 17.5 Upper row. Vascular linear signal voids in a non-secreting PitNET. (**a**) Coronal T2WI, (**b**) Sagittal CE T1WI. Lower row. Tiny calcifications (arrow) in a T2W hypointense prolactinoma resistant to cabergoline treatment. (**c**) Coronal T2WI. (**d**) Sagittal T1WI

Further Readings

Briet C, Suteau V, Illouz F, Rodien P. Thyrotropin-secreting tumor "TSH-PitNET": from diagnosis to treatment. Ann Endocrinol (Paris). 2023;84(4):407–12. https://doi.org/10.1016/j.ando.2023.01.004. Epub 2023 Jan 27.

Drummond J, Roncaroli F, Grossman AB, Korbonits M. Clinical and pathological aspects of silent pituitary adenomas. J Clin Endocrinol Metab. 2019;104(7):2473–89. https://doi.org/10.1210/jc.2018-00688.

Langlois F, Woltjer R, Cetas JS, Fleseriu M. Silent somatotroph pituitary adenomas: an update. Pituitary. 2018;21(2):194–202. https://doi.org/10.1007/s11102-017-0858-y.

18 Is Cavernous Sinus Space Invaded or Not?

This question certainly obtains less consensual answers, even among experts—at least when it comes to discrete cavernous sinus invasion. Yet, it is essential for patient management. Even if surgery has made improvements in this field, we need to accept that invasion of the cavernous sinus space by a secreting pituitary adenoma makes the functional prognosis of the disease uncertain. This is particularly true for Cushing disease and acromegaly where additional medical treatment or radiotherapy is frequently required to control residual hormonal hypersecretion.

Full cavernous sinus space invasion and discrete invasion must be described separately.

Full cavernous sinus invasion by PitNET is generally obvious. The lateral wall of the cavernous sinus is unilaterally swollen. The normal anterior pituitary is not shown between the pituitary adenoma and the cavernous sinus (Fig. 18.1). Veins are no longer visible and the cavernous sinus is replaced by a solid tissue whose T1 and T2 signals and enhancement are similar to those of the intrasellar compartment of the adenoma. Asymmetric tentorial enhancement is not specific to invasion and can be observed in cavernous sinus compression as well as in meningiomas. Sometimes, an anterolateral characteristic bulging signals a tumoral extension through the dural pocket of the third nerve (Fig. 18.2).

If the diagnosis of pituitary adenoma is not obvious or not known, the question of the differential diagnosis of a cavernous lesion can be asked and is discussed in Chap. 33. Two arguments—one clinical and the other radiological—favor, if necessary, the diagnosis of pituitary adenoma invading the cavernous sinus: the cavernous sinus lesion itself is not symptomatic, and, particularly, there is no symptom of intracavernous nerves compression—except in the case of hemorrhage—and the diameter of the intracavernous internal carotid artery is unchanged.

If cavernous sinus space invasion is less massive, several landmarks have been proposed based on the correlation between MRI and operative findings. For example, Cottier stated that invasion is certain when two-thirds of the intracavernous internal carotid artery diameter is encased by tumoral tissue. It has to be noted that

J.-F. Bonneville, *Tricks and Traps in MRI of the Pituitary Region*,
https://doi.org/10.1007/978-3-031-64710-9_18

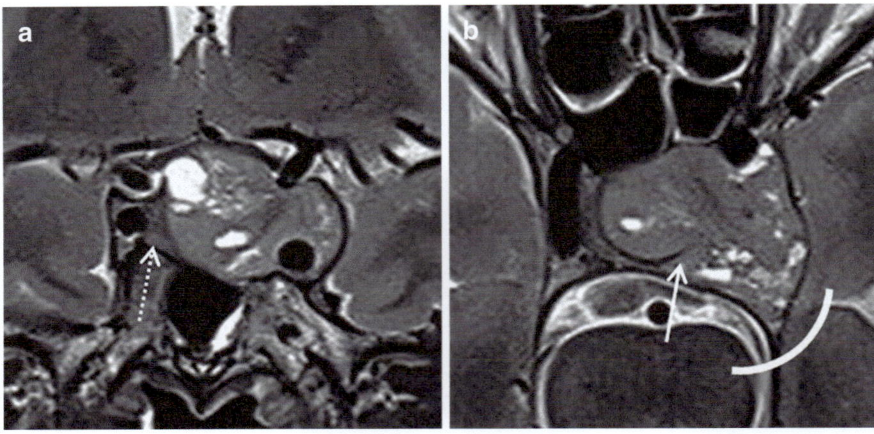

Fig. 18.1 Non-secreting pituitary adenomas with left cavernous sinus invasion. Rupture of the adenoma "capsule" (arrow). Note the preferential posterolateral extension (curved line). The normal anterior pituitary gland is compressed and displaced to the right (dotted arrow). (**a**, **b**) Coronal and axial T2WIs

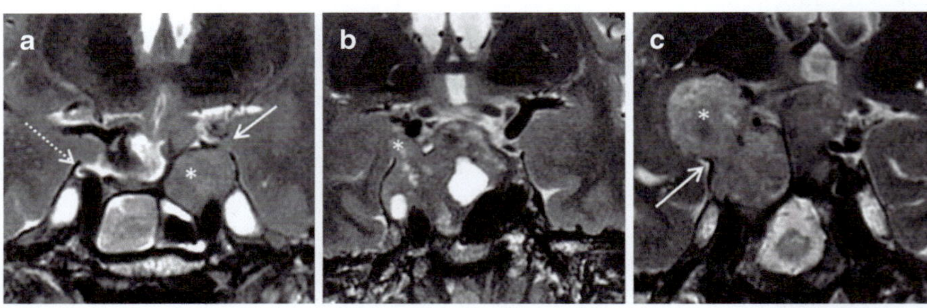

Fig. 18.2 Non-secreting pituitary adenomas with cavernous sinus invasion and tumoral extension through the porus of the dural pocket of the third nerve. (**a**) Light opening of the porus (arrow) preceding extra-dural tumoral extension of this pituitary adenoma recurrence. Normal contralateral pocket of the third nerve (dotted arrow). (**b**) Limited tumoral extension (*) through an enlarged porus. (**c**) Recurrent non-secreting pituitary adenoma. The porus of the dural pocket of the third nerve (arrow) is considerably enlarged and lets the tumor (*) pass through. (**a**–**c**) Coronal T2WIs

this work was conducted at a time when direct visualization of the internal wall of the cavernous sinus was not helped by recent endoscopic and optical improvements.

Knosp and Miko (also comparing MRI and surgical data) state that invasion is observed in about one-third of the cases when tumoral tissue passes a line joining the mid-diameter of intracavernous and supraclinoid internal carotid artery, but not the line joining their lateral surfaces. And they affirm cavernous sinus invasion in all cases when the tumor extends beyond a line joining the lateral surface of both segments of the internal carotid artery (Fig. 18.3). We think that, if these approaches can be useful for a statistical purpose when reporting a large series of patients, they are not so much for individual cases and above all in the case of limited cavernous sinus invasion.

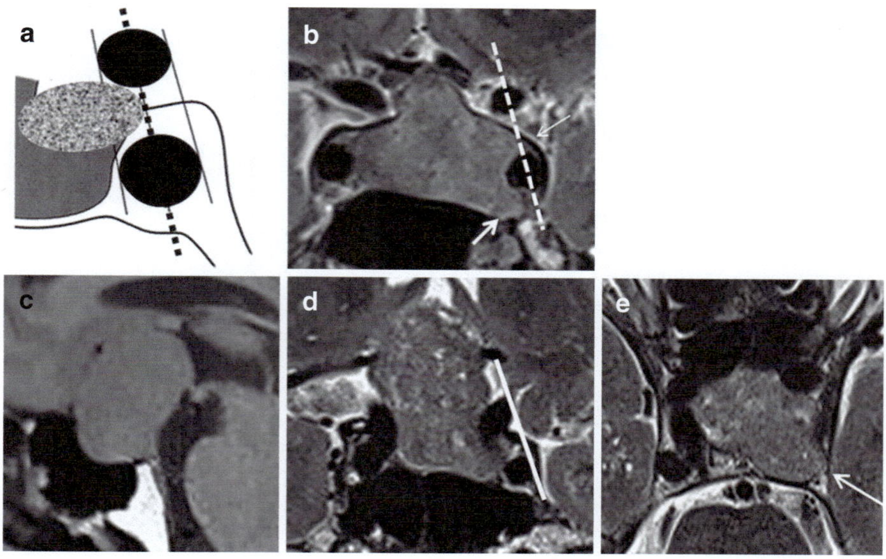

Fig. 18.3 (**a**) The Knosp landmark (simplified). If a tumor passes the lateral full line, cavernous sinus invasion is very likely. (**b**) Example: the pituitary adenoma passes barely (small arrow) the dotted line joining the mid diameters of intracavernous and intracisternal segments of the internal carotid artery. According to Knosp and Micko, there is a 30% chance that the cavernous sinus is truly invaded. Note the enlargement of the space normally occupied by the vein of the carotid sulcus (thick arrow). See Fig. 18.6. (**c**–**e**) Example of the Knosp landmark limitation. The lateral line is not crossed by the tumor, but posterior invasion of cavernous sinus is more than very likely on an axial T2W view (arrow)

In these last cases, the ultimate proof of invasion would be the demonstration of a tear of the thin dural wall separating the cavernous sinus space from the pituitary fossa on coronal or axial T2W images (Fig. 18.4). This finding is far from constant, the barrier being frequently totally destroyed when the cavernous sinus is invaded. If the dural wall is not completely torn, a floating curtain can be observed between the sellar content and the cavernous sinus. Conversely, demonstration of an intact internal wall from front to behind eliminates cavernous sinus invasion.

Other features can help, such as a shoulder-like extension of tumoral tissue above the C4 segment of the internal carotid artery visible on coronal sections (Fig. 18.5a, b).

A unilateral triangular posterolateral tumoral extension seen on axial sequences attests to the extreme thinness and fragility of the posterior part of the internal dural wall as opposed to its anterior part (Fig. 18.5c, d).

Obliteration of the venous inferolateral compartment constitutes another red flag (Fig. 18.6).

Generally speaking, it is noticeable that coronal and axial T2W sequences are more informative than gadolinium-enhanced sequences for the diagnosis of cavernous sinus invasion.

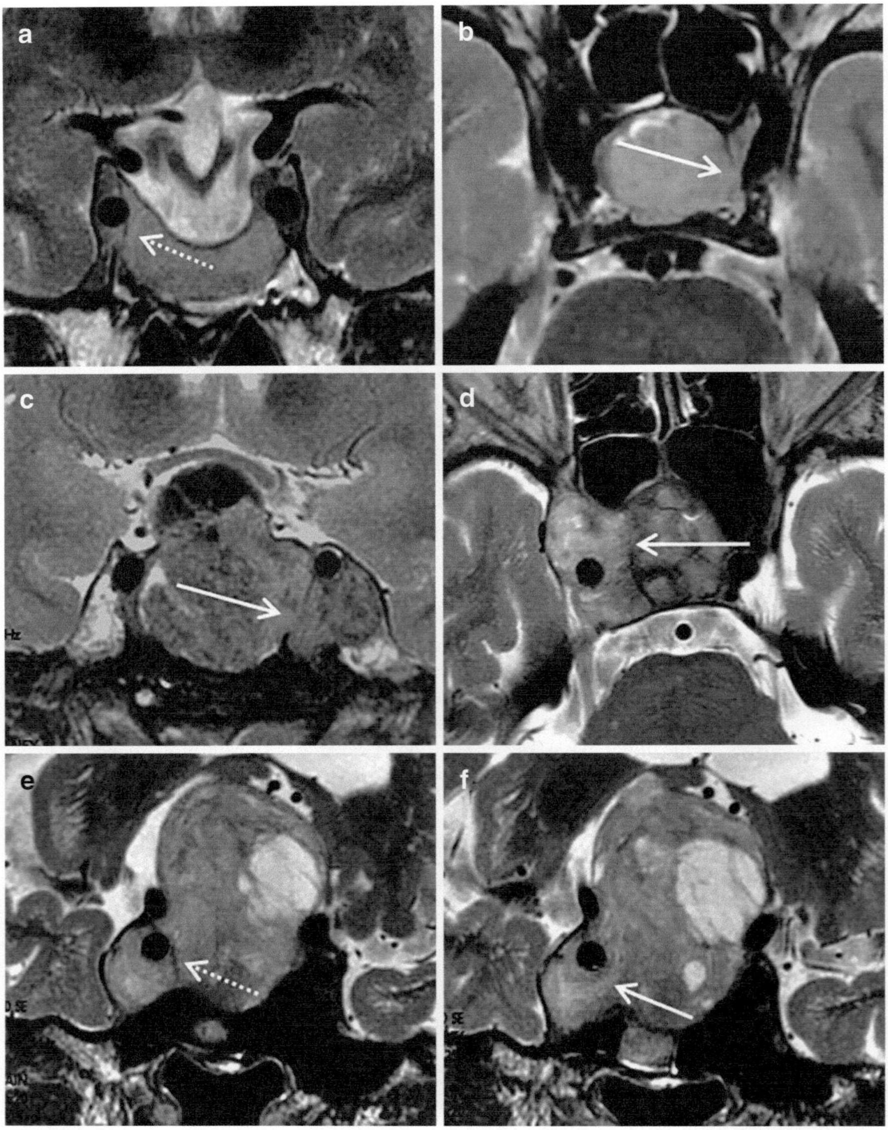

Fig. 18.4 The medial dural wall of the cavernous sinus. (**a**) Normal intact dural wall (dotted arrow). (**b**–**d**) Torn dural wall (full arrow). (**e**, **f**) The dural wall is intact anteriorly (dotted arrow) but destroyed on a section more posteriorly located. Note that the tumor infiltrates below the internal carotid artery which is remote from the sphenoid (arrow). Coronal (**a**, **c**, **e**, **f**) and axial (**b**, **d**) T2WIs

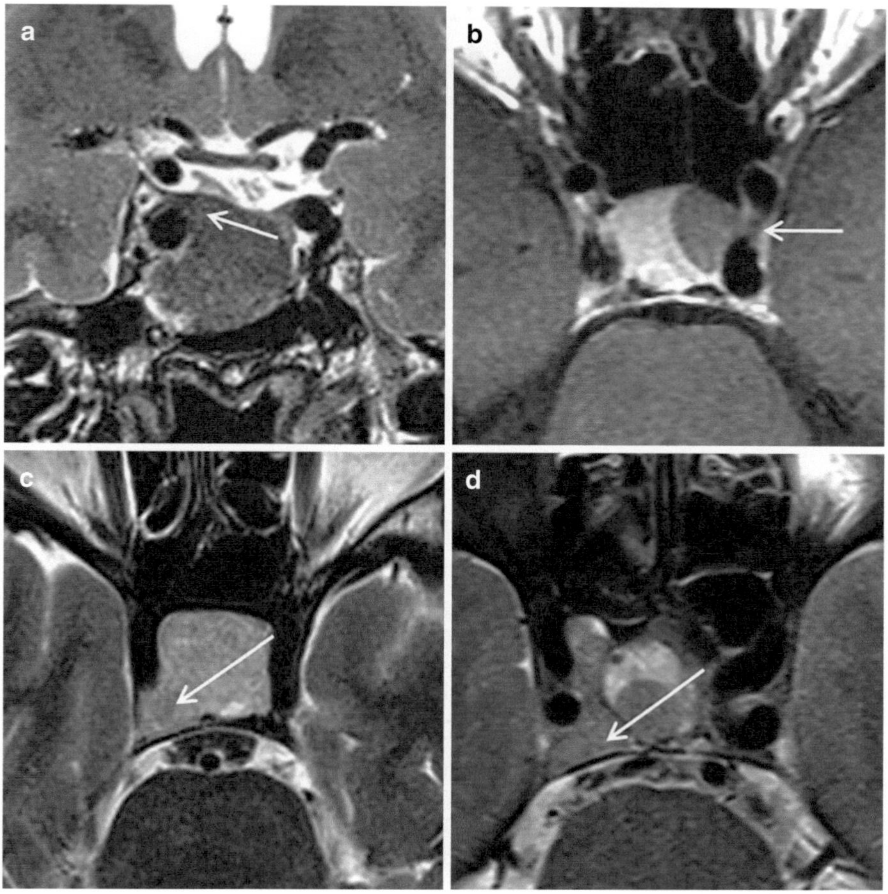

Fig. 18.5 Upper row. Discrete shoulder-like extension of tumoral tissue above the C4 segment of the internal carotid artery in two patients. (**a**) Coronal T2WI; (**b**) Axial CE T1WI. Lower row: Characteristic posterolateral tumoral extension related to the weakness of the posterior segment of the medial dural wall of cavernous sinus. (**c**, **d**) Axial T2WIs

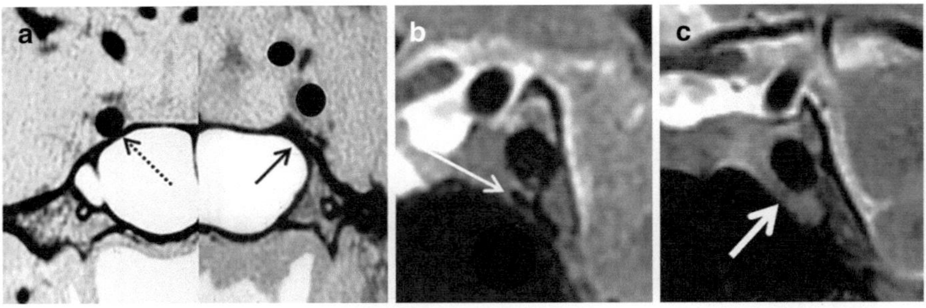

Fig. 18.6 The vein of the carotid sulcus. There are two normal anatomical situations: either the vein of the carotid sulcus does not exist and the internal carotid artery lies closely on the carotid sulcus of the sphenoid bone (dotted arrow), or the vein is visible between the sphenoid bone and the carotid artery (full arrow in **a** and **b**). When the internal carotid artery is remote from the sphenoid bone without visible vein (**c**), invasion of the cavernous sinus is highly likely. (**a**) schematic drawing of the two normal anatomical situations. (**b**, **c**) Coronal T2WIs

Further Readings

Dhandapani S, Singh H, Negm HM, Cohen S, Anand VK, Schwartz TH. Cavernous sinus invasion in pituitary adenomas: systematic review and pooled data meta-analysis of radiologic criteria and comparison of endoscopic and microscopic surgery. World Neurosurg. 2016;96:36–46. https://doi.org/10.1016/j.wneu.2016.08.088. Epub 2016 Aug 30.

Micko AS, Wöhrer A, Wolfsberger S, Knosp E. Invasion of the cavernous sinus space in pituitary adenomas: endoscopic verification and its correlation with an MRI-based classification. J Neurosurg. 2015;122(4):803–11. https://doi.org/10.3171/2014.12.JNS141083. Epub 2015 Feb 6.

Wu X, Xie SH, Tang B, Yang YQ, Yang L, Ding H, Bao YY, Lan SH, Zhou L, Hong T. Pituitary adenoma with posterior area invasion of cavernous sinus: surgical anatomy, approach, and outcomes. Neurosurg Rev. 2021;44(4):2229–37. https://doi.org/10.1007/s10143-020-01404-1. Epub 2020 Oct 2.

Aggressive or Invasive PitNETs? 19

If the vast majority of pituitary adenomas are benign tumors, a few do exhibit aggressive behavior which has been defined by the invasion of surrounding structures and resistance to conventional treatment. Recently, histological and molecular markers were added to define aggressive tumors. Therefore, invasion represents only one aspect of aggressiveness and radiologists must keep in mind that the term "aggressive pituitary adenoma" is improper in MRI reports unless evidence of tumor growth despite optimal treatment. Much more rarely, the occurrence of systemic or cerebrospinal metastases justifies the denomination of pituitary carcinomas.A five-tiered classification taking into account invasion, immunohistological type, and proliferative makers is today recognized as a useful tool to approach the prognosis of PitNETs and to propose the most appropriate treatment (Table 19.1).

We will briefly discuss first the diagnosis of invasive pituitary adenomas; we will then expose several semeiologic points which may suggest aggressiveness.

Invasion of the cavernous sinus is largely presented in Chap. 18. Let us simply recall that a subtle invasion can escape the Knosp criteria and that demonstration of the rupture of the cavernous sinus medial wall which positively attests to invasion is unfortunately far from constant (Fig. 19.1). This barrier has a point of weakness located posteriorly which explains that early invasion usually starts posteriorly as shown at best by axial sequences. Finally, if a cavernous sinus invasion is frequently present in aggressive tumors, it does not mean that all tumors with cavernous sinus invasion are aggressive. Male prolactinomas, for instance, tend to be large and invade the sphenoid sinus and the cavernous sinus but respond usually well to medical treatment and must not be considered aggressive (Fig. 13.5).

Invasion of the sphenoid bone and sphenoid sinus mucosa may be difficult to differentiate from the mere displacement of a thinned sellar floor. A localized acute change of the sellar contour is very suggestive of invasion (Fig. 19.2). Computerized tomography could be helpful here to show the integrity or the erosion of the sellar floor. The diagnosis of dura mater invasion is still reserved for pathologists.

Apart from invasion, several MRI features can evoke aggressiveness.

J.-F. Bonneville, *Tricks and Traps in MRI of the Pituitary Region*,
https://doi.org/10.1007/978-3-031-64710-9_19

Table 19.1 The five-tiered classification of PitNETs

1: Tumor diameter into micro (<10 mm), macro (≥10 mm) and giant (>40 mm) by MRI
2: Tumor type into somatotroph, lactotroph, corticotropin, gonadotroph, thyrotroph, plurihormonal, and immunonegative tumor by IHC
3: Tumor grade based on the following criteria:
Invasion defined as histological and/or radiological (MRI) signs of cavernous or sphenoid sinus invasion
Proliferation considered on the presence of at least 2 of the 3 markers:
Mitoses count: $n > 2/10$ HPF
Ki-67 index: ≥3%
P53 detection positive: >10 strongly positive nuclei/10 HPF
The 5 grades are the following:
Grade **1a**: non-invasive and non-proliferative tumor
Grade **1b**: non-invasive and proliferative tumor
Grade **2a**: invasive and non-proliferative tumor
Grade **2b**: invasive and proliferative tumor
Grade **3**: metastatic tumor (cerebrospinal or systemic metastases)

From Trouillas et al. (2020), with permission

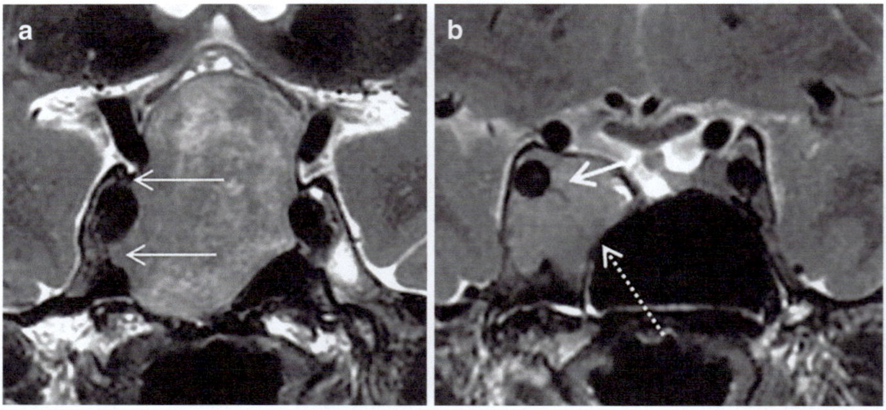

Fig. 19.1 Compression (**a**) versus invasion (**b**) of the cavernous sinus in two patients with a non-secreting PitNET. In (**a**), the dural wall is not visible excepted superiorly (short arrow). In (**a**), the dural wall (thin arrows) is displaced but not ruptured. In (**b**), the medial dural wall appears as a floating curtain (thick arrow). The space between the internal carotid artery and the carotid sulcus is enlarged (dotted arrow) and the vein of the carotid sulcus is invisible. (**a**, **b**) Coronal T2WIs

- Rapid growth of a pituitary adenoma or of a remnant can be recognized very early if the reproducibility of MR sequences is perfect as it is obtained by using coronal sections perpendicular to the subcallosal line (Fig. 19.3).
- Sleeve button exophytic nodules (Fig. 19.4c, d) or invasion of the clivus (Fig. 19.5) are considered as manifestations of aggressiveness.
- Intratumoral multiple small microcysts are frequently observed on T2W images in silent corticotropic pituitary adenomas and also in other types of PitNETs and are known to grow quickly and can recur after surgery (Fig. 19.4a).

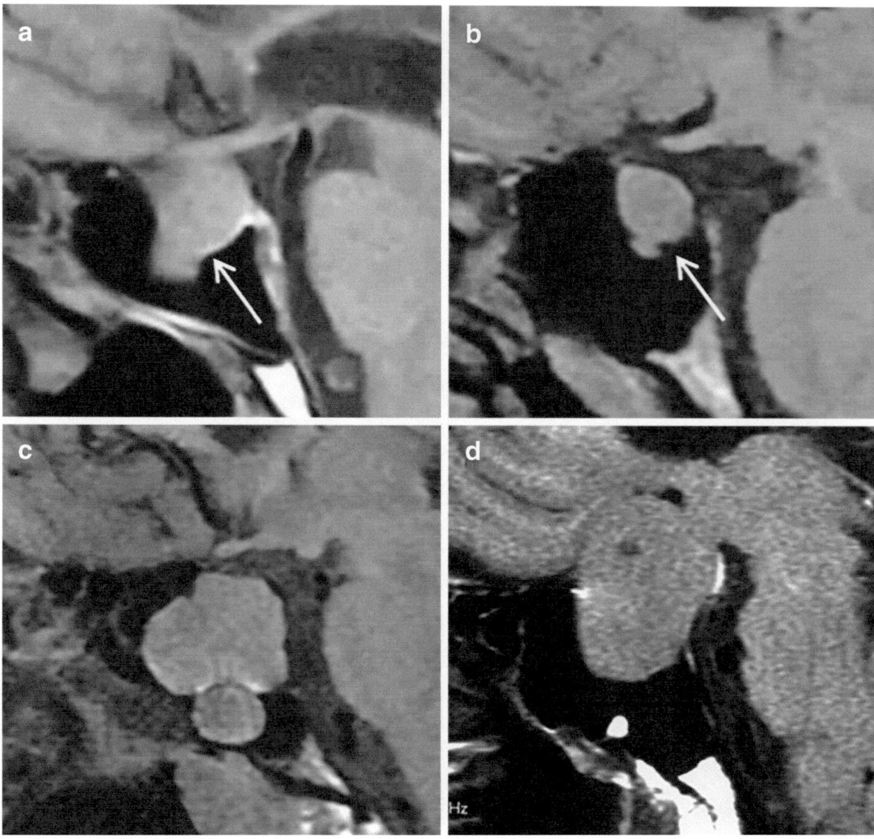

Fig. 19.2 Upper row. Short, acute brutal change of the contour of the sella in two patients presenting a prolactinoma signing true invasion (arrows). Lower row. Sphenoid invasion (**c**) versus no invasion (**d**). In (**d**), the sellar floor is simply pushed down by the tumor. (**a**–**d**) Sagittal T1IWs

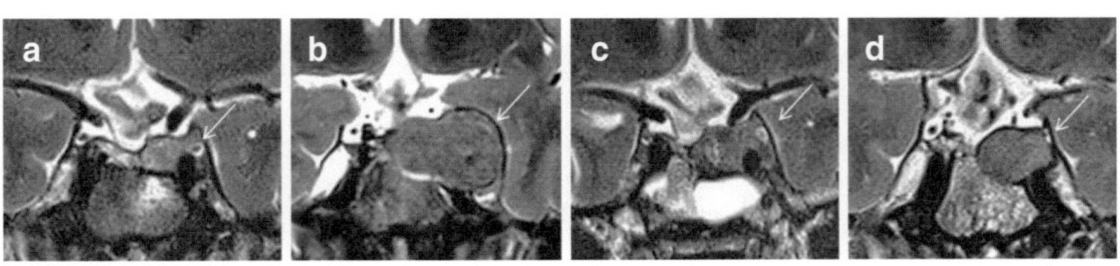

Fig. 19.3 Aggressive non-secreting PitNET invading the cavernous sinus. (**a**) Intrasellar left recurrence 2 years after surgery. (**b**) Two years later, huge tumoral extension to the cavernous sinus. The internal carotid artery diameter is severely narrowed. (**c**) One year after radiotherapy, a tumoral shrinkage is obvious. (**d**) Four more years later, new recurrence. Observe the changes of the sheath of the third cranial nerve (long arrows). (**a**–**d**) Coronal T2WIs

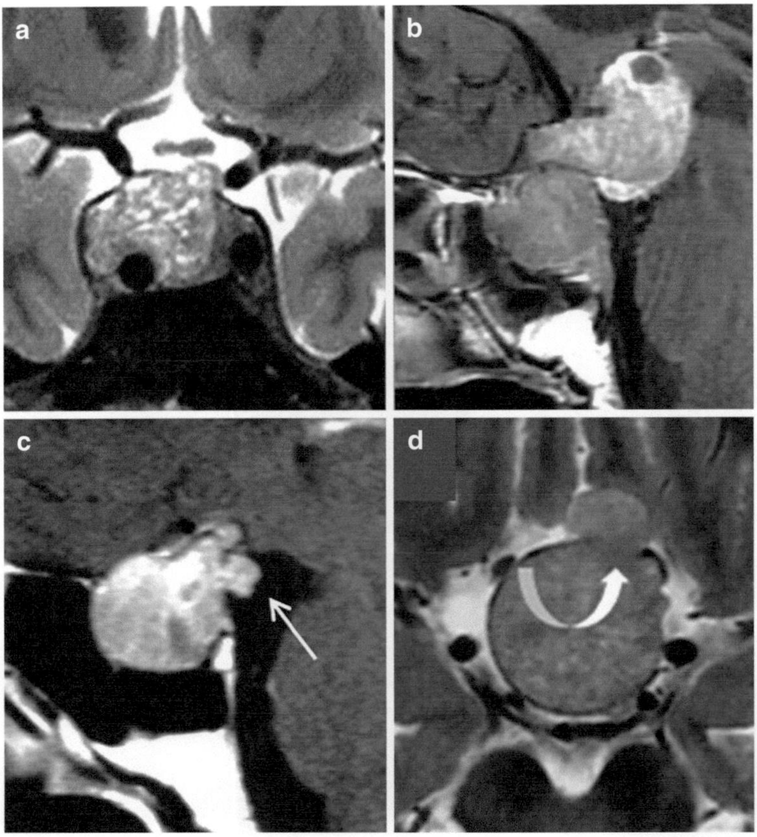

Fig. 19.4 Aggressive PitNETs. Upper row. (**a**) Microcystic pattern of a silent PitNET on coronal T2WI. (**b**) Appalling evolution of an aggressive prolactinoma despite multimodal treatment including temozolomide on sagittal CE T1WI. Lower row. Aggressive prolactinomas. (**c**, **d**) Sleeve button exophytic nodules (arrows). (**c**) Sagittal CE T1WI. d: Axial T2WI

- Pituitary adenomas revealed by apoplexy can be aggressive and may regrow after tumoral shrinkage.
- Giant pituitary adenomas—more than 40 mm in diameter—are considered aggressive (Fig. 19.5).
- Evidently, metastases are also a sign of aggressiveness.

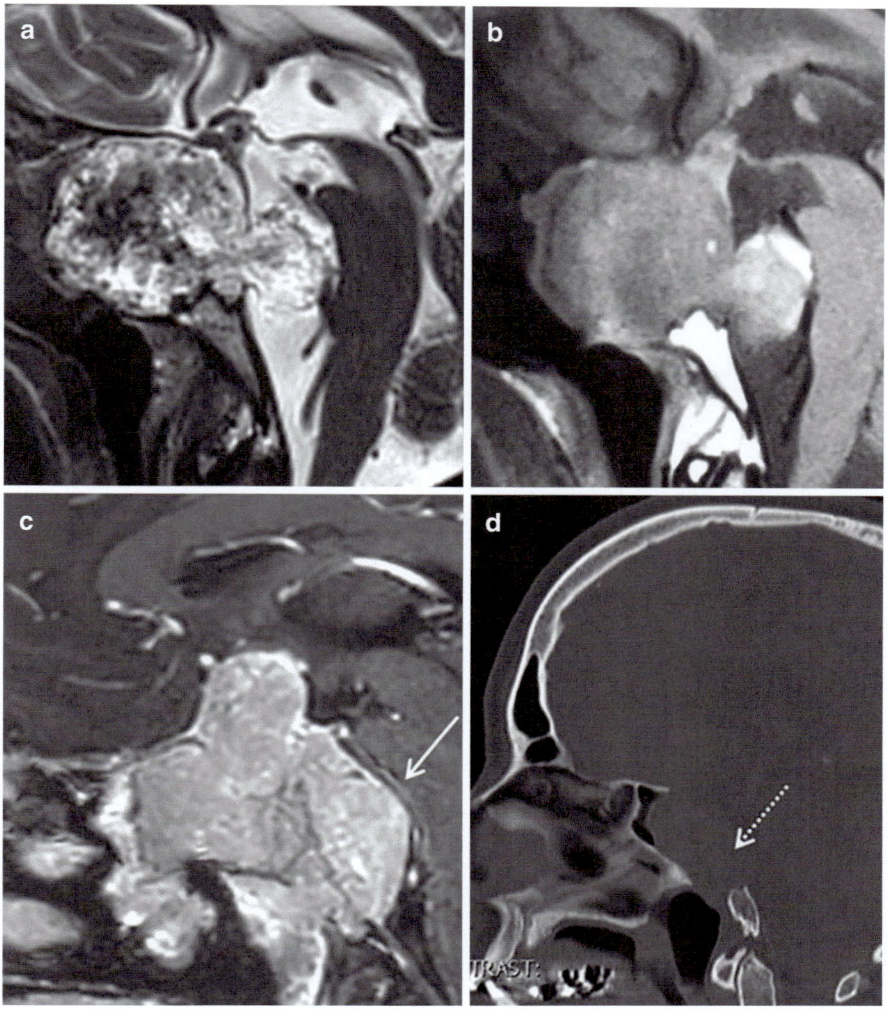

Fig. 19.5 Aggressive PitNETs with clivus erosion and brain stem compression in two patients. (**a**) Sagittal T2WI. (**b**, **c**) Sagittal CE T1WIs. (**d**) CT

Reference

Trouillas J, Jaffrain-Rea ML, et al. How to classify the pituitary neuroendocrine tumors (PitNET)s in 2020. Cancers (Basel). 2020;12(2):514. https://doi.org/10.3390/cancers12020514.

Further Readings

Bonneville JF, Potorac J, Beckers A. Neuroimaging of aggressive pituitary tumors. Rev Endocr Metab Disord. 2020;21(2):235–42. https://doi.org/10.1007/s11154-020-09557-6.

Chatzellis E, Alexandraki KI, Androulakis II, Kaltsas G. Aggressive pituitary tumors. Neuroendocrinology. 2015;101(2):87–104. https://doi.org/10.1159/000371806. Epub 2015 Jan 5. Review.

20 Apoplexy or Hemorrhage?

While a trend to replace outdated medical terms is emerging, it is curious that no one has proposed eliminating the term "pituitary apoplexy" from medical vocabulary yet. Apoplexy is a vague term used in the past to describe a sudden loss of vital functions regardless of the etiology and is not clearly appropriate to describe the complex phenomenon which sometimes occurs in pituitary adenoma. Using this term contributes to the confusion which could exist between true hemorrhage and apoplexy.

Pituitary apoplexy is either an ischemic or hemorrhagic sudden intratumoral event, associated with burning symptoms while a pituitary hemorrhage is usually a slow non-symptomatic process. Apoplexy almost always complicates a PitNET and frequently reveals the lesion. We have noted that most pituitary apoplexies complicate pituitary macroadenomas with a suprasellar extension approaching the optic chiasm, but rarely giant adenomas, as if hemorrhagic infarction preferentially occurs when the responsible pituitary adenoma is still contained by the sellar diaphragm (Fig. 20.1). Moreover, massive invasion of cavernous sinus is uncommon in this condition, the frequent oculomotor nerves palsy being related to a compression of the cavernous sinus by the increased volume of the pituitary without rupture of the medial cavernous sinus wall.

A variety of precipitating factors have been linked to the occurrence of pituitary apoplexy. The possible development of apoplexy during pregnancy has been recently highlighted. Symptomatology of pituitary apoplexy is acute and noisy. The sudden onset of headaches can simulate a subarachnoid hemorrhage which is easily eliminated on CT. Unilateral oculomotor palsy is almost the rule. An acute corticotropic deficit is responsible for intense sudden fatigue with pallor (Fig. 20.2). Despite its dramatic onset, pituitary apoplexy is considered today a medical emergency instead of a surgical one because the mass effect resolves spontaneously and because the pituitary deficit is not improved by surgery. Only severe chiasmatic or optic nerve compression requires immediate surgical decompression.

Differentiating apoplexy from pituitary adenoma hemorrhage is crucial.

J.-F. Bonneville, *Tricks and Traps in MRI of the Pituitary Region*,
https://doi.org/10.1007/978-3-031-64710-9_20

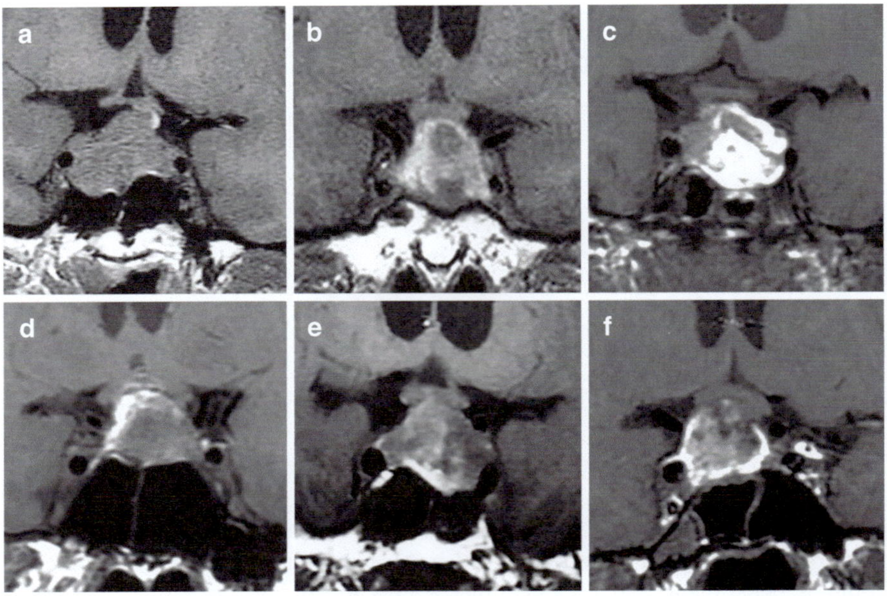

Fig 20.1 A series of pituitary apoplexies. (**a–f**) Coronal non-enhanced T1WIs. Note the very similar size of the responsible macroadenomas just abutting the optic chiasm

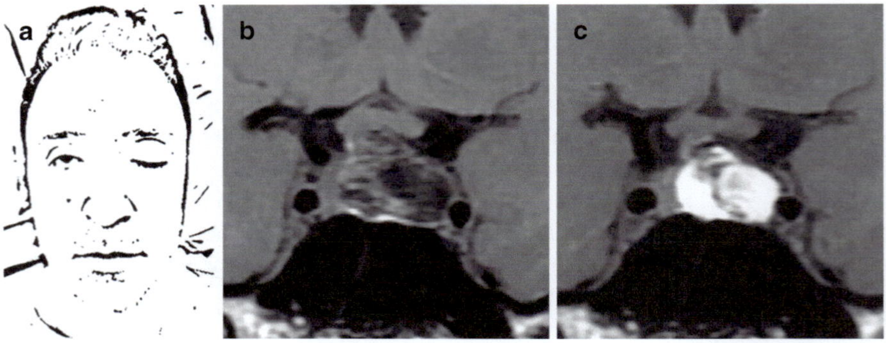

Fig 20.2 (**a**) Characteristic symptoms of acute apoplexy: asthenia, pallor, and left third nerve palsy. (**b**, **c**) Coronal T1WIs at 3 days (**b**) and 5 days (**c**). "Brushed pattern" in (**b**) followed by T1W hyperintensity corresponding to methemoglobin in (**c**)

Hemorrhage within a pituitary adenoma is usually detected on MRI without clinical manifestations.

The pattern is of a cystic pituitary mass. With recent hemorrhage, a fluid-fluid level is characteristic, with typically a posterior dark component well shown on sagittal T2WI and a T1-T2 hyperintense anterior component but both signals vary with the age of hemorrhage (Fig. 20.3). There are no signs of recent pituitary size increase or thickening of the sphenoid sinus mucosa. In case of old hemorrhage,

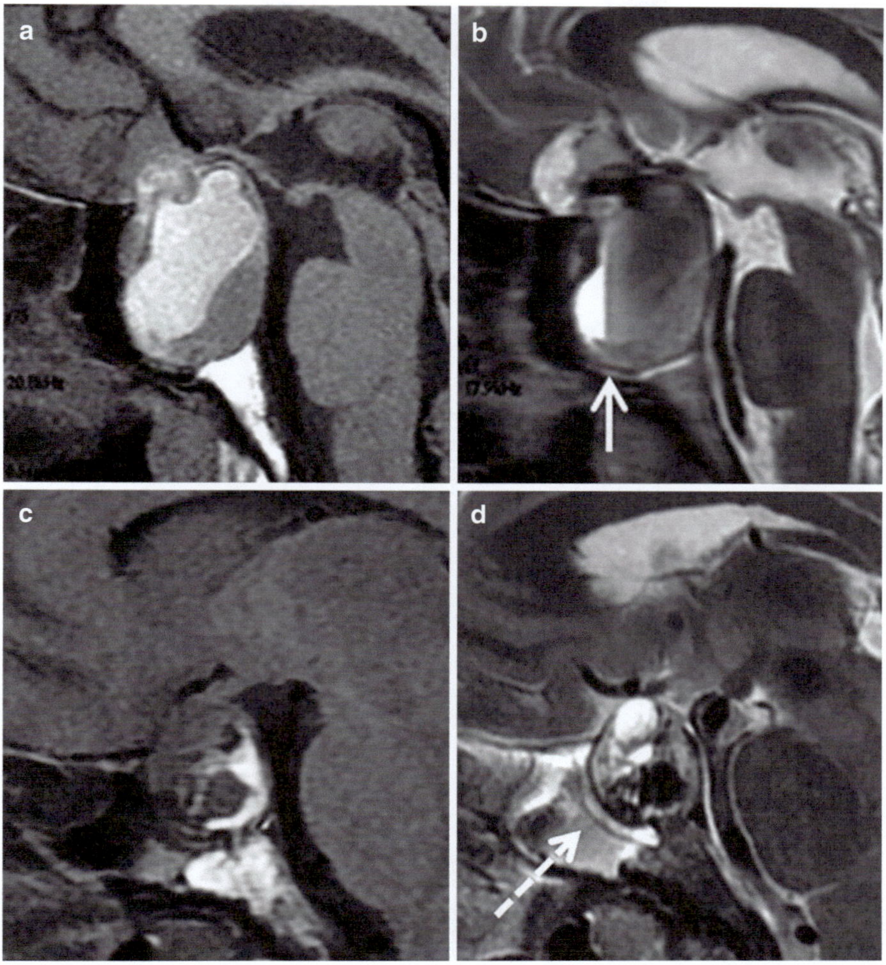

Fig 20.3 Typical pattern of a non-symptomatic PitNET hemorrhage (**a**, **b**) versus pituitary apoplexy (**c**, **d**). Fluid-fluid level (arrow) in benign hemorrhage with dark posterior component better demonstrated on sagittal T2WI (**b**). No thickening of sphenoid sinus mucosa. In apoplexy (**c**, **d**) mixture of various areas of T1 and T2W hypo- and hyperintensities. Marked thickening of the sphenoid sinus mucosa (dotted arrow)

PitNETs appear as a mass with an eccentric cyst with thick-walled enhancement and frequent septations (Fig. 28.6e). It is very likely that most cystic PitNETs have presented a hemorrhage or more rarely an infarct years before their discovery.

In *apoplexy* seen after a few days, MRI displays a mixture of T1 hyperintensities and T2W hypointensities with blurred contours (Fig. 20.3). We consider that the presence of a fluid-fluid level in the initial imaging study eliminates the diagnosis of apoplexy.

At the very early phase of apoplexy, i.e., in the first two days, T1W hyperintensity is frequently absent either because the event is purely ischemic or because hemorrhage is still in the form of deoxyhemoglobin. A "brushed" specific pattern of alternating subtle T1 hyperintense and hypointense lines within the sellar mass may suggest apoplexy before that the more characteristic T1hyperintense signal of blood becomes visible (Fig. 20.4). T2WI is more sensitive by demonstrating heterogeneous low signal intensity areas. Diffusion-weighted imaging can show an increased

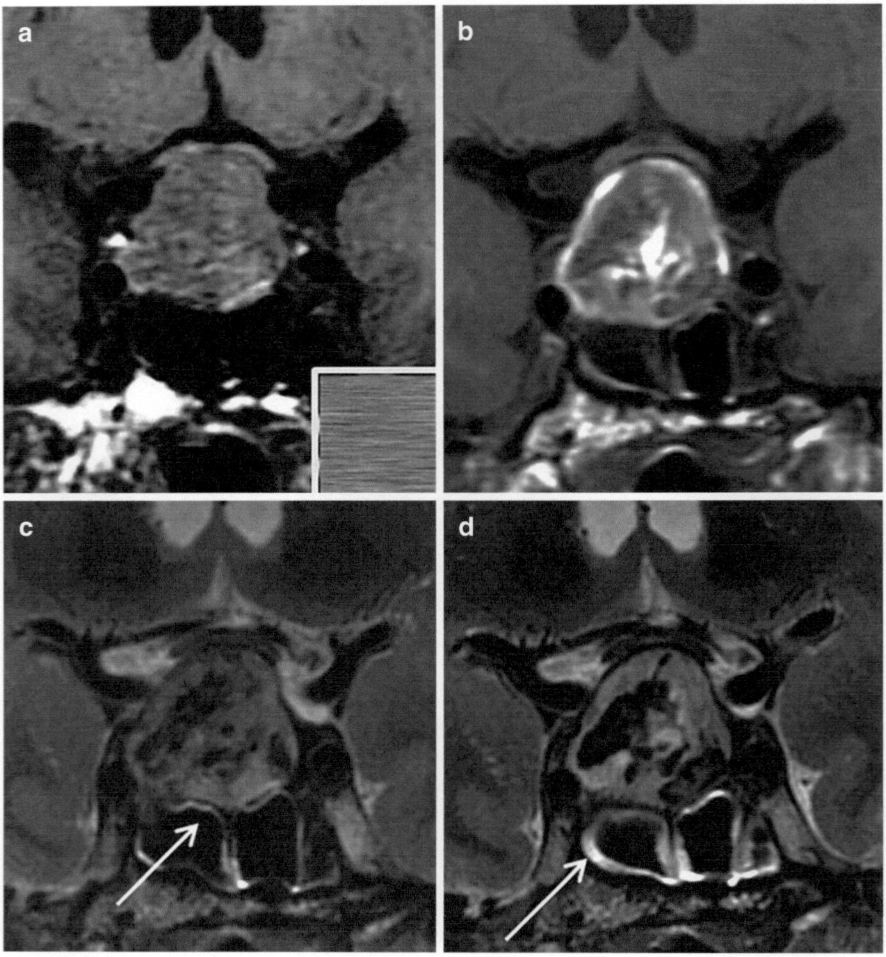

Fig 20.4 Serial coronal T1W (**a**, **b**) and T2WIs (**c**, **d**) of a patient with pituitary apoplexy. (**a**, **c**) 12 h after the onset of symptoms. Pituitary mass abutting the optic chiasm and yielding a heterogeneous signal with linear alternating areas of T1 hyper- and hypointensities, showing a general striated or "brushed aluminum" pattern (see insert in **a**). Irregular areas of T2 hypointensities and discrete thickening of the sinus mucosa (arrow) in (**c**): Coronal T2WI. (**b**, **d**) At 36h: peripheral and central areas of spontaneous T1W hyperintense signal. More obvious thickening of the sphenoid sinus mucosa (arrow) in (**d**): Coronal T2WI

signal intensity and a low apparent diffusion coefficient, consistent with restricted diffusion. This sequence has great value in the cases of ischemic pituitary necrosis without hemorrhage. Reactional thickening of sphenoid sinus mucosa is very sensitive and may attest to recent pituitary adenoma changes before any obvious signal change (Fig. 20.5). It is never observed in hemorrhagic adenoma. Dural enhancement is another early sign evoking pituitary apoplexy but is less reliable (Fig. 20.5). Compression and/or stenosis of the internal intracavernous carotid artery leading to stroke has been exceptionally described.

Sequential MRI will demonstrate a gradual increase in the T1 hyperintense signal, from the periphery toward the center of the mass, corresponding to the transformation of deoxyhemoglobin to methemoglobin. In parallel, T2WIs demonstrate irregular hypointense areas widening in the more central part of the mass (Fig. 20.4).

A wait-and-see management with corticoid supplementation is usually proposed. Shrinkage of the mass occurs in some weeks or months. Regrowth of pituitary

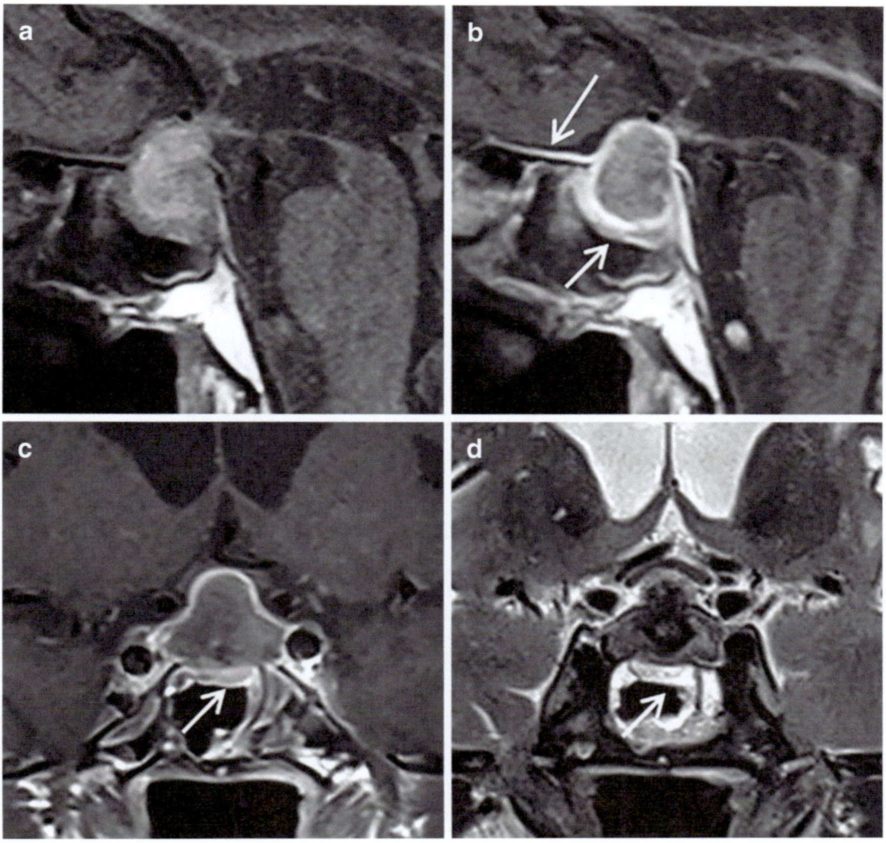

Fig 20.5 Pituitary apoplexy at 4 days. (**a**, **b**) Sagittal and sagittal CE T1Ws. (**c**, **d**) Coronal CE T1 and T2WIs. Spontaneous T1W hypersignal and peripheral enhancement of the sellar mass. Dural tail (long arrow) and thickening of the sphenoid sinus mucosa (short arrows)

adenoma may occur at some distance from the apoplectic episode. Consequently, apoplexy must be considered as a possible manifestation of tumoral aggressiveness and managed with a long-term follow-up.

Further Readings

Araujo-Castro M, Paredes I, Pérez-López C, et al. Differences in clinical, hormonal, and radiological presentation and in surgical outcomes in patients presenting with and without pituitary apoplexy. A multicenter study of 245 cases. Pituitary. 2023;26(2):250–8. https://doi.org/10.1007/s11102-023-01315-6.

Briet C, Salenave S, Bonneville JF, Laws ER, Chanson P. Pituitary apoplexy. Endocr Rev. 2015;36(6):622–45. https://doi.org/10.1210/er.2015-1042. Epub 2015 Sep 28.

Donegan D, Erickson D. Revisiting pituitary apoplexy. J Endocr Soc. 2022;6(9):bvac113. https://doi.org/10.1210/jendso/bvac113.

Pituitary Hyperplasia or Pseudo-hyperplasia?

21

For the pathologist, pituitary hyperplasia corresponds to an increased number of pituitary cells and not to an increased pituitary volume. The radiological definition could correspond to an increased pituitary volume without evidence of focal lesion or heterogeneity, and usually with a T1W signal close to that of the white matter or a T2W signal close to that of the cortex and a homogeneous enhancement after gadolinium injection. The limit of this definition is that there is no strict cut-off to determine if the pituitary gland is enlarged or not since the volume variations are large in individuals. For instance, the diagnosis of pituitary hyperplasia may be difficult in the elderly where a physiological shrinkage is observed.

Pituitary hyperplasia can be physiological or pathological and corresponds to an increased hormonal activity.

Physiological hyperplasia is observed in neonates and in adolescents in response to the increase in hormonal needs (Fig. 21.1). At puberty, pituitary

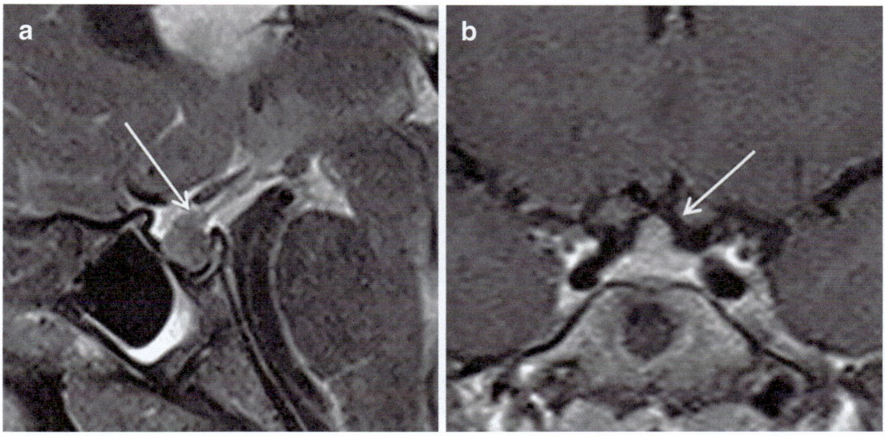

Fig. 21.1 Advanced puberty in a 8-year-old girl. Bulging pituitary. (**a**, **b**) Sagittal T2 and coronal CE T1WIs

J.-F. Bonneville, *Tricks and Traps in MRI of the Pituitary Region*,
https://doi.org/10.1007/978-3-031-64710-9_21

bulging may be so marked that it can simulate a tumoral process. In adolescents, particularly in girls, the observation of a bulging pituitary gland is common, and the gland can be 9 or 10 mm high with a symmetric tent-like configuration. T1 and T2W signals are normal as well as the enhancement pattern. If a dynamic sequence were obtained—but I will one more time remind you that this sequence is very rarely helpful and can be misleading—it post-gadolinium enhancement would be symmetric. This pattern in girl adolescents must be considered as normal and described as normal.

Coexistence of a small sella turcica with true physiological hyperplasia can occur in the adolescent girl and the young female and can lead to a possibly troubling image of an 11- or 12-mm high pituitary gland: In this non-pathological situation, the term pituitary hyperplasia must not be used by the radiologist to avoid additional costly examinations and possible anxiety (Fig. 21.2).

Another situation requiring increased hormonal needs is pregnancy: Pituitary hyperplasia is more obvious in the third trimester when the pituitary may reach and sometimes overcome 10 mm in height with a more or less discrete T1W hyperintensity of the anterior pituitary. Pituitary height is still increased during post-partum and during lactation and can reach 12 mm (Fig. 21.3).

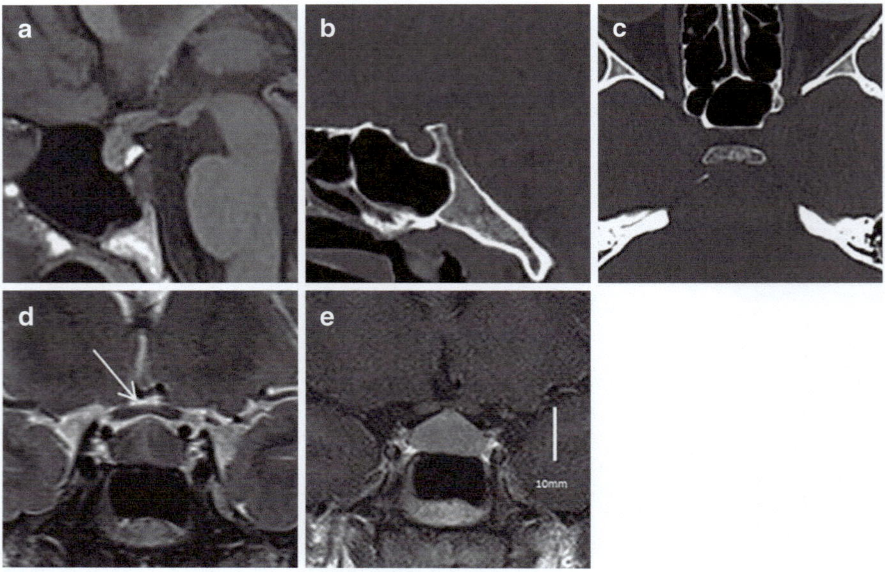

Fig. 21.2 Pseudo-hyperplasia in an 18-year-old female presenting with headache. Narrow sella turcica from front to behind and reduced sellar volume. (**a–c**) Sagittal T1, sagittal and axial CT. Homogeneous T2 signal and homogeneous enhancement of a 9 mm high pituitary. (**d, e**) Coronal T2 and CE T1WIs. There is no contact of this normal pituitary gland with the optic chiasm which is yet slightly deformed (arrow) despite the presence of a slice of CSF between both. Exceptionally, this presentation may become symptomatic with blurred vision during pregnancy

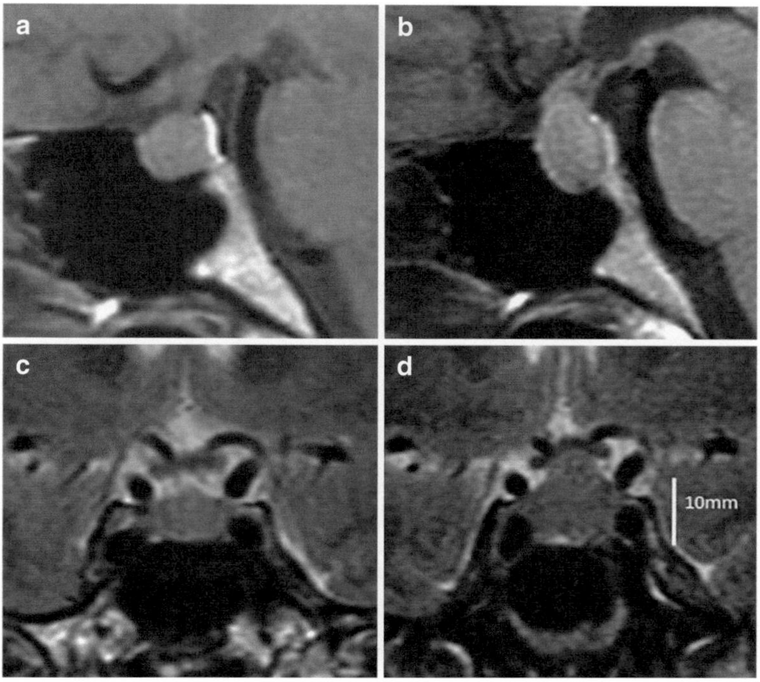

Fig. 21.3 Physiological pituitary hyperplasia in the third trimester of pregnancy. The pituitary gland is 12 mm high. Sagittal and coronal T1WIs before pregnancy (**a**, **c**) and 3 weeks before delivery (**b**, **d**)

A temporary small increased height of the pituitary gland may be observed during menopause, when FSH and LH synthesis is very important to answer to the drop in ovarian hormones (Fig. 21.4a–c). Exceptionally such a physiological image is so impressive that it can worry (Fig. 21.4d, e).

Pathological pituitary hyperplasia applies to the settings of end-organ insufficiency with loss of negative feedback and excess trophic hormone from the hypothalamus. The main manifestation of an organ failure is primary hypothyroidism. The resulting hyperplasia has been described as a cherry-like pituitary but in fact has no specific characteristics apart from sometimes a slightly T2W hyperintense signal. Optic chiasm threat may be present. A shrinkage of the pituitary content is observed very quickly after hormonal replacement therapy (Fig. 21.5). Other causes include primary hypogonadism as observed in Klinefelter and Turner syndromes and polycystic ovary syndrome.

True pituitary hyperplasia is also observed in rare acromegalic syndromes such as McCune-Albright syndrome and X-LAG syndrome which affects young children. It must be noted that pituitary adenoma and hyperplasia can coexist and that the adenomatous transformation from pituitary hyperplasia was described. Pituitary

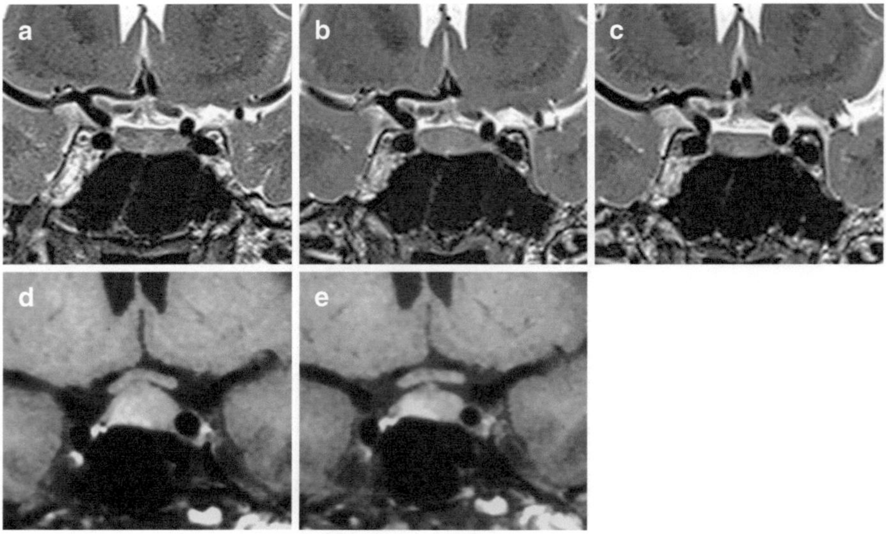

Fig. 21.4 Physiological pituitary hyperplasia related to menopause. It is rarely demonstrated and usually discrete (**a–c**) or unusually disturbing (**d, e**). (**a–c**) Coronal T2WIs before (**a**), during (**b**), and 1 year after menopause (**c**). Slight convexity of the upper aspect of the pituitary gland in (**b**). (**d, e**) Coronal T1WIs at menopause (**d**) and 4 months later in a 52-year-old asymptomatic woman

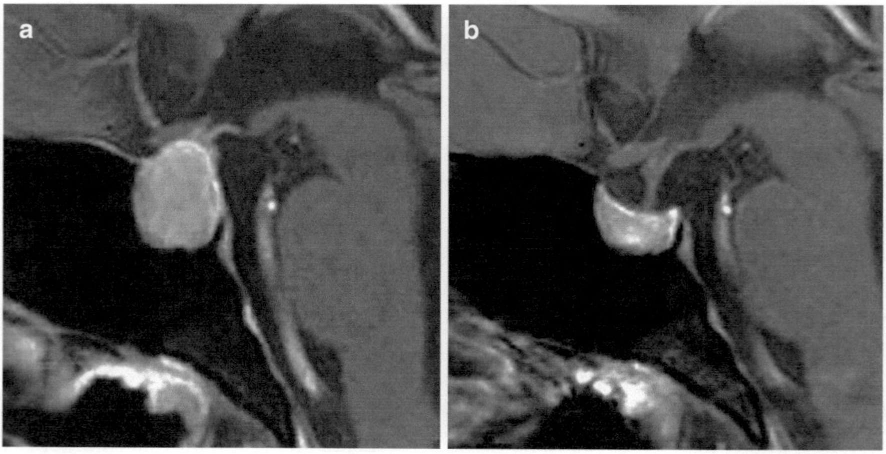

Fig. 21.5 Primary hypothyroidism before (**a**) and a 3 months after thyroxine replacement therapy (**b**). (**a, b**) Sagittal CE T1WIs

hyperplasia is also present with growth hormone-releasing hormone (GHRH) ectopic secretion from a neuroendocrine tumor. These conditions are developed in Chap. 15.

Pituitary hyperplasia could also be caused by medication, including estrogen, GNRH analogs, and antipsychotics.

The term pituitary hyperplasia is not appropriate for naming the enlargement of the pituitary gland observed in hypophysitis and other inflammatory conditions

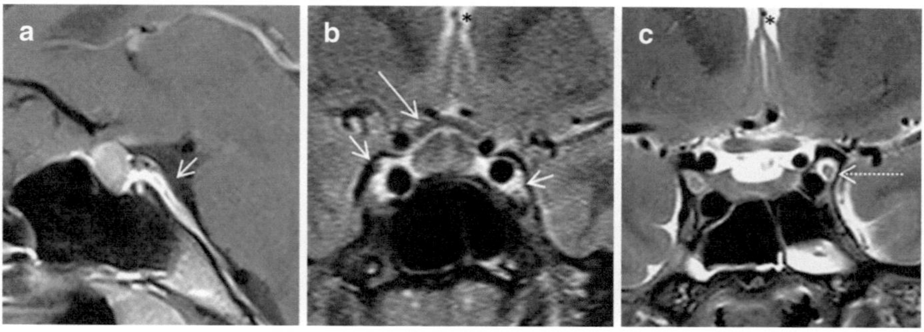

Fig. 21.6 Pseudo pituitary hyperplasia related to intracranial hypotension. (**a**, **b**) Engorgeous pituitary gland distorting the optic chiasm (long arrow). Distended parasellar veins (small arrows). Collapsed ventricles (*). (**c**) One month after blood patch. Shrinkage of the pituitary gland and shrinkage of parasellar veins. Enlarged third nerve sheath (dotted arrow). (**a**) Sagittal CE T1WI. (**b**, **c**) Coronal T2WIs

since additional changes are noted, such as the thickening of the pituitary stalk, dural tail, and strong enhancement after gadolinium injection.

The term pituitary hyperplasia is frequently erroneously used when there is a mismatch between the volume of the contents—the pituitary gland—and that of the container—the sella turcica, with no hormonal dysfunction. The image is that of a brioche overflowing its mold (Fig. 8.1).

The term *pseudo-hyperplasia* can also be applied to cavernous sinus fistula or to intracranial hypotension where the pituitary content is swelling in relation to a venous flow impairment. The intracranial hypotension syndrome—a frequently misdiagnosed condition—is usually caused by a spinal CSF leak. Pituitary bulging can be associated with dural enhancement and dural thickening, brain sagging, decreased ventricle size, collapsed cisterns, subdural collections, and venous distension. At the sellar level, enlargement of parasellar veins, for instance of the inferior intercavernous sinus below a bulging pituitary gland is obvious (Fig. 21.6). An associated calvarial hyperostosis, recently described, may also draw attention.

The differential diagnosis of pituitary hyperplasia or pseudo-hyperplasia is to be made with isointense pituitary adenoma or isointense Rathke cleft cyst.

Further Readings

Bonneville JF, Cattin F, Bonneville F. Enlargement of the inferior intercavernous sinus: a new sign for the diagnosis of craniospinal hypotension. AJNR Am J Neuroradiol. 2011;32(10):E194. https://doi.org/10.3174/ajnr.A2816. PMID: 22084192; PMCID: PMC7966023.

Han L, Wang J, Shu K, Lei T. Pituitary tumorous hyperplasia due to primary hypothyroidism. Acta Neurochir (Wien). 2012;154(8):1489–92. https://doi.org/10.1007/s00701-012-1342-0. Epub 2012 Apr 17. PMID: 22527578; PMCID: PMC3407554.

Sapkota S, Karn M, Sapkota S. Pituitary hyperplasia in childhood primary hypothyroidism: a review. Childs Nerv Syst. 2021;37(3):749–62. https://doi.org/10.1007/s00381-020-05014-6. Epub 2021 Jan 6.

22 In Pregnancy

Each time I give a presentation dealing with pituitary MRI and pregnancy in front of an audience of endocrinologists, it raises a wind of disapproval as if MRI in this condition was completely irrelevant when carrying an unclear risk and I was considered irresponsible. I have here the opportunity to clarify my position.

I have first to discuss the risk of MRI during pregnancy. For decades, the word imaging has been subconsciously associated to X-rays with their potential of devastating risk for the fetus. Just to be clear: provided that MRI is performed during the third trimester and without gadolinium, such a risk is considered null. The reluctance of many endocrinologists to prescribe an MRI during the last trimester of gestation is clearly unjustified *if the situation requires it.* Indications for pituitary MRI during pregnancy are very rare. But they exist, so then, it looks useful to know the appearance of the pituitary gland in this condition.

The normal pituitary gland height increases linearly by 0.08–0.1 mm/week, i.e., by 3–4 mm at term. The upper surface of the gland becomes more convex superiorly. The pituitary gland height can reach 10 mm during the last trimester and 12 mm in the immediate postpartum period, approaching the optic chiasm. Thus, a possible threat to the optic chiasm in late pregnancy must be considered in case of history of pituitary tumor or if a small sella with pituitary gland bulging has been incidentally observed before pregnancy. It has to be noted that the peak height of the pituitary gland observed during the early postpartum period is prolonged by breastfeeding. A visual blur may occur in these situations.

The T1W signal intensity of the pituitary gland increases during pregnancy (Fig. 22.1b, d), particularly during the last trimester and if breastfeeding. This is made clear when comparing the T1W signal of the anterior pituitary with that of the white matter of the temporal lobe on coronal views or with that of the pons on sagittal views. This is an interesting feature when hypophysitis is suspected because the pituitary gland which is enlarged in hypophysitis does not display a spontaneous T1W hyperintense signal.

During the third trimester, the posterior lobe may be slightly compressed and thinned by the enlarged anterior pituitary gland and pressed against the dorsum

J.-F. Bonneville, *Tricks and Traps in MRI of the Pituitary Region*,
https://doi.org/10.1007/978-3-031-64710-9_22

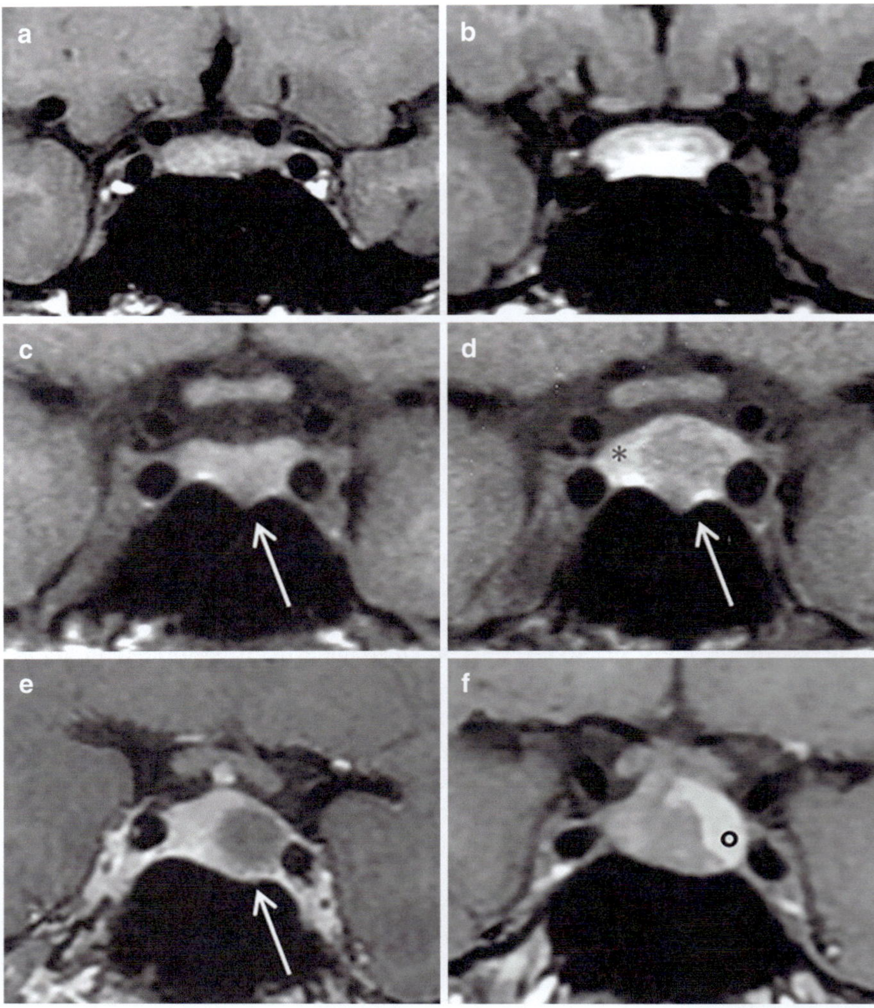

Fig. 22.1 Upper row. Normal pituitary gland before (**a**) and in late pregnancy (**b**). Increased size and T1W hyperintensity of the pituitary gland. Middle row. Microprolactinoma after cabergoline treatment (**c**) and in late pregnancy (**d**). Marked increased size of the prolactinoma (arrow). Note the T1W hyperintense signal of the normal gland (*). Lower row. Microprolactinoma before treatment (**e**). Prolactin level is 50 μG/L. The medical treatment has been stopped as soon as the pregnancy was known. The patient complains of blurred vision and dizziness at 30 weeks of pregnancy. MRI revealed a pituitary adenoma hemorrhage (°). Spontaneous evolution was favorable. (**a**–**f**) Coronal T1WIs. (**e**) is enhanced

sellae (Fig. 5.1). Moreover, the posterior lobe is less T1 hyperintense than outside pregnancy and may be barely visible on a sagittal view. Axial projection is useful here for its demonstration for instance in the case of a polyuro-polydipsic syndrome.

Monitoring microprolactinomas changes during pregnancy is rightfully considered unjustified. We will just point out a few exceptions to this rule. Apart from the increase in the size of the normal pituitary, a pituitary microadenoma theoretically grows to reach twice its initial size in late pregnancy if dopaminergic treatment has been suspended, as is usually the case. Therefore, the optic chiasm may be exceptionally threatened for instance if the microprolactinoma initial size approaches 10 mm, in the case of small sella (Fig. 21.3) or with the occurrence of a prolactinoma hemorrhage during pregnancy (Fig. 22.1f).

Furthermore, we have observed that the rare T2W hypointense prolactinomas (Fig. 22.2a, b) which are correlated to a higher prolactin level than the common T2W hyperintense ones and those which display a microcystic pattern on T2WI (Fig. 22.2c, d) tend to increase in size in a larger proportion.

Therefore, it seems not unreasonable to consider pituitary unenhanced MRI if unexplainable symptoms—such as severe headache, polyuro-polydipsic syndrome or blurred vision—occur in the third trimester of pregnancy particularly in the context of small sella, T2W hypointense, microcystic or hemorrhagic prolactinoma and obviously if an apoplexy is suspected. Demonstration of a threat of the optic chiasm could then consider resuming medical treatment in some rare circumstances.

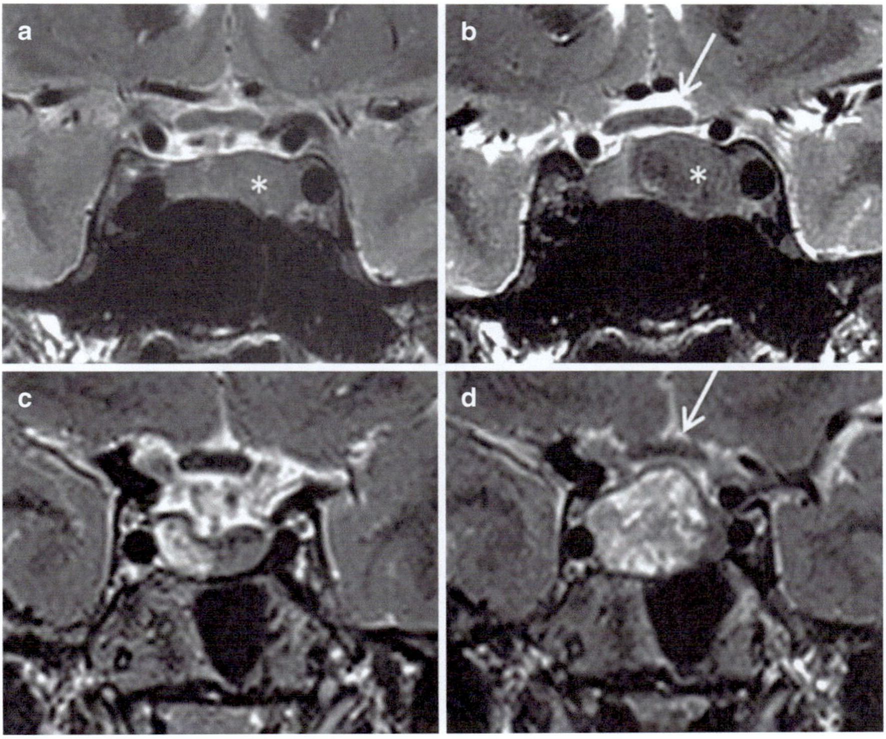

Fig. 22.2 Evolution of two prolactinomas in late pregnancy. (**a**, **b**) Marked increased size with slight optic chiasm tilt (arrow) of a T2W hypointense adenoma (*). (**c**, **d**) Identical evolution of a T2W microcystic adenoma (*) seen is after cabergoline treatment (**c**) and in late pregnancy (**d**). (**a**–**d**) Coronal T2WIs

A coexisting Rathke cleft cyst (Fig. 22.3) or a craniopharyngioma (Fig. 22.4) could also be an indication for MRI follow-up since we have observed noticeable changes of these lesions in late pregnancy or postpartum. Visual troubles during pregnancy may reveal a centimetric RCC.

In addition, it has to be remembered that the context of a high progesterone plasmatic level can lead to an increase in meningioma volume during pregnancy. Thus pregnancy can be revealing of meningiomas. At last, unusual headache during pregnancy can be related to a thrombophlebitis, for instance at the cavernous sinus level (Fig. 33.4). Therefore, if an MRI is indicated during pregnancy, it must cover not only the hypophyseal-hypothalamic region but also the whole brain.

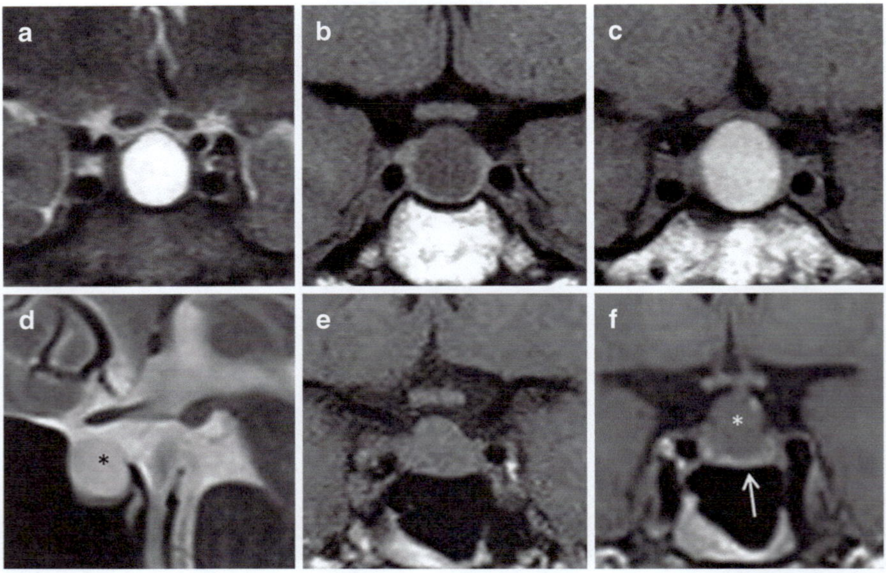

Fig. 22.3 Upper row. T2W hyperintense (**a**), T1W hypointense serous RCC before pregnancy (**b**). In late pregnancy (**c**), the RCC whose T1W signal has turned from hypo- to hyperintense abuts the optic chiasm. This signal change is not related to hemorrhage but to increased protein concentration. The RCC has changed from serous to mucoid. (**a**) Coronal T2WI. (**b**, **c**) Coronal T1WIs. Lower row: Serous RCC (*) before (**d**, **e**) and during pregnancy (**f**). The cyst is slightly enlarged but mostly raised by the thickened T1W hyperintense normal pituitary gland (arrow) (**d**) Sagittal T2WI. (**e**, **f**) Coronal T1WIs

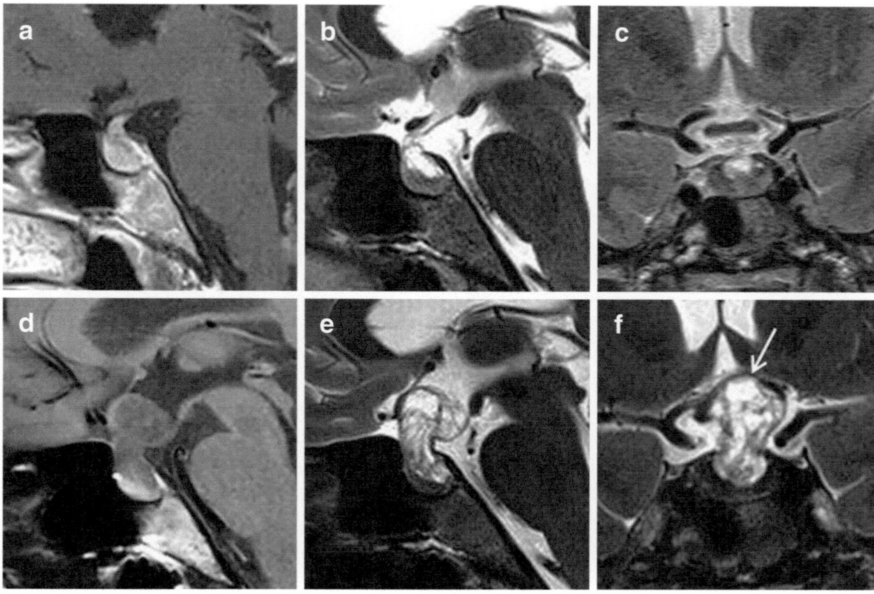

Fig. 22.4 Marked increased size of a previously asymptomatic craniopharyngioma (**a–c**) with severe optic chiasm compression (arrow) during pregnancy (**d–f**). (**a**) Sagittal T1WI. (**d**) Sagittal CE T1WI. (**b**, **c**, **e**, **f**) T2WIs

Further Readings

Araujo PB, Vieira Neto L, Gadelha MR. Pituitary tumor management in pregnancy. Endocrinol Metab Clin N Am. 2015;44(1):181–97.

Bonneville JF, et al. Normal pituitary gland and pregnancy in MRI of the pituitary gland. 2016; https://doi.org/10.1007/978-3-319-29043-0_8.

Molitch ME. Prolactinomas and pregnancy. Clin Endocrinol (Oxf). 2010;73(2):147–8.

23 Intrasellar Rathke Cleft Cyst/Pars Intermedia Cyst

With high-quality MRI and particularly T2W sequence, the incidence of posteriorly located intrasellar cysts is almost as high as in autopsy studies where their presence has been reported in one in three persons. This raises the question of the necessity to mention them in the radiological report: is it a lesion or an anatomical variant (Fig. 23.1)?

We will present here the intrasellar cysts located precisely between the anterior and posterior lobes of the pituitary. Other pituitary cysts are described in Chap. 26. These cysts present different patterns. The most frequent are mucinous: When small, less than 5 mm, their aspect is that of a T2W hypointense nodule or more rarely a hypointense T2W vertical band demonstrated at the posterior edge of the anterior pituitary (Fig. 23.1). They are more or less hyperintense on T1W images, but can be invisible (Fig. 23.2). Their signal intensity varies with the concentration of cholesterol and proteins. If these concentrations are high, the cyst can display the same signal as the posterior lobe on T1W, mimicking a thickened posterior lobe. Axial images would best show their specific midline location between the anterior and posterior lobes (Figs. 23.2d, g, h and 23.3).

Serous cysts are rarer. They are more or less T1 hypointense and T2 hyperintense (Fig. 23.4) and can escape diagnosis if isointense on T1 and T2W sequences but are hyperintense on FLAIR and do not enhance after gadolinium injection. T1 and T2W signals can be modified with time so that serous cysts can be changed into mucous cysts.

Are these mucinous or serous cysts RCCs or pars intermedia cysts? It has been arbitrarily proposed to reserve the term pars intermedia cysts to those less than 3 mm in diameter. Others name nodular images "Rathke cleft cyst" and the band-like ones "pars intermedia cysts"—even if, from an embryological point of view, the pars intermedia is located dorsal to the Rathke cleft. T2W hypointense band-like mucinous cysts—vertically positioned—must be differentiated from a band-like inferior intercavernous sinus—horizontally positioned on sagittal T1WIs (Fig. 23.5).

All these images are non-symptomatic and do not change a lot with time. They may shrink (Fig. 23.4c, d) or even vanish particularly when seen in children.

J.-F. Bonneville, *Tricks and Traps in MRI of the Pituitary Region*,
https://doi.org/10.1007/978-3-031-64710-9_23

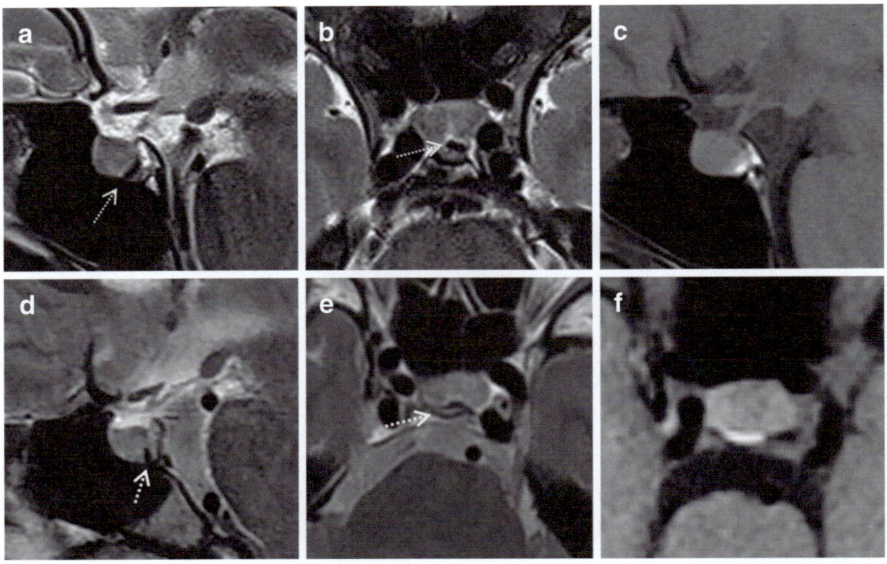

Fig. 23.1 T2W hypointense microcysts (dotted arrows) invisible on T1WIs. (**a**, **d**) Sagittal T2WIs. (**b**, **e**) Axial T2WIs. (**c**, **f**) Sagittal and axial T1WIs

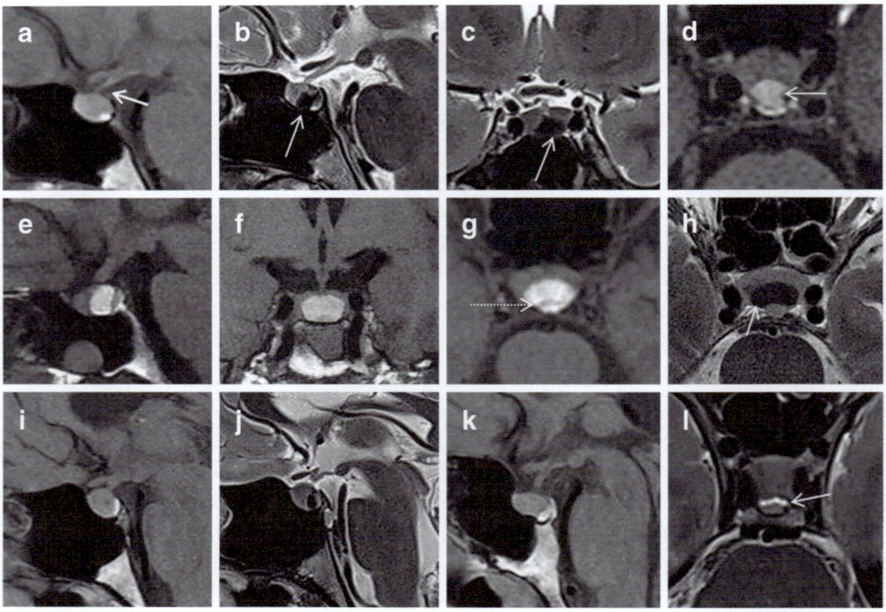

Fig. 23.2 Patient 1. Isointense RCC on sagittal T1W (**a**), hypointense on sagittal T2WI (**b**). The pituitary stalk is displaced forward (arrow in **a**). Patient 2. RCC hypointense on coronal T2WI (**c**), hyperintense and well separated from the posterior lobe in (**d**), axial T1W Fatsat image. Patient 3. (**e–h**) Sagittal and coronal T1WIs, axial TIW Fatsat and T2WI. The T1W hyperintense RCC is clearly separated from the posterior lobe in (**g**) (dotted arrow) and in (**h**). Patient 4. (**i, j**) RCC invisible in (**a**), sagittal T1WI, well seen on T2WI (**j**), responsible of a slight bulging of the pituitary content which could be intriguing without a T2W image. Patient 5. (**k, l**) Small serous RCC invisible in (**k**), sagittal T1WI, hyperintense in (**l**), axial T2WI (arrow)

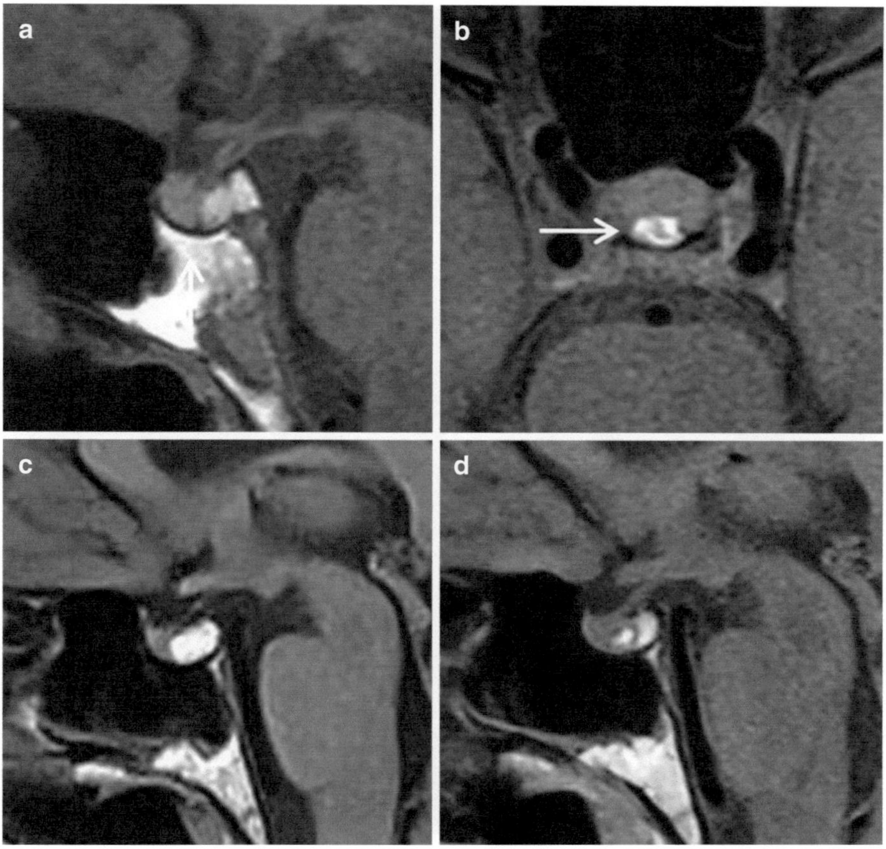

Fig. 23.3 Upper row: RCC mimicking a posterior lobe on sagittal T1WI (**a**). The diagnosis is corrected in (**b**), axial T1W Fatsat image. A thin line separates both structures (arrow). Lower row. Spontaneous shrinkage of an RCC in 5 years. (**c**, **d**) Sagittal T1WIs

To avoid unnecessary follow-ups, we propose to precise in the MRI report that the image—if it is less than 5 mm—is so frequent that it has to be considered as a normal variant, or even to simply disregard it, which is perhaps better. Finally, this latter approach permits to avoid a passionate and unresolved debate between pathologists: is it a Rathke cleft cyst or a pars intermedia cyst?

When they measure more than 5 mm, intrasellar Rathke cleft cysts are usually oval-shaped, vertically oriented and have a characteristic midline location in front of the posterior lobe. They displace the pituitary stalk forward (Fig. 23.2a, b). RCCs are sometimes originally located off-midline and they can be displaced or distorted by a concomitant pituitary microadenoma (Fig. 34.2). It is remarkable that in the case of such collision lesions, the microadenoma not only displaces but deforms the RCC whose internal pressure is low (Fig. 34.1). Another RCC location is remote from the original Rathke pouch, at the level of the sellar diaphragm, in front of the distal pituitary stalk. These cysts are small, well rounded, and can be centered by a

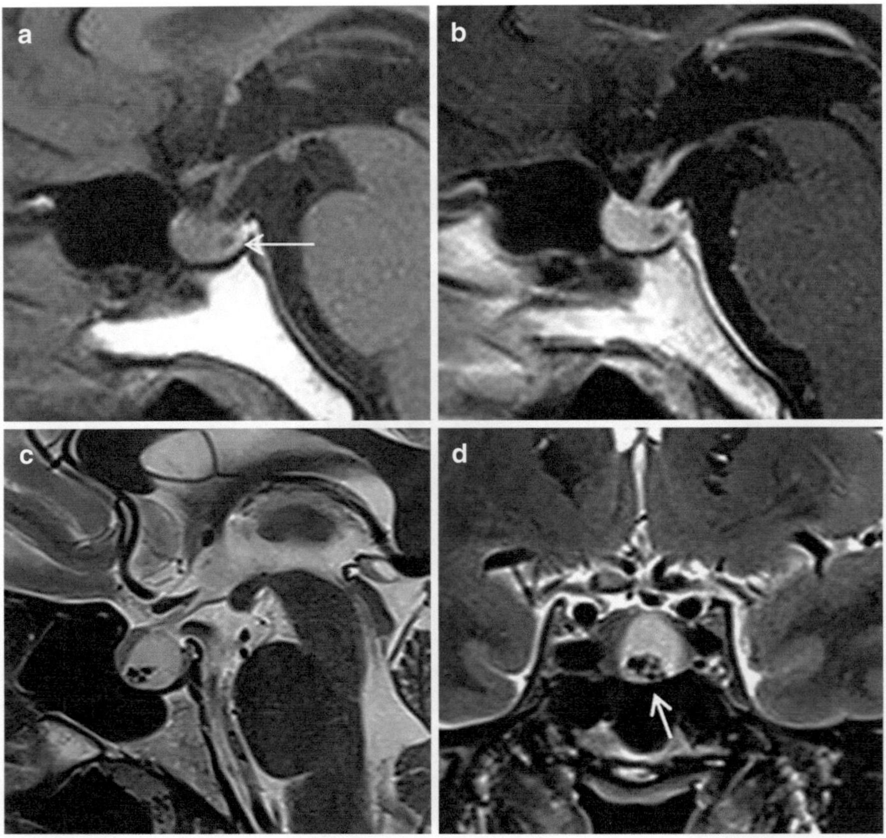

Fig. 23.4 Upper row. Tiny T1W hypointense serous RCC on sagittal and CE sagittal T1WIs. Lower row. Intrasellar serous T2W hyperintense RCC in sagittal and coronal T2WIs. T2W hypointense nodules (arrow)

T2 hypointense nodule. Double localization for instance in the suprasellar area and at the stalk level is not exceptional (Fig. 27.4).

From a general point of view, it must be recalled that axial T1 and sagittal T2W sequences are the most informative for the diagnosis of intrasellar Rathke cyst. Gadolinium-enhanced sequences are usually less informative.

Intrasellar RCCs rarely progress but some can grow significantly, extend within the suprasellar area, and threaten the optic chiasm. Changes in size, signal, or location mean that the cyst is active and must be followed (see Chap. 25). No other risk factor for their progression has been identified except perhaps their presence in older adults.

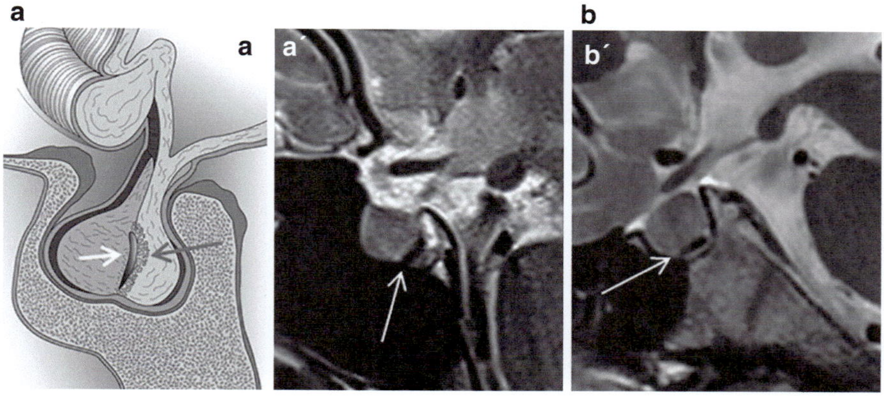

Fig. 23.5 (**a**) Schematic representation of Rathke pouch (white arrow) and pars intermedia (grey arrow). (**a′**) Rathke pouch (or pars intermedia cyst). (**b′**) Differential diagnosis. Inferior intercavernous sinus. (**a′**, **b′**) Sagittal T2WIs

Further Readings

Byun WM, Kim OL, Kim D. MR imaging findings of Rathke cleft cysts: significance of intracystic nodules. AJNR Am J Neuroradiol. 2000;21(3):485–8.

Gobara A, Katsube T, Asou H, Yoshida R, Yoshizako T, Kitagaki H. T2 hypointense signal discovered incidentally at the posterior edge of the adenohypophysis on MRI: its prevalence and morphology and their relationship to age. Neuroradiology. 2022;64(9):1755–61. https://doi.org/10.1007/s00234-022-02935-8. Epub 2022 Mar 31.

Kinoshita Y, Taguchi A, Yamasaki F, Tominaga A, Arita K, Horie N. Natural course of Rathke's cleft cysts and risk factors for progression. J Neurosurg. 2022;138(5):1426–32. https://doi.org/10.3171/2022.7.JNS22716.

Rathke Cleft Cysts or PitNET?

24

Most Rathke cleft cysts (RCCs) originate intrasellarly and may extend into the suprasellar region; pure suprasellar RCCs are rare. When extended into the optochiasmatic cistern, an RCC can mimic a pituitary adenoma, particularly if the latter presents a hemorrhage. We will discuss here the fundamental differences between both. Complicated RCCs and cysts of the pituitary stalk will be discussed and illustrated separately (see Chaps. 25 and 27).

Several multivariable models using MRI have been proposed but are not really useful in front of an individual case. Machine learning approach to differentiate PitNET and RCC is still in the field of research. MRI characteristics facilitate the differential diagnosis although each characteristic taken separately is not always decisive.

- The shape of an RCC is usually smooth, while that of a pituitary adenoma when large is more often irregular or lobulated.
- PitNETs are often asymmetrical and displace the pituitary stalk laterally while intrasellar RCCs are located on midline, but can be observed off-midline when extended superiorly (Fig. 24.1).
- Presence of a non-T2W hypointense solid component within a cystic lesion advocates the diagnosis of pituitary adenoma.
- A peripheral T2W hypointense rim may be seen in PitNETs, not in RCCs.
- A fluid–fluid level usually related to hemorrhage supports the diagnosis of pituitary adenoma (Fig. 20.2) even if a hemorrhage can be observed but extremely rarely in RCCs.
- Intracystic septations can be seen in pituitary adenomas and are very unusual in RCCs (Fig. 24.2a, b).
- If mucoid RCCs appear classically hyperintense on T1WI and serous RCCs hyperintense on T2WI, different combinations of T1 and T2W signals may be observed as well in RCC as in PitNET. A hyperintense T1W signal of a hemorrhagic pituitary adenoma can mimic the signal of a mucoid RCC (Fig. 24.3).

J.-F. Bonneville, *Tricks and Traps in MRI of the Pituitary Region*,
https://doi.org/10.1007/978-3-031-64710-9_24

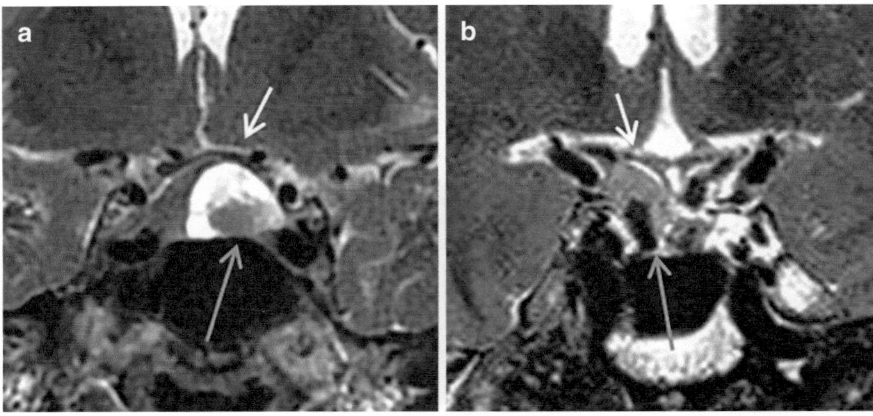

Fig. 24.1 Off-midline RCCs deforming the optic chiasm (small arrows). Hyperproteinic nodules (long arrows). (**a**, **b**) Coronal T2WIs

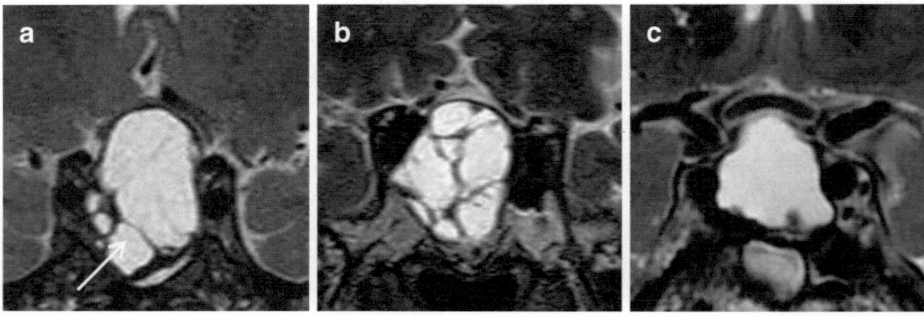

Fig. 24.2 PitNETs (**a**, **b**) versus serous RCC (**c**). Presence of septations (arrows) distinguishes PitNETs. (**a**–**c**) Coronal T2WIs

- But is noticeable that if an intrasellar hemorrhagic pituitary adenoma gives mass-effect, an RCC does not or less so (Fig. 24.3).
- The location of the normal pituitary gland can also help: it is frequently visible below the RCC, but not with PitNET (Fig. 24.4).
- Cavernous sinus invasion is never seen with RCCs.
- The wall of uncomplicated RCCs is not enhanced after gadolinium injection. A band of enhanced normal pituitary tissue displaced by the cyst can be misleading and mimic a thickened RCC wall, but this strip is thin and incomplete and enhances theoretically earlier than the RCC wall. Flair can also help (Fig. 25.5).
- Altogether, MRI features can help but are not all absolutely reliable except for one: a T2W hypointense hyperproteinic intracystic nodule which can be tiny or occupy the whole cyst is present in a large number of RCCs but is never seen in pituitary adenomas (Fig. 24.5). This nodule frequently changes in size and in position within the cyst (Fig. 24.6).

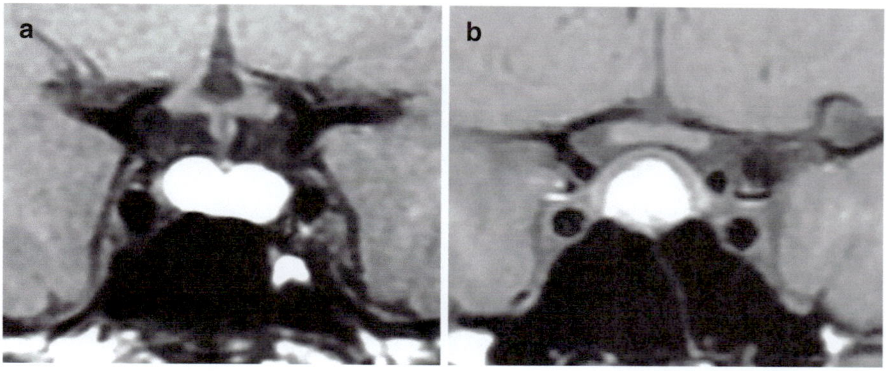

Fig. 24.3 Mucoid RCC (**a**) versus hemorrhagic PitNET (**b**). Both lesions are hyperintense on T1WIS (**a**, **b**). Mass effect is more pronounced PitNET: depressed sellar floor, bulging pituitary gland

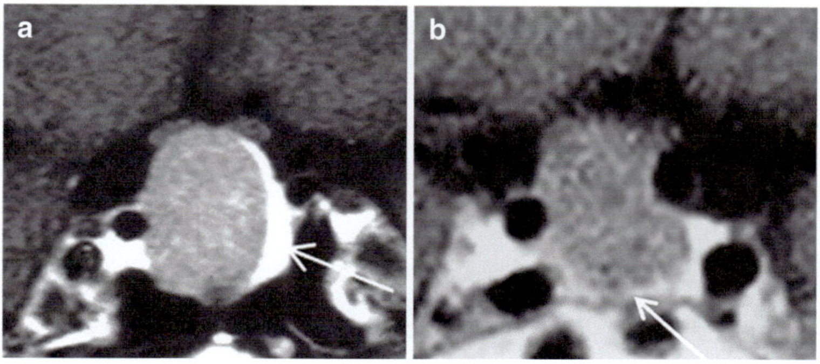

Fig. 24.4 PitNET (**a**) versus RCC (**b**) in coronal CE T1 WIs. The normal pituitary gland (arrow) is displaced unilaterally in PitNET, inferiorly and bilaterally in RCC

- Volume and MR signal of RCCs may vary during follow-up, more rarely with pituitary adenoma. The progression of RCCs can sometimes alternate with regression. Regression can be preceded by an acute headache which is generally attributed to intracystic hemorrhage or to a rupture with leakage of cyst content. These features are not observed in pituitary adenomas.
- Volume and T1 and T2 MR signals of RCC are not predictive factors of the progression or regression of the cyst, nor the presence of a T2 hypointense intracystic nodule. It has only been noted that cyst progression was more frequent in older patients who consequently must be observed more closely than middle-aged patients. A 5-year follow-up period seems reasonable to verify RCC inactivity.
- When surgery of an RCC is indicated, a regrow of the RCC is seen in more than one in three patients after cyst puncture and aspiration.

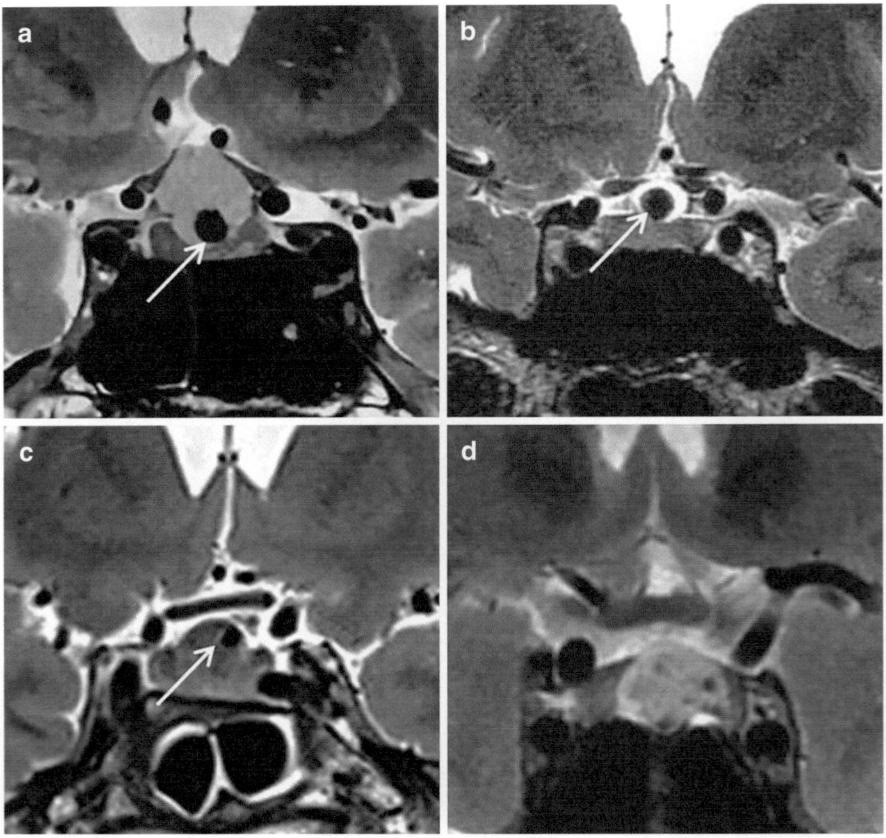

Fig. 24.5 Various pathognomonic aspects of T2W hypointense hyperproteinic nodules in RCCs. (**a–d**) Coronal T2WIs

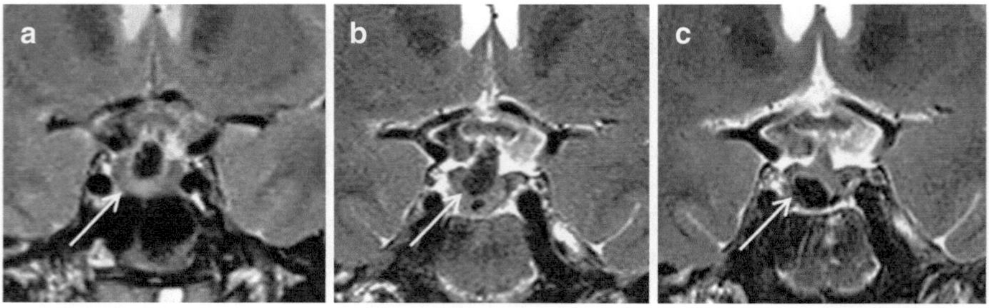

Fig. 24.6 Spontaneous changes of hyperproteinic nodules in an asymptomatic RCC. (**b**) is 6 months after (**a** and **c**) 3 years after (**b**). (**a–c**) Coronal T2WIs

- Non-secreting pituitary adenomas and Rathke cleft cysts are frequently discovered incidentally. When symptomatic, the manifestations are related to mass effect, mainly visual field defects, and more rarely headaches. Unlike non-secreting adenomas, RCCs if uncomplicated are rarely responsible for a pituitary deficit. In a large series of patients presenting a cystic lesion of the sella, it has been noted that obesity was more prevalent in patients harboring a pituitary adenoma.
- In the presence of a cystic mass of the sellar region, hyperprolactinemia must be interpreted with caution: in cystic macroprolactinoma with minimal solid component, there is a mismatch between adenoma size and prolactin levels; a prolactin level of around 100 µG/L can correspond to a cystic prolactinoma as well as to a hyperprolactinemia by stalk effect.

Further Readings

Bonneville JF. Hemorrhagic pituitary adenoma versus Rathke cleft cyst: a frequent dilemma. AJNR Am J Neuroradiol. 2016;37(3):E27–8. https://doi.org/10.3174/ajnr.A4653. Epub 2015 Dec 17. PMID: 26680456; PMCID: PMC7960133.

Park M, Lee SK, Choi J, Kim SH, Kim SH, Shin NY, Kim J, Ahn SS. Differentiation between cystic pituitary adenomas and Rathke cleft cysts: a diagnostic model using MRI. AJNR Am J Neuroradiol. 2015;36(10):1866–73. https://doi.org/10.3174/ajnr.A4387. Epub 2015 Aug 6. PMID: 26251436; PMCID: PMC7965051.

Tavakol S, Catalino MP, Cote DJ, Boles X, Laws ER Jr, Bi WL. Cyst type differentiates Rathke cleft cysts from cystic pituitary adenomas. Front Oncol. 2021;11:778824. https://doi.org/10.3389/fonc.2021.778824. PMID: 34956896; PMCID: PMC8702518.

Complicated Rathke Cleft Cysts 25

Most Ratke cleft cysts are silent and are managed conservatively. Their size and their MR signals frequently vary and they can spontaneously vanish. Some RCCs produce a mass effect if mucus production exceeds absorption: headaches and visual symptoms can occur.

Other RCCs, not necessarily the largest, can become symptomatic through complications such as hemorrhage, infection, or rupture with leakage of cyst content.

The latter may cause secondary pituitary inflammation and may result in anterior pituitary deficit and/or AVP deficiency. It is today admitted that xanthomatous hypophysitis (or xanthomatous granuloma) is most of the time secondary to a RCC rupture. Xanthomatous hypophysitis is characterized by an intrasellar mass with cystic components and peripheral enhancement while the thin cyst wall of a non-complicated RCC is either invisible or incompletely enhanced (Fig. 25.1). Nevertheless, a band of normal pituitary tissue displaced upward by the RCC can mimic a RCC wall enhancement. But this band of pituitary gland wraps only partially the upper contour of the RCC (Fig. 25.1c). A dynamic sequence could demonstrate an early peripheral enhancement of the compressed pituitary versus a delayed enhancement of the RCC wall in case of non-symptomatic and symptomatic RCC respectively (Figs. 25.2 and 25.3). Another ingenious trick has been recently proposed: on CE 3D T2-FLAIR images with high gadolinium concentration, the pituitary gland appears unenhanced whereas the wall of a symptomatic RCC is strongly enhanced (Fig. 25.4). On the opposite, the thin layer of pituitary tissue overlaying a non-symptomatic RCC is non-enhanced on CE 3D FLAIR (Fig. 25.5). An abnormal thickening of an RCC wall can also be discernable on T2WIs (Fig. 25.2). At last, enhancement and edema of the bone marrow of the sphenoid bone below the sella may be observed in complicated RCC (Fig. 25.6).

Apart from wall rupture, an RCC can be affected by hemorrhage or infection. Intracystic hemorrhage is rare and can be seen principally in patients with coagulation disorders. The proof of bleeding is not always obvious on MRI, but enhancement and thickening of the cyst wall confirm that something is wrong in the RCC. The term RCC apoplexy has been inopportunely proposed when the symptoms simulate

J.-F. Bonneville, *Tricks and Traps in MRI of the Pituitary Region*,
https://doi.org/10.1007/978-3-031-64710-9_25

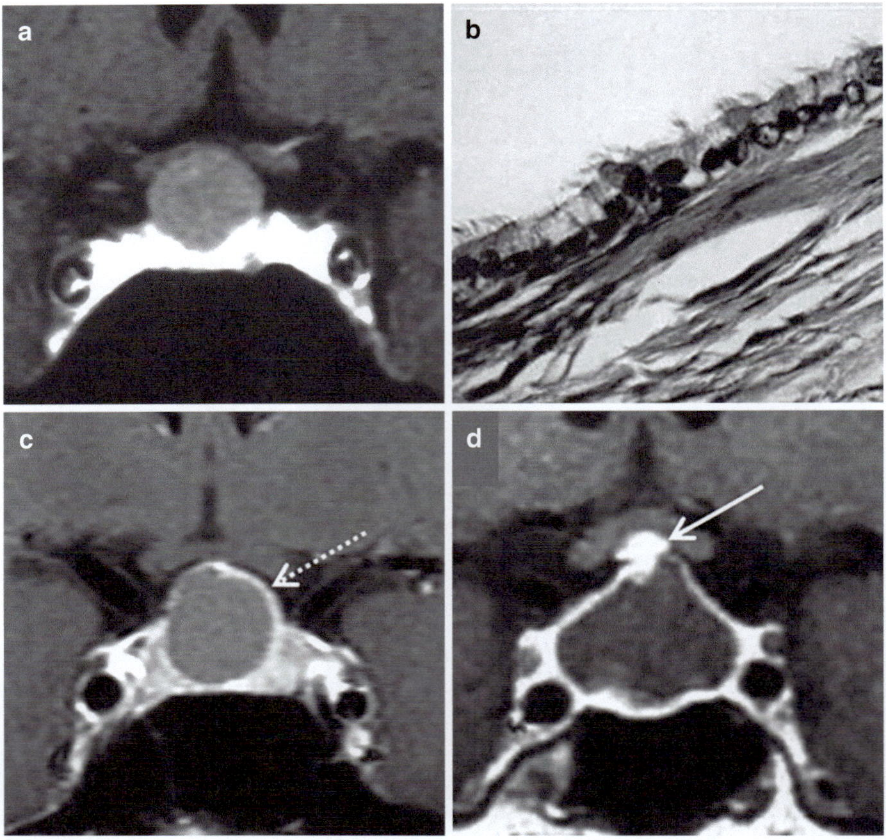

Fig. 25.1 The wall of RCC on coronal CE T1WIs (**a**, **c**, **d**). (**a**) Usual pattern. The cyst wall is invisible. (**c**) Normal variant. A band of pituitary gland covers incompletely the RCC (dotted arrow). (**d**) Complicated RCC. Thick enhancement of its wall and nodular enhancement of the infundibulum (arrow). (**b**) Monocellular wall of a non-symptomatic RCC under the microscope

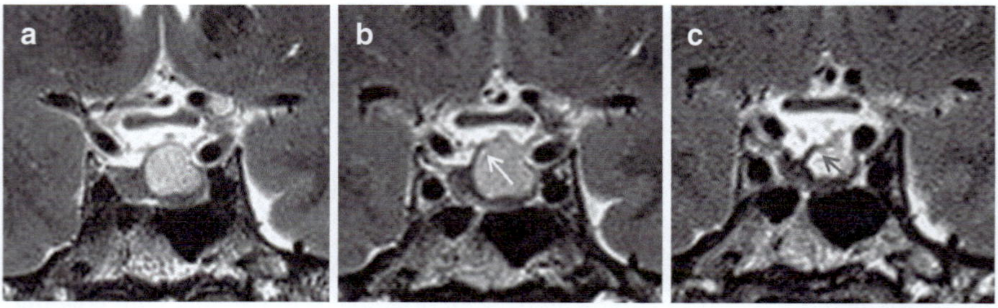

Fig. 25.2 Evolution of a ruptured RCC over the years. Increased size and thickening (arrows) of the RCC wall (**b**), then shrinkage (**c**). (**a–c**) Coronal T2WIs

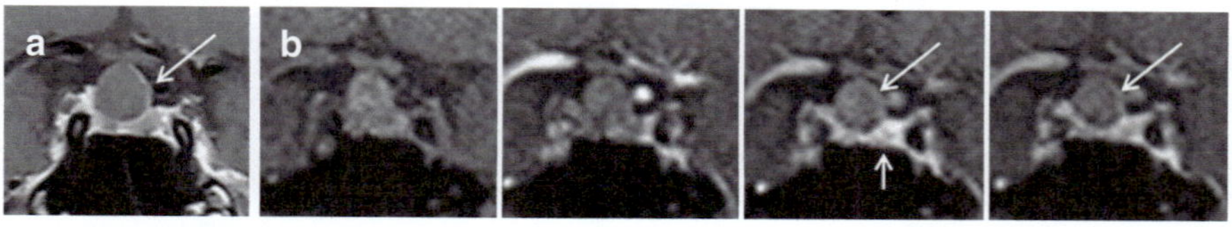

Fig. 25.3 Dynamic MRI (**b**) of a non-symptomatic RCC. The shell partially covering the RCC (arrow) is enhanced together with the pituitary gland (short arrow): it is not the wall of the RCC. (**a**) Coronal CE SE T1WI

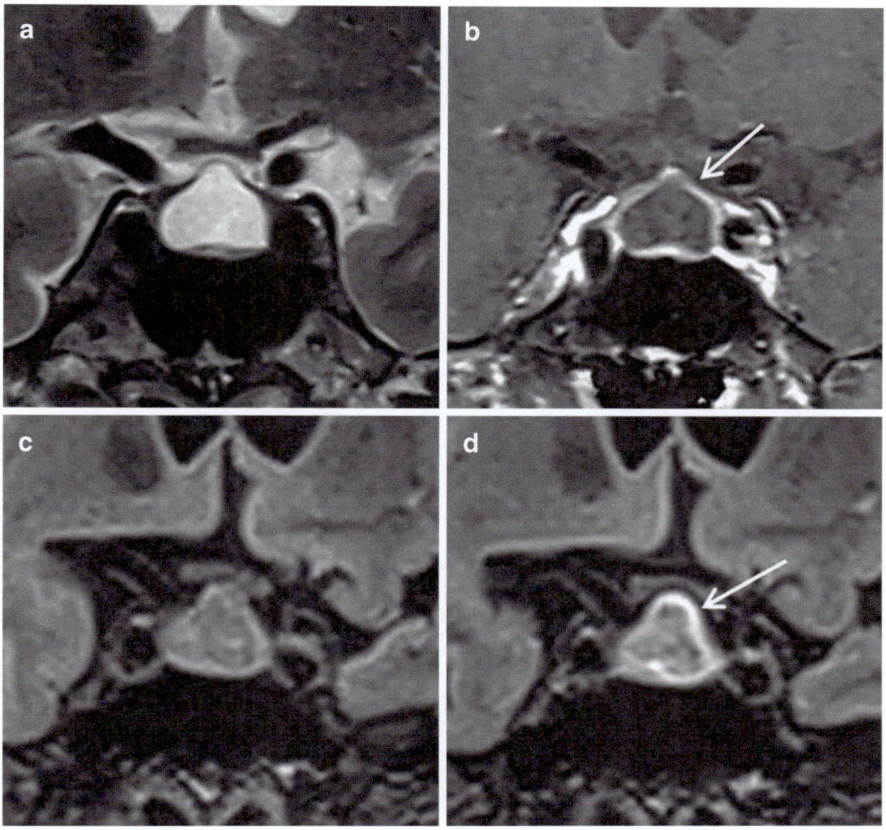

Fig. 25.4 Complicated RCC with anterior pituitary deficit. Thick enhanced cyst wall (arrows) in (**b**), better seen on CE FLAIR (**d**). (**a**, **b**) Coronal T2 and CE T1WIs. (**c**, **d**) 3D FLAIR before and after a high dose (0.3 mmol/kg) of gadolinium (to eliminate the pituitary signal)

a PitNET apoplexy with sudden onset of a severe headache. Cyst infection occurs principally in mucinous RCC. Imaging features of an abscess within an RCC are not specific and diffusion-weighted imaging (DWI) is not helpful because restriction diffusion can be seen in any lesions with viscous content. Sinus mucosa enhancement can be observed but no feature of sinus infection can generally be found.

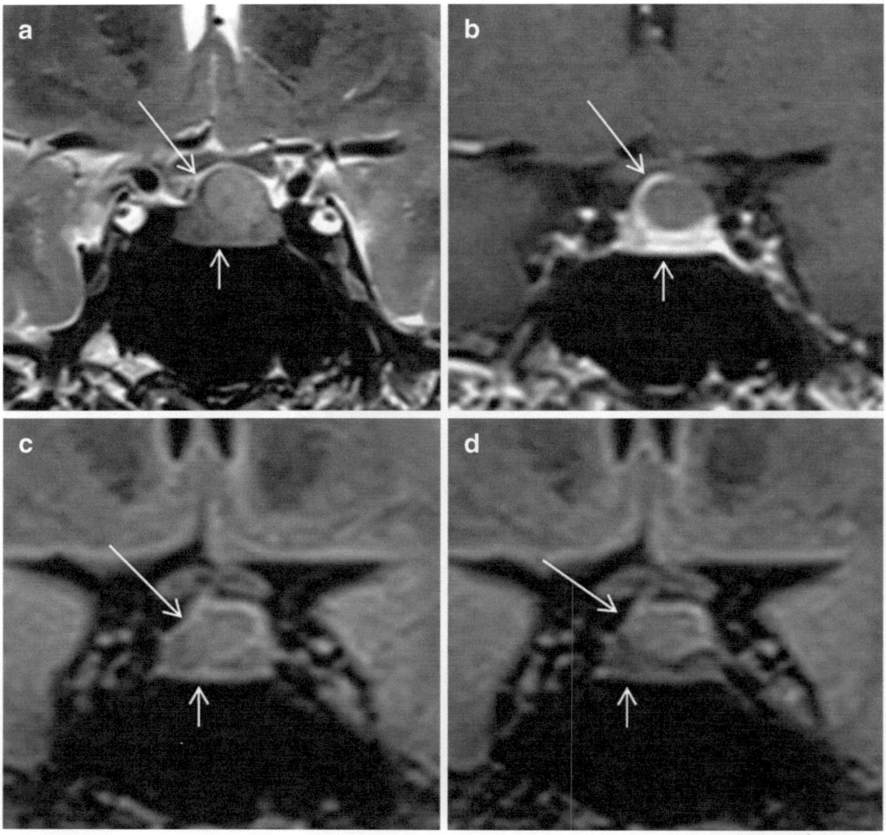

Fig. 25.5 Non-symptomatic RCC. Partial enhancement of the cyst wall (long arrow) together with enhancement of the pituitary (short arrow). On 3D CE FLAIR (**d**), the normal pituitary tissue is unenhanced as well above the sellar floor as above the RCC. (**a**) Coronal T2WI. (**b**) Coronal CE T1WI. (**c**, **d**) 3D CE FLAIR before and after gadolinium (0.3 mmol/kg)

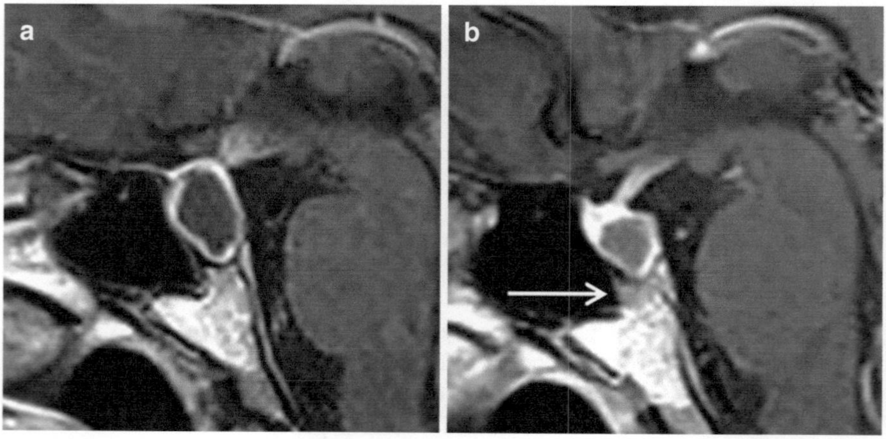

Fig. 25.6 Complicated RCC with thick wall enhancement (**a**). Partial shrinkage 2 months later (**b**) supporting cyst rupture. Focal sphenoid bone marrow enhancement (arrow). (**a**, **b**) Sagittal CE T1WIs

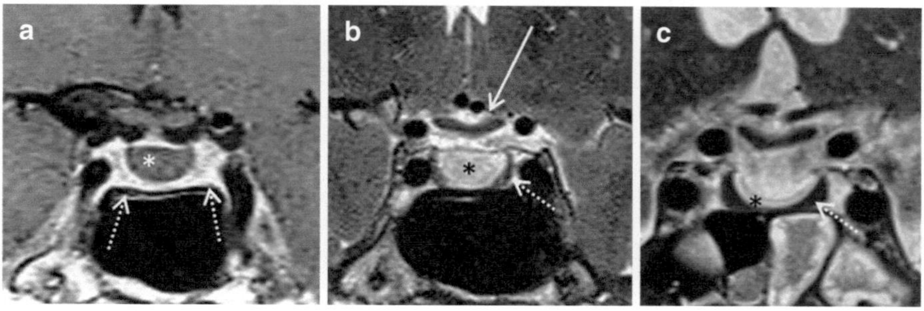

Fig. 25.7 Sudden pituitary deficit 2 months ago. (**a**, **b**) Coronal CE T1 and T2WIs. Intrasellar RCC (*). The normal pituitary gland (dotted arrow) encircles the cyst. The shape of the optic chiasm (long arrow) corresponds to a slight ptosis testifying that the sellar mass has shrunk previously. (**c**) Coronal T2WI in another patient seen long after RCC puncture. The normal pituitary gland (dotted arrow) encircles a tiny residual T2W hyperintense cyst (*)

Complications can result in partial or nearly complete cyst shrinkage. In the latter case, in the absence of initial diagnosis, the diagnosis of shrunk RCC can be difficult. The features mimic an empty sella but with a sellar content presenting a mixture of MR signals: the central part—the RCC remnant—is usually slightly hyperintense on T1WI and T2WI if compared with the peripheral part, i.e., the normal residual pituitary tissue. The same pattern is seen after RCC puncture (Fig. 25.7). Demonstration of a hyperproteinic T2 hypointense nodule can also help. Optic chiasm ptosis may attest to a previously large suprasellar mass. Spontaneous shrinkage of an RCC must be evoked in front of a so-called empty sella in a patient presenting a hypopituitarism of unknown origin, especially with a history of headache.

Further Readings

Han SJ, Rolston JD, Jahangiri A, et al. Rathke's cleft cysts: review of natural history and surgical outcomes. J Neuro-Oncol. 2014;117(2):197–203.

Kinoshita Y, Taguchi A, Yamasaki F, Tominaga A, Arita K, Horie N. Natural course of Rathke's cleft cysts and risk factors for progression. J Neurosurg. 2022;138:1–7. https://doi.org/10.3171/2022.7.JNS22716. Epub ahead of print.

Mark IT, Glastonbury CM. MR imaging appearance of ruptured Rathke cleft cyst and associated bone marrow enhancement. AJNR Am J Neuroradiol. 2023;44(11):1314–7. https://doi.org/10.3174/ajnr.A8009. Epub 2023 Oct 5. PMID: 37798112; PMCID: PMC10631529

Trifanescu R, Ansorge O, Wass JA, et al. Rathke's cleft cysts Clin Endocrinol (Oxf). 2012;76(2):151–60.

26 Non-Rathke Cleft Cysts

Various cyst-like lesions of different sizes can be observed in the sellar area. Some—particularly the smallest—cannot be formally identified but others are relatively easily diagnosed, such as the pituitary cystic adenomas (Chap. 24), the intrasellar Rathke cleft cysts/pars intermedia cysts (Chap. 23), the arachnoid cysts, or the cysts of the posterior lobe.

Arachnoid cysts are usually asymptomatic but can be responsible for headaches or visual disturbances. If silent, they are not candidates for surgery (Fig. 41.1). They can be intrasellar with often a suprasellar extension that displaces the pituitary stalk posteriorly. They can be suprasellar and push the floor of the third ventricle upward and the pituitary stalk forward. They are filled with CSF and appear as well-defined, sharply marginated purely cystic lesions with homogeneous T1-low signal intensity and T2-high signal intensity, with no solid portion, no contrast enhancement, and no calcification. The FLAIR sequence is key in demonstrating the signal suppression of the cyst content (Fig. 26.1).

Bleeding is rare. Presence of a T1W signal slightly more intense than that of CSF and a non-suppressed signal on FLAIR can make the diagnosis more elusive and a serous Rathke cleft cyst or a cystic pituitary adenoma cannot be totally eliminated.

The main differential diagnosis of arachnoid cyst is the empty sella because both display the same signal on FLAIR.

- Unlike empty sella, arachnoid cysts have no communication with the subarachnoid spaces and heavy T2W sequences are able to demonstrate the thin cyst wall which of course does not exist in an empty sella.
- The pituitary stalk is entirely visible from the infundibulum to the bottom of the sella in empty sella while it is not visible below the sellar diaphragm level in arachnoid cysts. Flow artifacts from the CSF pulsations are not seen in arachnoid cysts.

Cysts in the posterior lobe are not infrequent and may be troublesome on sagittal or coronal views but their diagnosis is easy on axial T1W sequence where it appears

J.-F. Bonneville, *Tricks and Traps in MRI of the Pituitary Region*,
https://doi.org/10.1007/978-3-031-64710-9_26

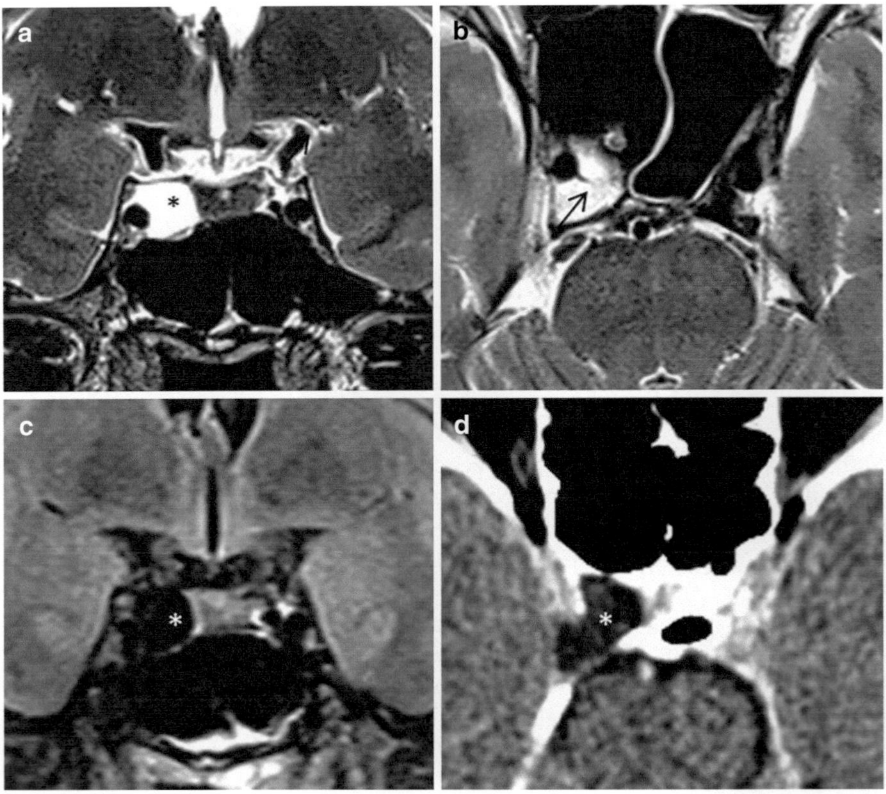

Fig. 26.1 Arachnoid cyst (*) extended from the sella to the cavernous sinus. Torn cavernous sinus medial wall (arrow in **b**, axial T2WI). The lesion is hyperintense on T2WIs (**a**, **b**), hypodense on CT (**d**), and its signal is suppressed on FLAIR (**c**)

as a more or less large T1W hypointense-T2W hyperintense area totally surrounded by the T1W hyperintense normal signal of the vasopressin storage (Fig. 26.2). The same axial T1W sequence easily eliminates a serous Rathke cleft cyst which is located in front of the posterior lobe. On FLAIR, the signal of the cyst content is not suppressed. This pattern is pathognomonic. Curiously cysts of the posterior lobe have not been described in pathology nor reported apart from our group in the radiological community. Radiologically, the described cystic formation totally surrounded by a T1W hyperintense peripheral rim cannot accept a different origin. Most of these cysts are small and respect the global volume of the posterior lobe. Some are large enough to be a cause of concern but demonstration of the distinctive peripheral T1W hyperintense rim on axial images is essential for the diagnosis of this benign variant (Fig. 26.3).

Posterior lobe cysts are silent and are never correlated with AVP deficiency. Multiple intrasellar cysts of different nature may be observed in the same patient (Fig. 26.4).

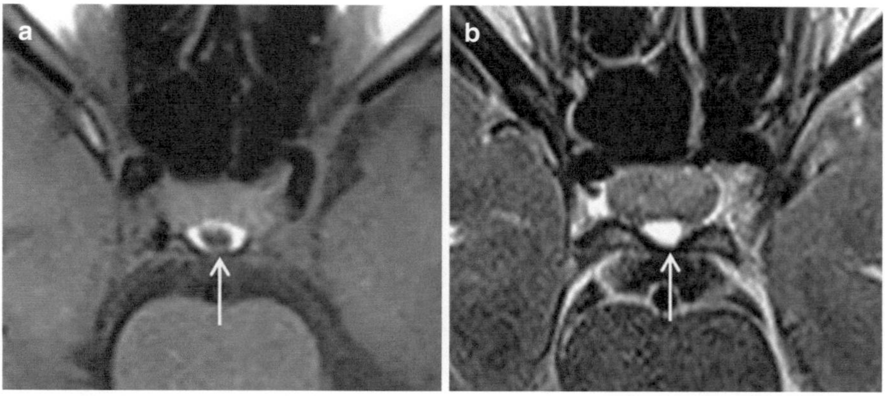

Fig. 26.2 Characteristic image of an asymptomatic posterior lobe cyst. The cyst is hyperintense on axial T2WI (**b**) and hypointense with a peripheral hyperintense ring on axial T1WI (**a**). Its location strictly applied to the concave dorsum sellae eliminates an RCC

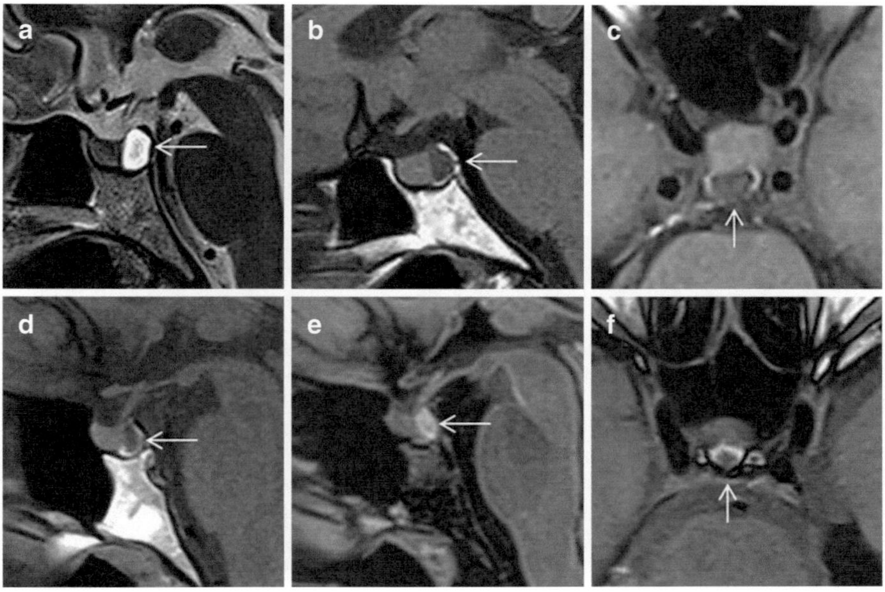

Fig. 26.3 Asymptomatic posterior lobe cysts followed for years. Upper row: Large T2W hyperintense image (**a**). On T1WIs (**b**, **c**), the cyst appears hypointense with a hyperintense flange on axial Fatsat T1WI (**c**). Lower row: Characteristic pattern of a posterior lobe cyst on sagittal (**d**) and axial (**f**) T1WIs. The cyst is hyperintense on FLAIR (**e**)

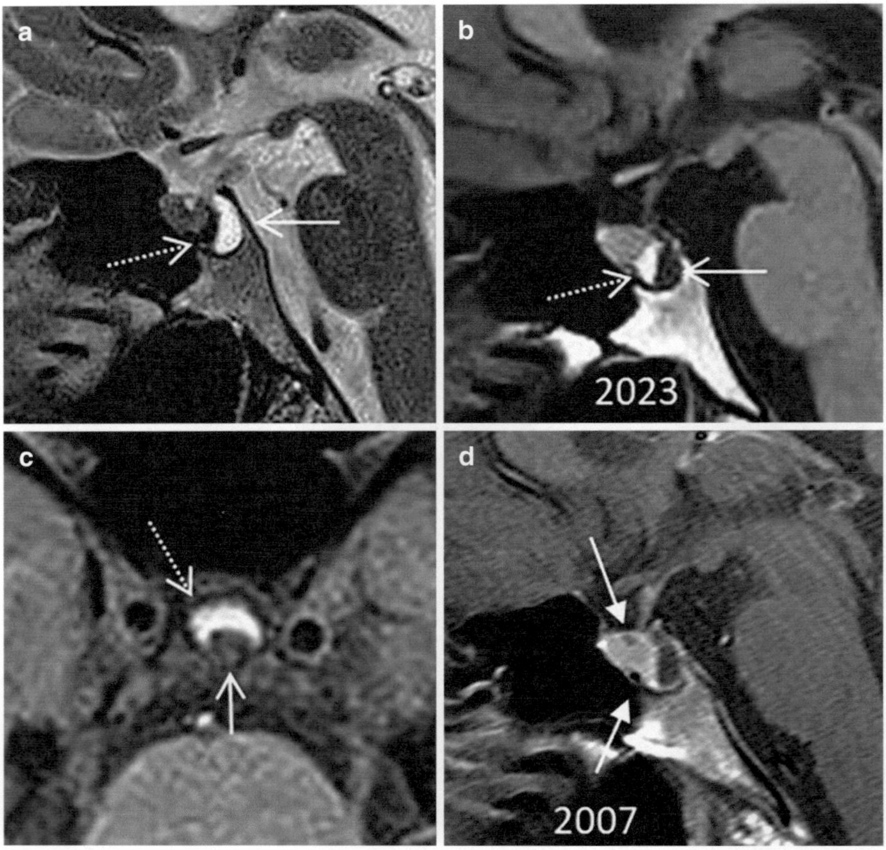

Fig. 26.4 Multiple asymptomatic intrasellar cysts followed for 15 years. Two tiny cysts of the anterior lobe are demonstrated after contrast injection only (arrows in **d**). The posterior image is more complex. Its dorsal component hyperintense on T2WI (**a**), hypointense on T1WI (**b**), and strictly applied to the dorsum sellae on axial Fatsat T1WI (c) advocates for a cyst of the posterior lobe (full arrow). The ventral component (dotted arrow) is hypointense on T2WI (**a**) and hyperintense on T1WIs (**b**, **c**) and looks like an RCC. But the image of vasopressin storage seems here missing. It is very likely that the T1W hyperintense signal of the posterior lobe is mixed up with the T1W hyperintense signal of the mucoid RCC. This difficult case illustrates the major role of the axial T1W sequence together with the T1 and T2W sequences as well as FLAIR (Fig. 26.7) to elucidate cystic sellar lesions

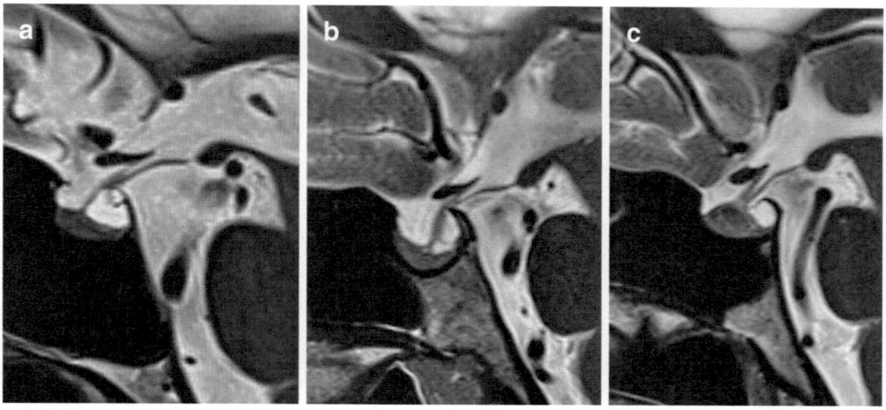

Fig. 26.5 Large asymptomatic cysts of the posterior part of the sella on sagittal T2WIs (**a**–**c**) (non-Rathke cleft cysts). The precise diagnosis is impossible without the help of T1WI, axial T1WI, and FLAIR (Fig. 26.6)

Other intrasellar posterior cysts can also be seen above the posterior lobe or at its upper extremity; they usually display a T1W hypo-T2W hyperintense signal on sagittal views (Fig. 26.5). They can mimic a limited posterior extension of the subarachnoid space through a defect of the sellar diaphragm (Fig. 26.6g–i).

Some cystic lesions display a high signal on FLAIR and eventually enhance after gadolinium injection potentially mimicking a pituitary microadenoma (Figs. 26.6a–f and 26.7). These cysts are not described elsewhere and are therefore unnamed. Their location being different from that of RCC, the term of no-Rathke cleft cysts (nRCC) could be proposed to define them.

Apart from RCC, nRCC, arachnoid cysts, and posterior lobe cysts, *small cyst-like images* can be demonstrated in the sella, since sagittal T2W sequences as well as 3D CE FLAIR sequence are more frequently performed.

When they are T2W hypointense, the diagnosis of serous Rathke cleft cyst or pars intermedia cyst must be retained (Fig. 23.1). When they are T2W hyperintense, these images could correspond to *mini infarcts or hemorrhagic scars* whose presence has been frequently reported in ancient autopsy reports.

However, when located in the anterior lobe, such cyst-like images raise the issue of a pituitary microadenoma. It has been suggested that 3D CE FLAIR could demonstrate a late enhancement. On the other hand, the presence of a tiny T2W hypointense nodule centering the cyst-like image orients more toward an RCC, even if it is non-midline.

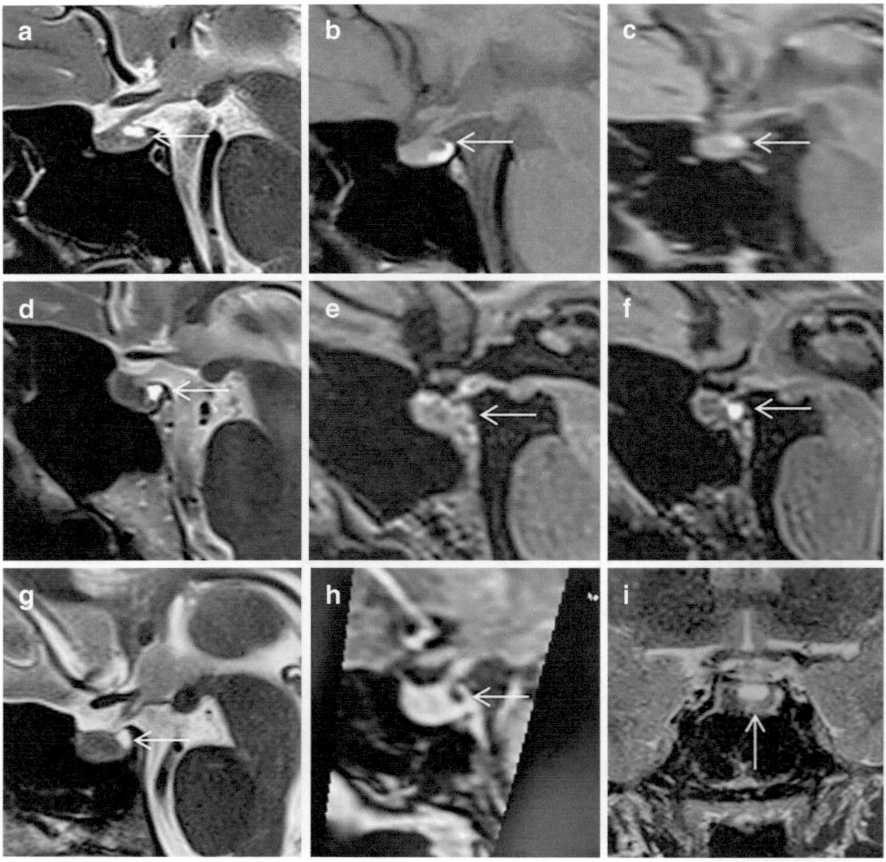

Fig. 26.6 Asymptomatic microcysts of the postero-upper part of the sella (nRCCs). Different aspects. Upper row: The cyst looks like an intrasellar extension of the suprasellar cistern on sagittal T1 and T2WIs (**a**, **b**), but its FLAIR hyperintensity (**c**) corrects the diagnosis. Middle row: Microcyst in the same location on sagittal T2WI (**d**). Its signal is not suppressed on FLAIR (**e**). Its enhancement on 3D CE FLAIR (**f**) eliminates the presence of CSF. Lower row: Intrasellar extension of CSF through an incomplete sellar diaphragm. (**g**, **i**) Sagittal and coronal T2WIs. No enhancement in **h**, sagittal reformatted CE 3D T1WI

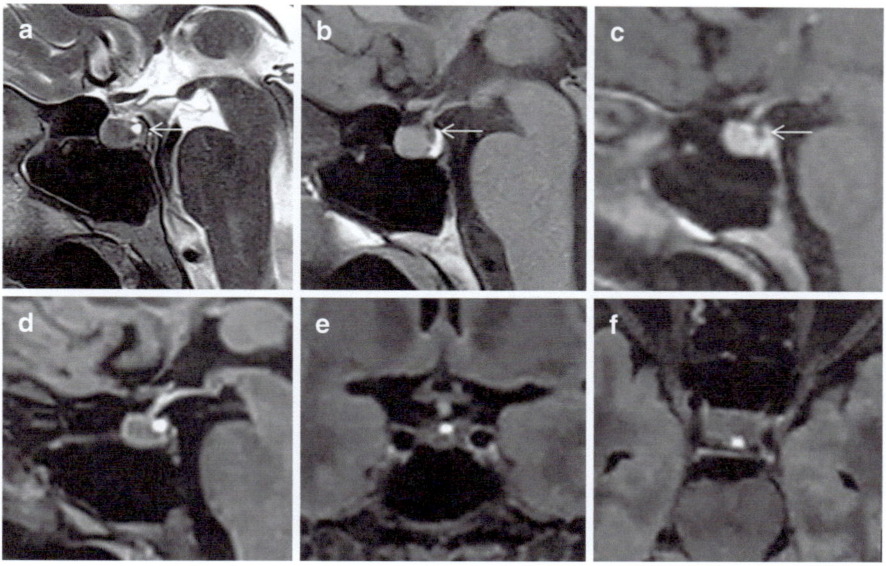

Fig. 26.7 Characteristic "non Rathke cyst". This small cyst displays a T2W hypersignal (**a**), a T1W hyposignal (**b**), and is not enhanced on sagittal 3D CE T1WI (**c**). It is hyperintense on FLAIR (not shown) and enhanced on delayed 3D CE FLAIR (**d**–**f**)

Further Readings

Meyrignac O, Idir IS, Cognard C, Bonneville JF, Bonneville F. 3D TOF MR angiography to depict pituitary bright spot and to detect posterior pituitary lobe cyst: original description at 3T MR imaging. J Neuroradiol. 2015;42:321–5. pii: S0150-9861(15)00113-3. https://doi.org/10.1016/j.neurad.2015.04.009.

Shanklin W. On the presence of cysts in the human pituitary. Anat Rec. 1949;104(4):379.

Teramoto A, Hirakawa K, Sanno N, Osamura Y. Incidental pituitary lesions in 1000 unselected autopsy specimens. Radiology. 1994;193(1):161–4.

Pituitary Stalk Cysts

27

Cysts originating from the Rathke pouch can develop everywhere along the hypothalamic-pituitary axis. Most are located in the sella and frequently extend to the chiasmatic cistern. Some extend to the pituitary stalk and the continuity between the sella and the stalk compartments of the cyst is well demonstrated on sagittal and coronal T2W images (Fig. 27.1a–d). Other cysts are strictly detected at the pituitary stalk level without any contact with the pituitary gland (Fig. 27.1e–g). They are poorly described in textbooks and rarely reported. And yet, they represent the major differential diagnosis of the thickened pituitary stalk.

Cysts of the pituitary stalk are oval with very regular contours and displace the neural tissue peripherally as seen on T2W or T1-enhanced images (Fig. 27.2). They usually demonstrate a T2W hyperintensity, more rarely a T2W hypointensity and are isointense or slightly hyperintense on T1W images. Hyperintensity on FLAIR is a useful clue to eliminate a deep posterior recess of the third ventricle (Figs. 27.1d and 27.2c). Some pituitary stalk cysts are very tiny and/or present a punctiform T2 hypointense nodule (Fig. 27.3e–f). Discrete changes in size and signal may be observed (Fig. 27.2d–f). The diagnosis of benign pituitary cysts must be severely questioned if irregular contours or unusual signals or in case of hormonal disturbance. A light hyperprolactinemia by stalk effect can be observed. An MRI follow-up is highly advised especially in atypical cases.

Another frequently observed location of pituitary stalk cysts is just in front of the distal end of the stalk, as sitting on the anterior part of the sellar diaphragm or just above. These cysts are round and usually tiny. They are mostly more or less hyperintense on T1W images or visible only on T2WI where they appear typically hyperintense with possibly a hypointense characteristic hyperproteinic nodule (Fig. 27.4). They are hyperintense on FLAIR. A double localization of the cysts at the pituitary stalk level and in the sella is not infrequent (Fig. 27.4a, b). Collision lesions with pituitary adenomas are not uncommon (Fig. 27.4c, d).

J.-F. Bonneville, *Tricks and Traps in MRI of the Pituitary Region*,
https://doi.org/10.1007/978-3-031-64710-9_27

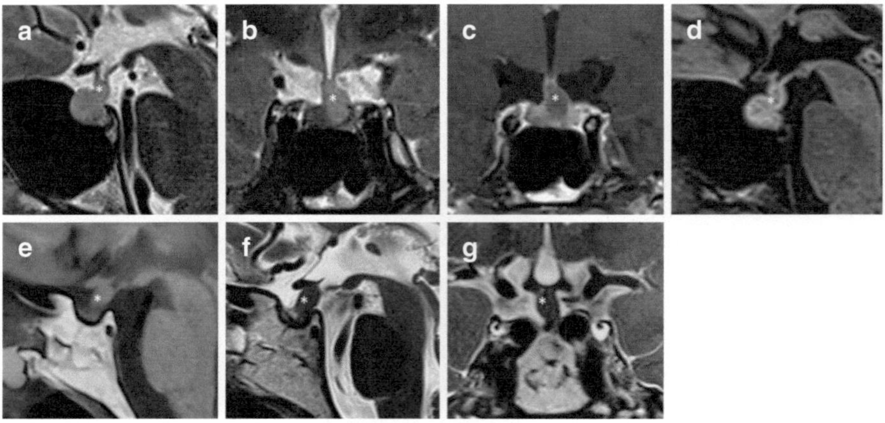

Fig. 27.1 Upper row: Pituitary stalk cyst extended from the pituitary gland. The cyst is hyperintense on T2WIs (**a**, **b**), is not enhanced after contrast injection (**c**), and is hyperintense on FLAIR (**d**). Lower row: Pituitary stalk cyst remnant 20 years after surgery with fluctuating size. The cyst is hyperintense on T1WI (**e**) and hypointense on T2WIs (**f**, **g**)

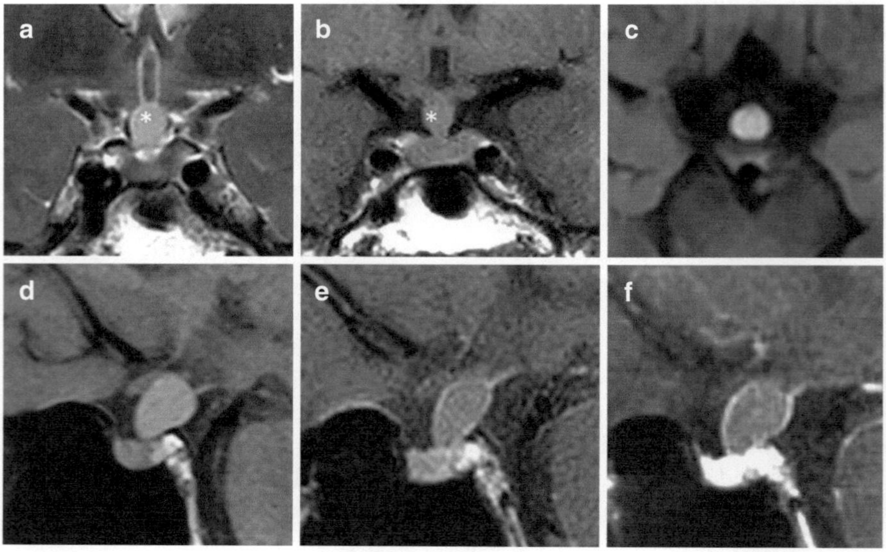

Fig. 27.2 Upper row: The T2W hyperintense cyst (**a**) displaces the neural tissue peripherally. It is isointense if compared with the pituitary gland on T1WI (**b**) and hyperintense on axial FLAIR sequence (**c**). Lower row: Changes in shape and size of an asymptomatic pituitary stalk cyst followed for 15 years. (**d**) Sagittal T1WI; (**e**, **f**) Sagittal CE T1WIs

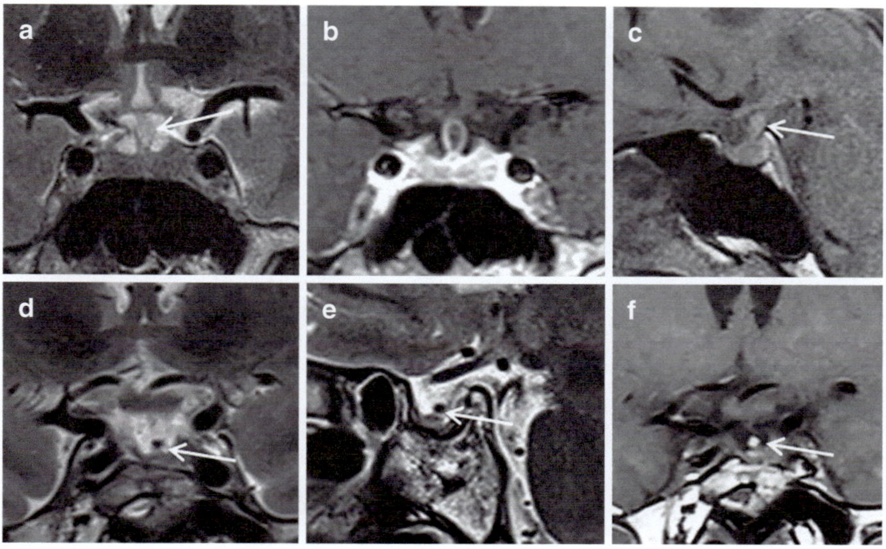

Fig. 27.3 Upper row: Characteristic small cyst of the pituitary stalk displacing the neural tissue laterally. It is hyperintense on T2WI (**a**), slightly hyperintense on T1WI (**c**), and is not enhanced (**b**). Lower row: Tiny cyst at the pituitary gland- pituitary stalk junction. The cyst is hypointense on coronal and sagittal T2WIs (**d**, **e**) and hyperintense on coronal T1WI (**f**)

The differential diagnosis of pituitary stalk cysts includes all causes of thickened pituitary stalk, mainly beginner craniopharyngioma (Fig. 28.1), ectopic posterior lobe, inflammatory diseases, ectopic pituitary adenoma or elongation of the infundibular recess of the third ventricle and what we have named an Infundibular Unidentified Object (IUO) (Chap. 6).

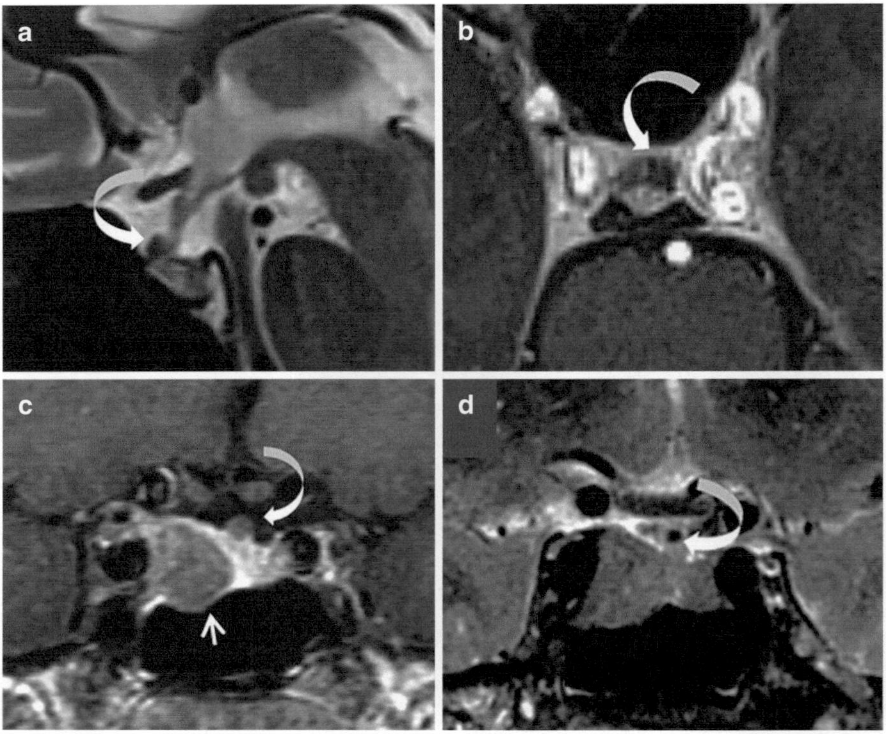

Fig. 27.4 Collision lesions. Upper row. Double localization of a Rathke pouch cyst. (**a**) Sagittal T2WI and (**b**) axial CE T1WI. Lower row. Tiny pituitary stalk cyst presenting a T2W micronodule (curved arrows) and coexisting GH-secreting PitNET (small arrow). (**c**) Coronal CE T1WI. (**d**) Coronal T2WI

Further Readings

Bonneville JF, Tshibanda L, Beckers A. An infundibular unidentified object (IUO): a new pituitary stalk marker? Pituitary. 2021;24(6):964–9. https://doi.org/10.1007/s11102-021-01169-w. Epub 2021 Jul 12. PMID: 34254253.

Glezer A, Paraiba DB, Bronstein MD. Rare sellar lesions. Endocrinol Metab Clin North Am. 2008;37(1):195–211, x. PMID: 18226737. https://doi.org/10.1016/j.ecl.2007.10.003.

Rupp D, Molitch M. Pituitary stalk lesions. Curr Opin Endocrinol Diabetes Obes. 2008;15(4):339–45. https://doi.org/10.1097/MED.0b013e3283050844. PMID: 18594274.

28 Craniopharyngiomas: Topography and Prognosis

Craniopharyngiomas (CPs) are derived from the remnants of the Rathke pouch and can occur anywhere along the course of the craniopharyngeal duct, from the nasopharynx to the third ventricle. They are characterized by a bimodal age distribution, with a main peak in children and a second peak in adults between the fifth and the seventh decade. They most commonly involve the suprasellar and sellar area, where they are more frequently anterior than posterior to the optic chiasm. Pure intraventricular craniopharyngiomas represent only 5% of CPs.

There are two histologic subtypes: the adamantinous type, the most common form, is typically seen in children and adolescents, while the papillary type is seen almost exclusively in adults. It has been hypothesized that papillary craniopharyngiomas originate from the pars tuberalis, the anterior pituitary tissue which wraps around the pituitary stalk, while adamantinous craniopharyngiomas arise from remnants of the Rathke pouch in the pituitary stalk. Autopsies studies taught us that a majority of CPs primarily develop in the infundibulum and in the tuber cinereum, that is in the floor of the third ventricle. A personal case has confirmed this hypothesis (Fig. 28.1).

Adamantinous craniopharyngiomas typically present with three components: solid, cystic, and calcified. The cystic component is single or multiple. Its signal is variable, usually hyperintense on T1 and FLAIR and hypo or hyperintense on T2WI (Fig. 28.2) because of the presence of proteinaceous liquid. At the difference of what is observed in hemorrhagic pituitary adenoma, there is no fluid-fluid level. The solid component has variable signal intensities and shows contrast enhancement. Unlike non-complicated Rathke cleft cysts, craniopharyngiomas display a thick wall enhancement, as it is observed in pituitary abscess (Fig. 28.6c, d). Hypothalamic T2 signal change and irregular contrast enhancement may predict a higher-grade subtype.

Papillary craniopharyngiomas are generally well-circumscribed, predominantly solid tumors. The solid component may contain small cystic areas or calcifications. The third ventricle is a common location of this subtype (Fig. 28.3).

J.-F. Bonneville, *Tricks and Traps in MRI of the Pituitary Region*,
https://doi.org/10.1007/978-3-031-64710-9_28

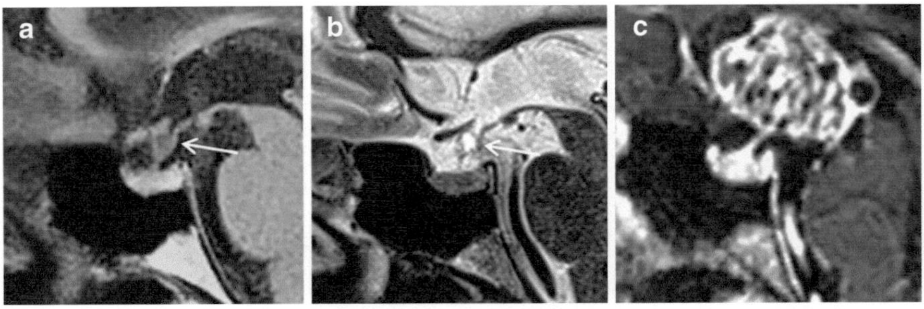

Fig. 28.1 Hypogonadotropic hypogonadism in a 52-year-old man. Nodular thickening of the infundibulum. The lesion which is T2W hyperintense and demonstrates irregular margins (arrow) was erroneously diagnosed as a Rathke cleft cyst. (**a**, **b**) Sagittal T1 and T2WI. The patient is out of sight. Two years later, he is admitted in emergency in a comatous state. A large CP has extended to the third ventricle. (**c**) Sagittal CE T1W

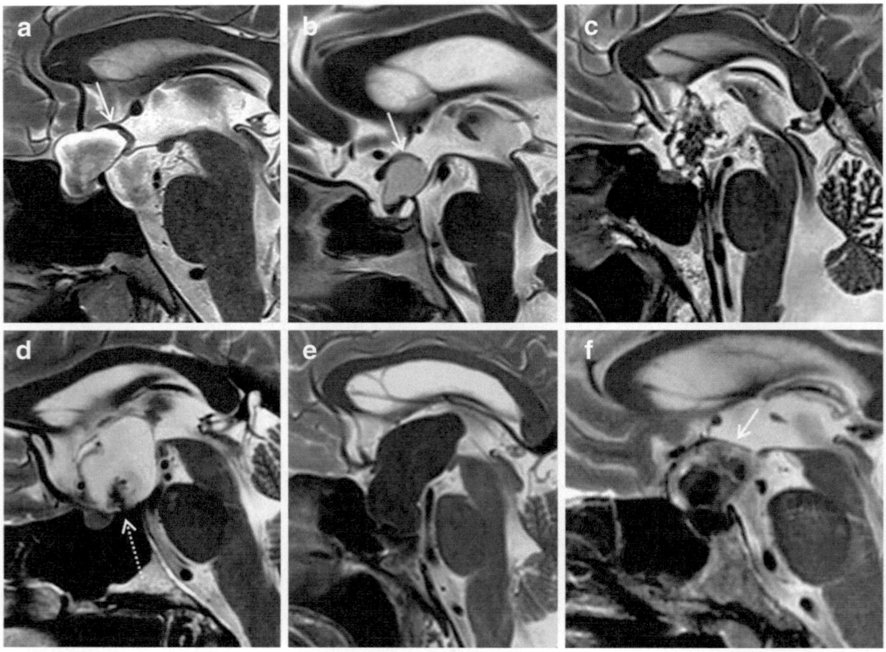

Fig. 28.2 Adamantinous craniopharyngiomas. Various appearances. (**a**–**f**) Sagittal T2WIs. T2W signal varies from hyper (**a**, **b**, **d**) to hypointense (**c**, **e**, **f**). Calcifications in **d** (dotted arrow). Note in **a**, **b**, and **f** that the floor of the third ventricle is perfectly respected (arrows). in **c**, **d**, **e** the tumor originates outside the third ventricle and extends secondarily to the ventricle

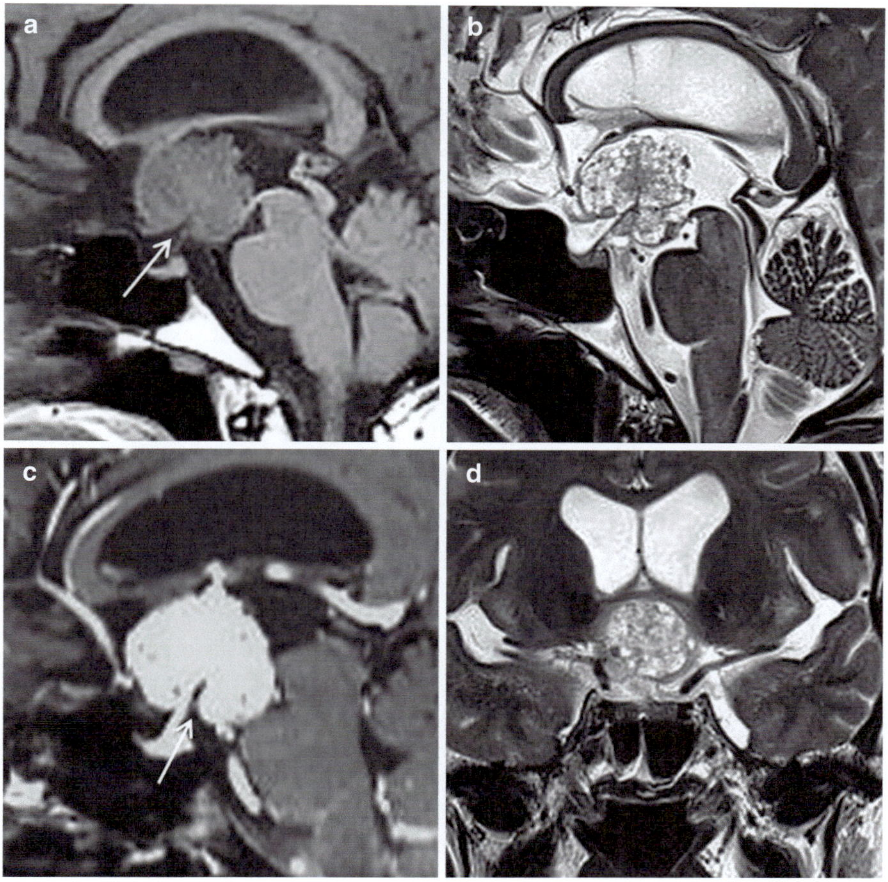

Fig. 28.3 Intraventricular papillary craniopharyngioma. Duct-like recess in the infundibular portion of the craniopharyngioma (arrow), characteristic of the papillary type. The pituitary stalk is preserved. (**a**, **c**) Sagittal TIW and CE T1WIs. (**b**, **d**) Sagittal and coronal T2WIs

Some statistically significant parameters have been proposed to differentiate the two subtypes:

- T1W hyperintense cysts, lobulated shape, and encasement of vessels in adamantinous CPs.
- T1W hypointense cysts, round shape, and solid appearance in papillary CPs.

The role of MRI is to define precisely the relationships between the tumor and the third ventricle floor and to detect the pure intraventricular form. The management of craniopharyngiomas depends greatly on these precisions.

A short reminder of the complex regional anatomy is needed.

- The anterior hypothalamus is defined by a line extending from the anterior commissure to the optic chiasm including the lamina terminalis and to the level of the mammillary bodies (Fig. 28.4a).
- The posterior hypothalamus is defined by a line drawn from the level of the mammillary bodies to the level of the posterior commissure.
- The third ventricle floor is the lamina terminalis anteriorly, the infundibulum, and the tuber cinereum inferiorly and posteriorly.
- The hypothalamic nuclei are located in the very thin walls of the third ventricle, particularly its floor.

The possibility of achieving tumoral resection without extremely severe sequelae—such as morbid obesity—depends on the relationship of the tumor with hypothalamus, for adamantinous as well as for papillary types. Posterior hypothalamic involvement could be associated with a higher body mass index after surgery.

- Five topographies according to the degree of hypothalamic distortion have been proposed: sellar-suprasellar, pseudo intraventricular, secondary intraventricular, not strictly intraventricular, and strictly intraventricular. In the first three categories, the pituitary stalk is usually not visible while it appears normal in strictly intraventricular CPs.
- An association between CP topography and optic chiasm distortion can also be noted: a chiasm displaced forward points to a not strictly intraventricular CP while a downward displacement of the chiasm indicates a strictly intraventricular CP.
- The interest of a mammillary body angle (MBA)—when this structure is recognized—has been emphasized: it is formed by the intersection of a line tangential to the base of mammillary bodies and the floor of the fourth ventricle (Fig. 28.4b, c).

  The normal MBA value ranges between 50 and 70°.

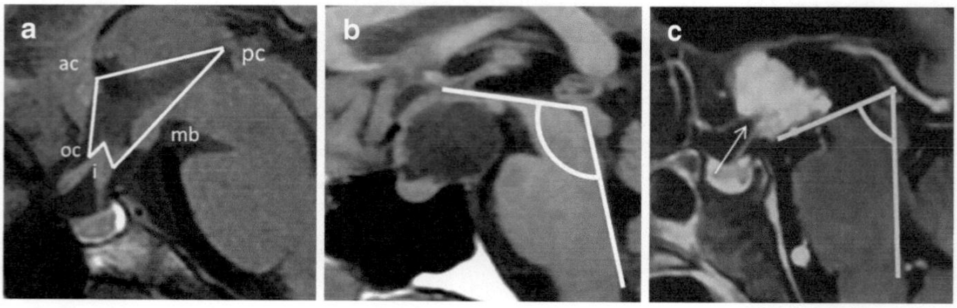

Fig. 28.4 Schematic representation of the limits of the hypothalamus on a sagittal view (**a**). *ac* anterior commissure, *pc* posterior commissure, *oc* optic chiasm, *mb* mammillary bodies, *i* infundibulum. The mammillary bodies angle is obtuse in a suprasellar CP (**b**), acute in an intraventricular CP (**c**). It is formed by the intersection of a line tangential to the base of mammillary bodies and the floor of the fourth ventricle. Note in **c** a duct-like recess (arrow) in this papillary intraventricular CP

An obtuse MBA indicates an upward displacement of the third ventricle floor and mammillary bodies and denotes a primary suprasellar CP position.

An acute MBA is observed with downward displacement of the mammillary bodies and is indicative of a primarily intraventricular topography.

A hyperacute MBA (30°) is indicative of a CP originated within the third ventricle floor itself.

- The presence of a duct-like recess at the infundibular portion of a third ventricle tumor representing a distinctive hallmark of papillary craniopharyngiomas located within the third ventricle has been recently described. It corresponds to a tubular-shaped recess of CSF invaginated at the midline bottom of the tumor, following the same angled trajectory as the pituitary stalk (Figs. 28.3 and 28.4c).

There is a major benefit to recognizing the different CP locations: for instance, a safer surgical approach through the corpus callosum or by opening the lamina terminalis can be proposed to remove the pure intraventricular forms. Non-strictly intraventricular tumors and particularly the infundibulo-tuberal topography have tighter adhesions to third ventricle walls and are associated with a worse outcome.

Differential diagnosis of CP with pituitary adenoma is usually easy (Figs. 28.5 and 28.6). It can be less easy with ependymomas, chordoid gliomas, or germinomas. The latter display a rectangular shape while papillary CPs usually affect a rounded configuration (Figs. 28.1c and 29.1d). Pilocytic astrocytomas of the suprasellar region also can mimic adamantinous craniopharyngiomas (Chap. 29).

If the duct-like recess of CPs is never seen in other third ventricle tumors, perifocal edema along the optic tracts (the mustache sign) is not specific. In CPs, it is frequently associated with post-operative hypothalamic dysfunction and worse visual functions.

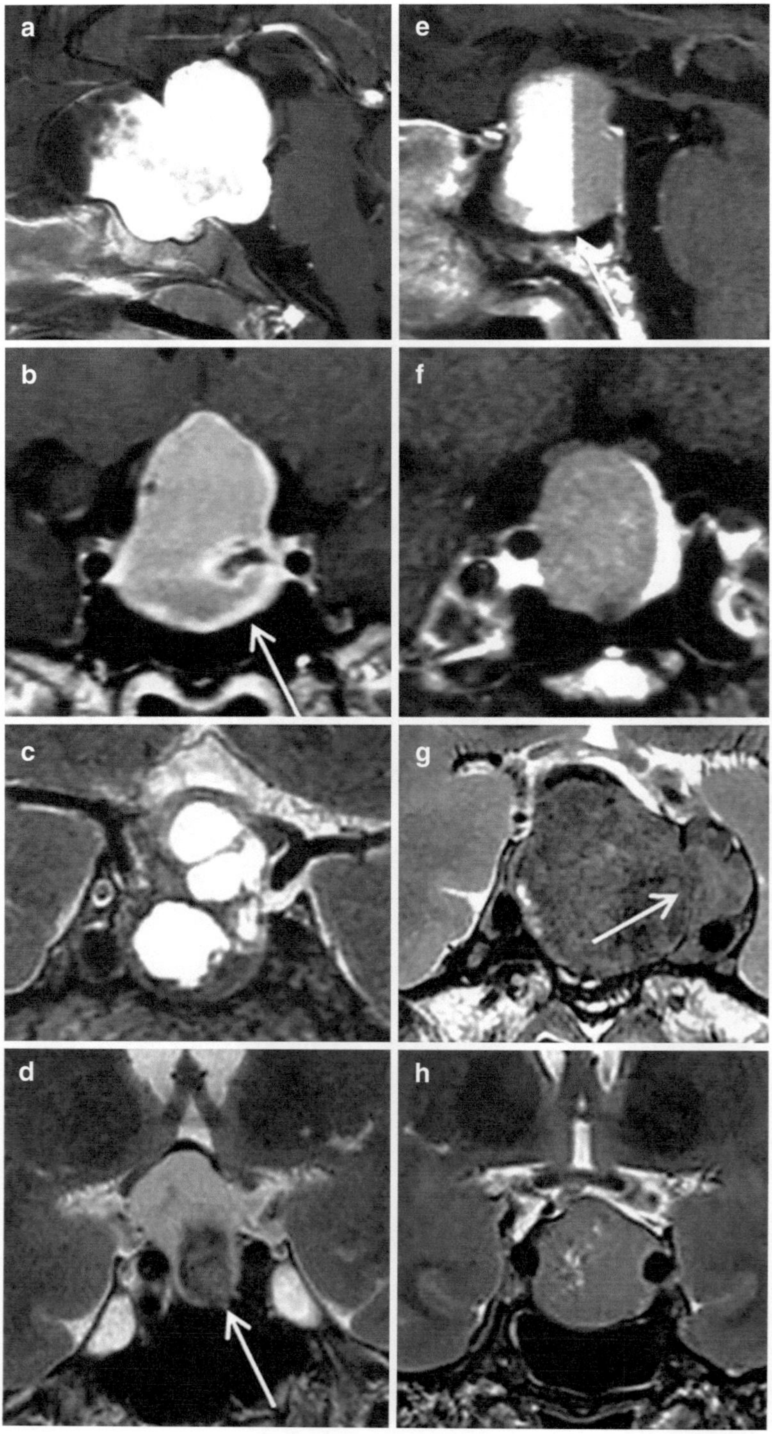

Fig. 28.5 Differential diagnosis of CPs (**a–d**) versus PitNETs (**e–h**). From top to bottom. Fluid level present in hemorrhagic PitNET, not in CP. Location of the normal pituitary: below the tumor in CP, not in PitNET. Cavernous sinus invasion: possible in PitNET, not in CP. Calcifications, frequent in CP, rare in PitNET

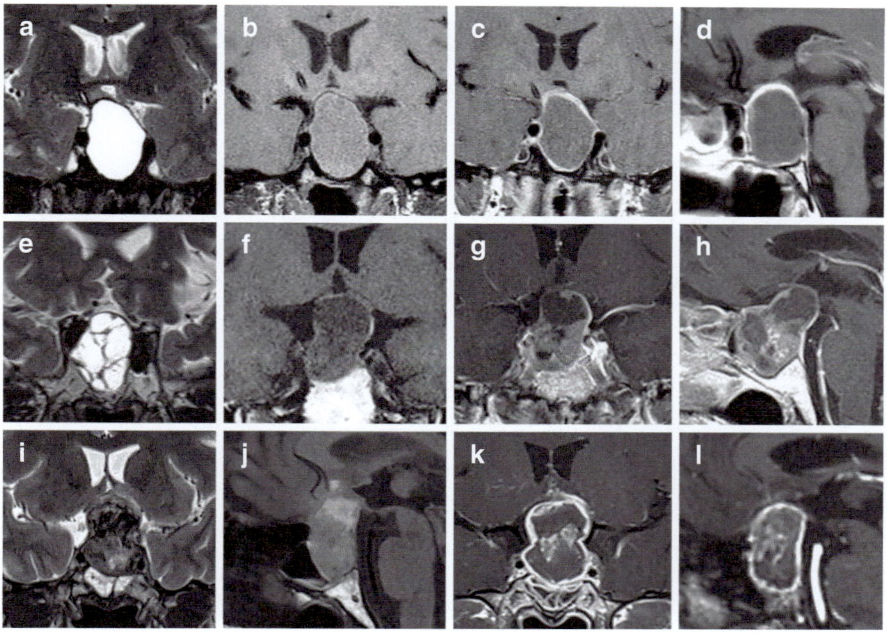

Fig. 28.6 Differential diagnosis. Upper row. Adamantinous CP with thick wall enhancement (**c**, **d**). Middle row. Cystic-hemorrhagic PitNET with septations, eccentric cysts, and thin wall enhancement (**h**). Lower row. Pituitary abscess. Heterogeneous T1 and T2W signal and thick wall enhancement (**k**, **l**). (**a**, **e**, **i**) T2WIs. (**b**, **f**, **j**) T1WIs. (**c**, **d**, **g**, **h**, **k**, **l**) CE T1WIs

Further Readings

Pascual JM, Carrasco R, Barrios L, R. Prieto duct-like recess in the infundibular portion of third ventricle craniopharyngiomas: an MRI sign identifying the papillary type. Am J Neuroradiol. 2022;43(9):1333–40. https://doi.org/10.3174/ajnr.A7602.

Prieto R, Barrios L, Pascual JM. Preoperative MRI diagnosis of papillary craniopharyngiomas: the revealing clues. Neurosurg Rev. 2023;47(1):8. https://doi.org/10.1007/s10143-023-02232-9. PMID: 38066315.

Rachmasari KN, Strauss SB, Phillips CD, Lantos JE, An A, Cisse B, Ramakrishna R, Schwartz TH, Dobri GA. Posterior hypothalamic involvement on pre-operative MRI predicts hypothalamic obesity in craniopharyngiomas. Pituitary. 2023;26(1):105–14. https://doi.org/10.1007/s11102-022-01294-0. Epub 2022 Dec 3. PMID: 36462067.

29 Germ-Cell and Other Bad Tumors

Germinoma is the most frequent intracranial germ-cell tumor and requires quick treatment. It arises along the midline from the pituitary stalk or the pineal gland or from both in a limited number of cases. Other tumors which belong to the same group are teratomas, embryonal carcinomas, and choriocarcinomas. Two out of three germinomas are diagnosed between 10 and 21 years of age with a peak frequency in early puberty. If boys are more affected than girls at the pineal level, both genders are equally affected in the suprasellar area. The first manifestation is usually arginine vasopressin deficiency (previously diabetes insipidus) and the thickening of the pituitary stalk may be equivocal at this stage. Classical tumor markers can be detected in serum and cerebrospinal fluid, but their absence does not eliminate the diagnosis.

Thereby, in the presence of a polyuro-polydypsic syndrome in a child, an adolescent, or a young adult, the rule is:

- To confirm the central origin of the symptoms by checking the missing bright spot on an axial T1W sequence.
- To observe meticulously the pituitary stalk, its morphology, and not only its size.
- To repeat the MRI at 3 and 6 months if the first examination is negative.

Later on, if the diagnosis is not made, the disease progression can result in hypothalamic-pituitary dysfunction, such as growth failure, precocious puberty, and visual disturbances.

The germ-cell tumor appears as a well-delineated round or lobulated mass without any specific T1 or T2W signal except in some cases where a T2W slightly hypointense signal may attest to a high nuclear to cytoplasmic ratio. Intratumoral cysts and rarely calcifications may be present. Less rarely, punctiform T2W hyperintense images can be seen (Fig. 29.1). Furthermore, a T2W FLAIR sequence may reveal peritumoral edema that mimics an inflammatory process, such as sarcoidosis or histiocytosis. After gadolinium injection, an unusual speckled and marked

J.-F. Bonneville, *Tricks and Traps in MRI of the Pituitary Region*,
https://doi.org/10.1007/978-3-031-64710-9_29

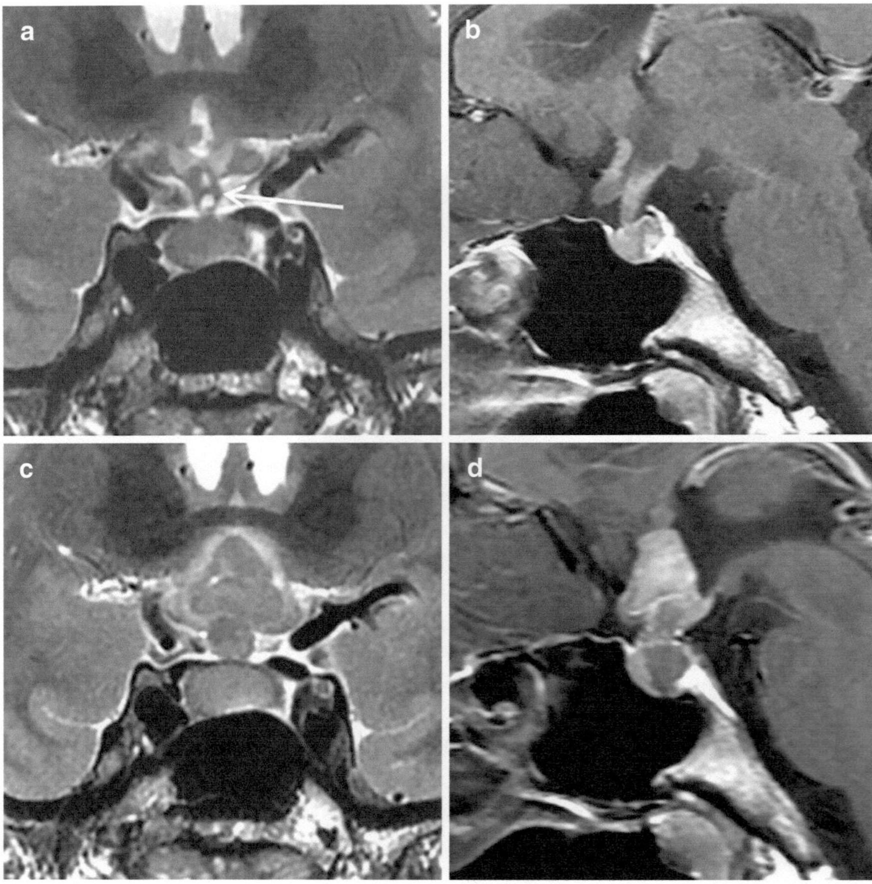

Fig. 29.1 Diabetes insipidus for one year in a young man. Upper row: Thickened pituitary stalk with small spots of T2 hyperintensity (arrow). Heterogeneous enhancement in front of the dorsum sellae. Lower row. Six months later, large intra- and suprasellar mass which is slightly T2 hyperintense and enhanced and involves the optic chiasm and the hypothalamus. (**a**, **c**) Coronal T2WIs. (**b**, **d**) Sagittal CE T1WIs

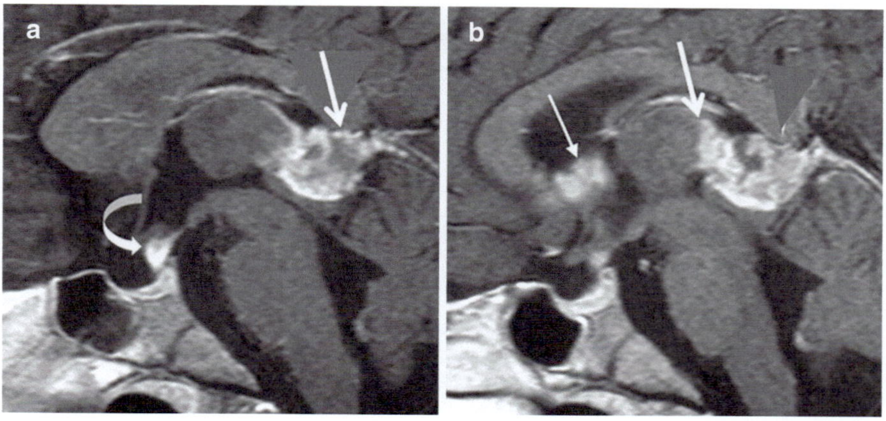

Fig. 29.2 (**a**) Slight enlargement of the pituitary stalk (curved arrow) and enhancing mass of the pineal region (arrow) in a bifocal germinoma. (**b**) Six months later, tumoral extension to the caudate nucleus and lamina terminalis (thin arrow). Extension of the pineal tumor to the third ventricle (thick arrow). (**a**, **b**) Sagittal CE T1WIs

enhancement can draw attention. Spinal cord MRI is mandatory since leptomeningeal spread with drop metastases has been reported.

Demonstration of an associated pineal localization when present makes the diagnosis easier, but differentiation from a benign pineal cyst can be challenging (Fig. 29.2). Benign pineal cysts are liquid lesions less than 2 cm in diameter, homogeneous with a FLAIR signal different from the signal of CSF and a thin peripheral enhancement after contrast injection.

Susceptibility-weighted (SWI) and diffusion-weighted imaging (DWI) using the ADC ratio value can help to differentiate germinomas from other tumors in the pineal region. A machine learning-based classification of pineal germinomas has also been proposed.

The prognosis *of non-germinomatous germ cell tumors (NGGCT)* is considered worse than that of germinomas. They secrete alpha-fetoprotein which can be detected in serum or CSF. These tumors present usually as posterior third ventricular masses with hydrocephalus and midbrain compression. They are larger than germinomas and can cause hydrocephalus (Fig. 29.3).

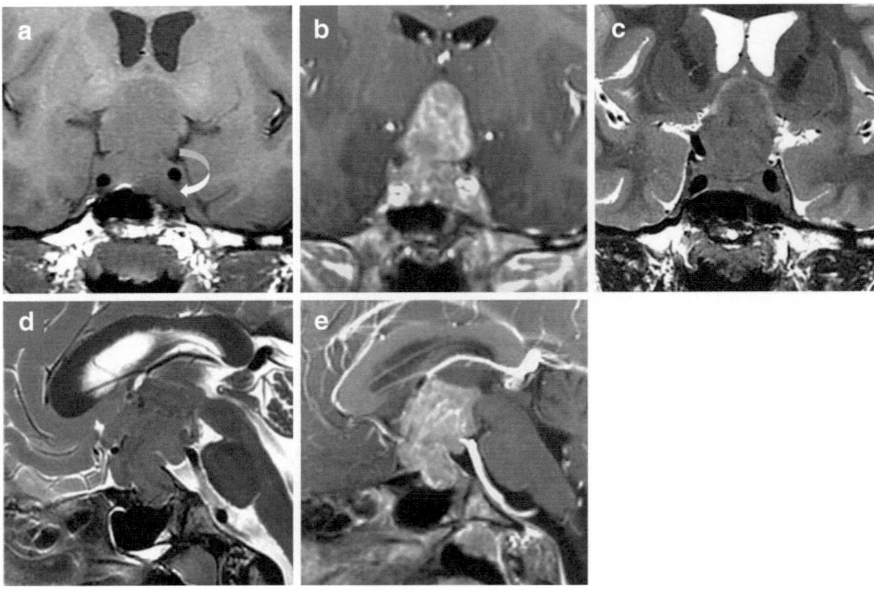

Fig. 29.3 Diabetes insipidus, headache and visual deficit in a 13-year-old boy. A non-germinomatous germ cell tumor has been suspected. Huge lobulated intra- and suprasellar homogeneous tumor with cavernous sinus invasion (curved arrow). The mass is clearly hypointense on T2WI. (**a–c**) Coronal T1, CE T1, and T2WIs. (**d**, **e**) Sagittal T2 and CE T1WIs

NGGCTs are more heterogeneous than germinomas: teratomas may present cysts, calcification, or even teeth (Fig. 29.4). Foci of hemorrhage evoke choriocarcinoma. But actually, differentiating pure germinomas from NGGCT remains difficult. Very recently, the specific role of T2 gradient echo MRI or susceptibility weighted imaging (SWI) has been emphasized: when on-midline located, NGGCTs show SWI or T2W gradient echo hypointensity whereas germinomas appear isointense or hyperintense to normal parenchyma.

Even if most germ cell tumors are radiosensitive and respond to chemotherapy, it must be recalled that an early diagnosis is fundamental but difficult and that it requires a high-quality MRI and a deep knowledge of the pituitary stalk radioanatomy, especially for the diagnosis of germinomas.

Pilocytic astrocytomas of the suprasellar region may have clinical presentation and MRI features similar to adamantinous craniopharyngiomas. They present as a cystic-solid mass with heterogeneous enhancement. Both tumors can have calcifications. Recently, the "cut green pepper sign" has been proposed to help to differentiate CPs from pilocytic astrocytomas. This sign is defined as irregular peripheral rim enhancement, or ground-glass-like appearance enhancement, with or without a strongly enhancing nodule in the lesion. The appearance is similar to that of the flesh of a cut green pepper (Fig. 29.5).

Primary central nervous system lymphoma (PCNSL) is rarely limited to the sellar region. The mean age of patients is 55 years, 60% of patients are males. PCNSL

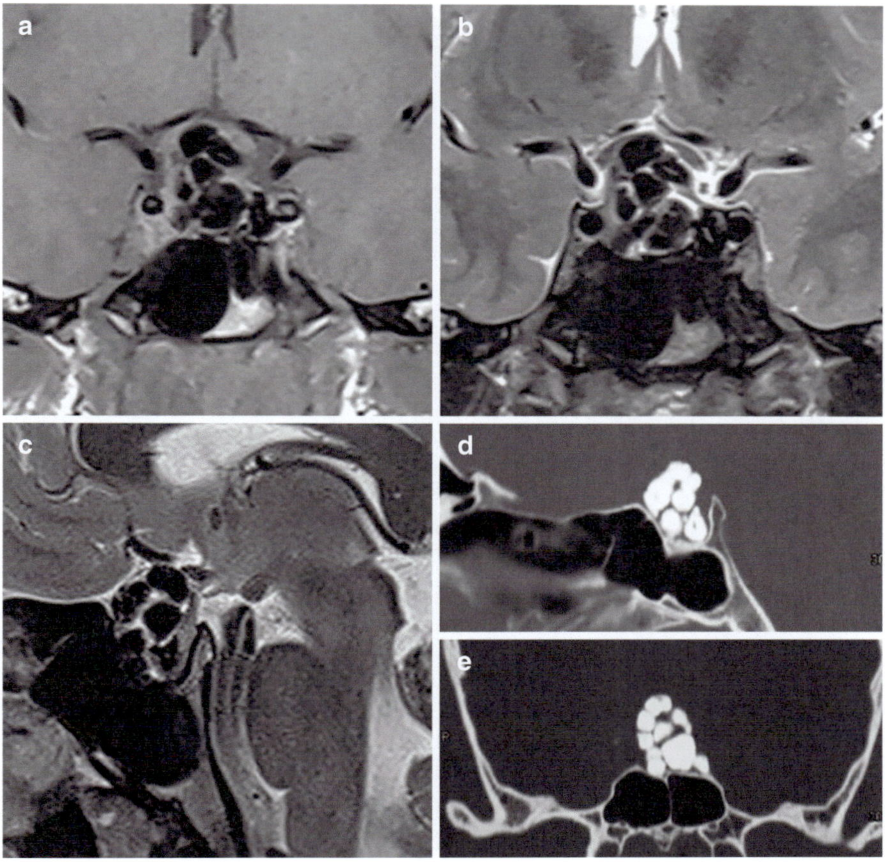

Fig. 29.4 Teratoma in a non-symptomatic 29-year-old man. Previous partial surgery years before for visual field deficit. Characteristic image of teeth in a sellar/suprasellar mass. (**a–c**) Coronal T1, T2, and sagittal T2WIs. (**d**, **e**) CT

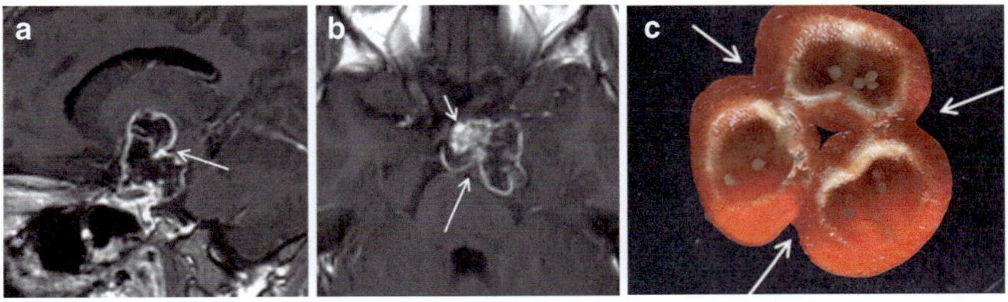

Fig. 29.5 Pilocytic actrocytoma showing the cut pepper sign. Indentations on the surface of the lesion (long arrows) and marked enhancing mural nodule (short arrow) on axial CE T1WI (**b**). The sagittal CE TI WI (**a**) shows discrete point-like enhancement inside the tumor, that resembles scattered pepper seeds. (**c**) Cut section of a red pepper (Adapted from S Xu, BMC Medical Imaging (2023) 23: 191)

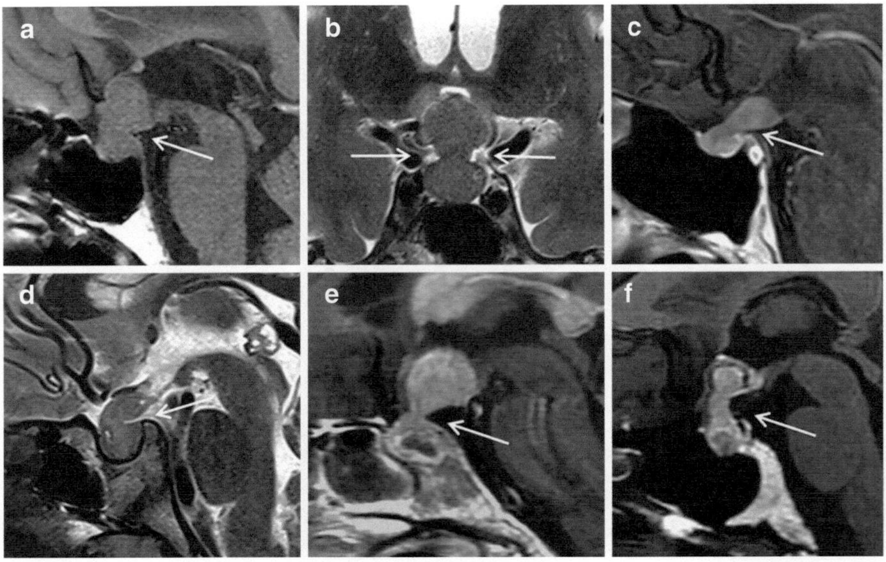

Fig. 29.6 Posterior notch at the sellar diaphragm suggestive of malignant lesions: in germinoma (**a**, **b**, **d**), in lymphoma (**c**), in metastasis (**e**), or in melanoma (**f**)

can mimic a pituitary adenoma or arise from the suprasellar and hypothalamic regions. Spread to the infundibular region and cavernous sinus is noticed. The common MRI finding is a sellar or suprasellar mass that is hypointense on T2WIs and presents a strong contrast enhancement. Diffusion-weighted imaging exhibits hyperintensity and FLAIR shows a vasogenic oedema. Nevertheless, these features are inconstant. A mass of the pituitary region with a propensity for perineural spread and an infiltrative growth pattern, particularly when the patient is immunocompromised or old is suggestive of lymphoma.

As in other malignant diseases such as *metastases,* a rapid tumoral growth on two successive MRIs, a posterior notch at the sellar diaphragm level or a dumbbell pattern (Fig. 29.6), may be observed.

Further Readings

Takase R, Nakano Y, Otsuka F. Malignant lymphoma developed in the hypothalamus. Intern Med. 2020;59(7):1009–10. https://doi.org/10.2169/internalmedicine.3655-19. Epub 2019 Dec 26. PMID: 31875635; PMCID: PMC7184080.

Xu S, Yang W, Luo Y, Wang X, Li Y, Meng X, Zhang Y, Zeng H, Huang B. A novel MRI feature, the cut green pepper sign, can help differentiate a suprasellar pilocytic astrocytoma from an adamantinomatous craniopharyngioma. BMC Med Imaging. 2023;23:191.

Yeo KK, Nagabushan S, Dhall G, Abdelbaki MS. Primary central nervous system germ cell tumors in children and young adults: a review of controversies in diagnostic and treatment approach. Neoplasia. 2023;36:100860. https://doi.org/10.1016/j.neo.2022.100860. Epub 2022 Dec 13. PMID: 36521378; PMCID: PMC9772847.

The Empty Sella Is Not Empty 30

An empty sella is in fact a sella turcica filled with CSF because of a large opening or an absence of the sellar diaphragm or after pituitary tumor removal. When present, the pituitary gland is flattened at the bottom of the sella.

The term “empty sella” is sometimes improperly used in medical reports for instance in the elderly in whom the physiological reduction of the volume of the anterior pituitary allows intrasellar penetration of the CSF. For general practitioners, the term “empty sella” could suggest a pathological condition and result in unuseful tests. If discovered incidentally, it could be suggested to prefer here the term “intrasellar penetration of subarachnoid spaces”, —which reflects a more or less physiological aspect—in the descriptive part of the MRI report without repeating it in the conclusion, implying that this observation does not require any hormonal test or further monitoring if the patient is non-symptomatic. Generally speaking, we suggest mentioning an empty sella in the radiological report when more than 50% of the sella is filled with CSF and especially when the pituitary gland thickness is less than 2–3 mm.

If it is admitted for a long time that most cases of empty sella are non-symptomatic, a recent study has found a high percentage of pituitary deficits, mainly central hypogonadism in a cohort of patients with a mean age of 55 years and presenting an empty sella. Therefore, a hormonal testing could be recommended in this specific category of patients, particularly in men. A moderate hyperprolactinemia, usually less than 50 μg/L and attributed to stalk effect, can be noted.

It is usual to distinguish the primary empty sella where the sellar diaphragm is constitutively absent or largely open and the secondary empty sella which appears after removal or shrinkage of the sellar content.

In *primary empty sella,* the sella turcica is more or less enlarged due to the repeated pulsations of the CSF against the walls of the sella. The pituitary stalk is elongated to reach the flattened pituitary gland and frequently pressed along the dorsum sellae, then sometimes invisible within the sella on sagittal as well as on coronal images. In this situation, an incorrect diagnosis of arachnoid cyst could be made (Fig. 30.1a, b). The diagnosis is corrected by the demonstration of the

J.-F. Bonneville, *Tricks and Traps in MRI of the Pituitary Region*,
https://doi.org/10.1007/978-3-031-64710-9_30

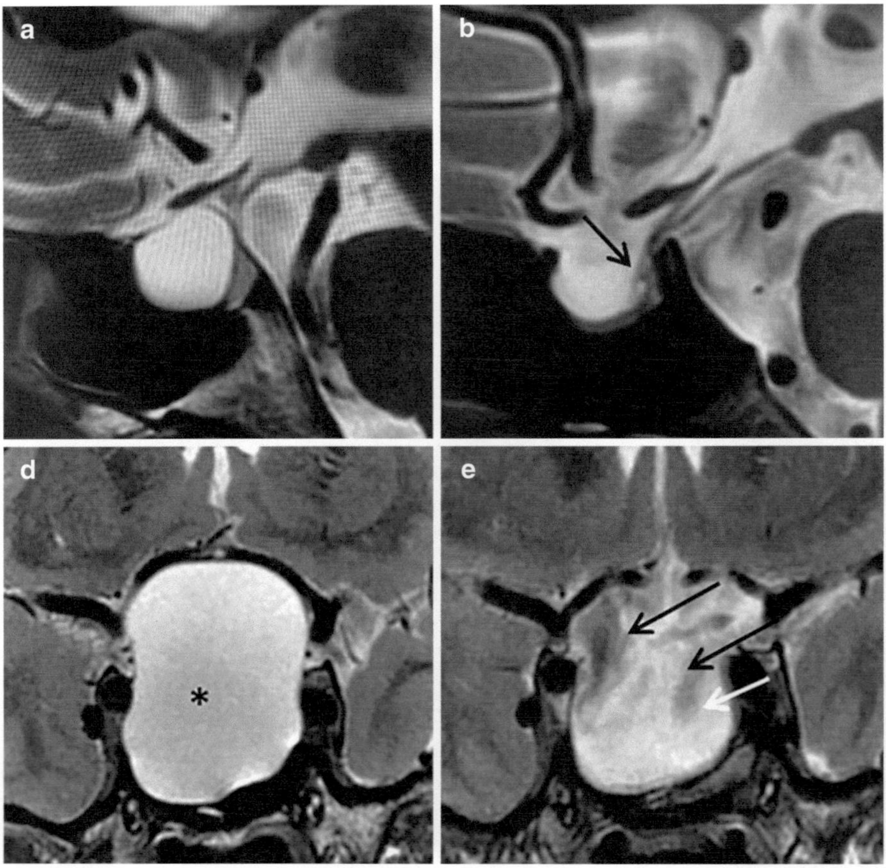

Fig. 30.1 Upper row. Arachnoid cyst (**a**) versus empty sella (**b**). In a, the pituitary stalk is invisible in the sella. Lower row. Secondary empty sella. Rathke cleft cyst * before (**c**) and after surgery (**d**). Flow artifacts (arrows). (**a, b**) Sagittal T2WIs. (**c, d**) Coronal T2WIs

pituitary stalk within the sella on an axial view. In addition, CSF flow artifacts are shown intrasellarly on T2W images in empty sella, not in sellar cysts (Fig. 30.1c, d). Visualization of a large opening of the sellar diaphragm on T2W images sometimes confirms the diagnosis.

An empty sella can be a marker of idiopathic intracranial hypertension when associated with optic nerve protrusion, distension of the optic nerve sheath, optic nerve tortuosity, or posterior globe flattening (Fig. 30.2).

Empty sella in the context of Cushing's disease can make the demonstration of the responsible corticotropic microadenoma more uncertain (Fig. 16.1c, d).

The physiological dehiscence of the sellar diaphragm is very common and one may wonder why an empty sella is not more frequently observed. We have hypothesized that the non-pneumatization of the posterior part of the sphenoid bone could be an adjunctive contributing factor: the deepening of the sella below the pulsating CSF could be facilitated when the sellar floor is adjacent to cancellous bone and not

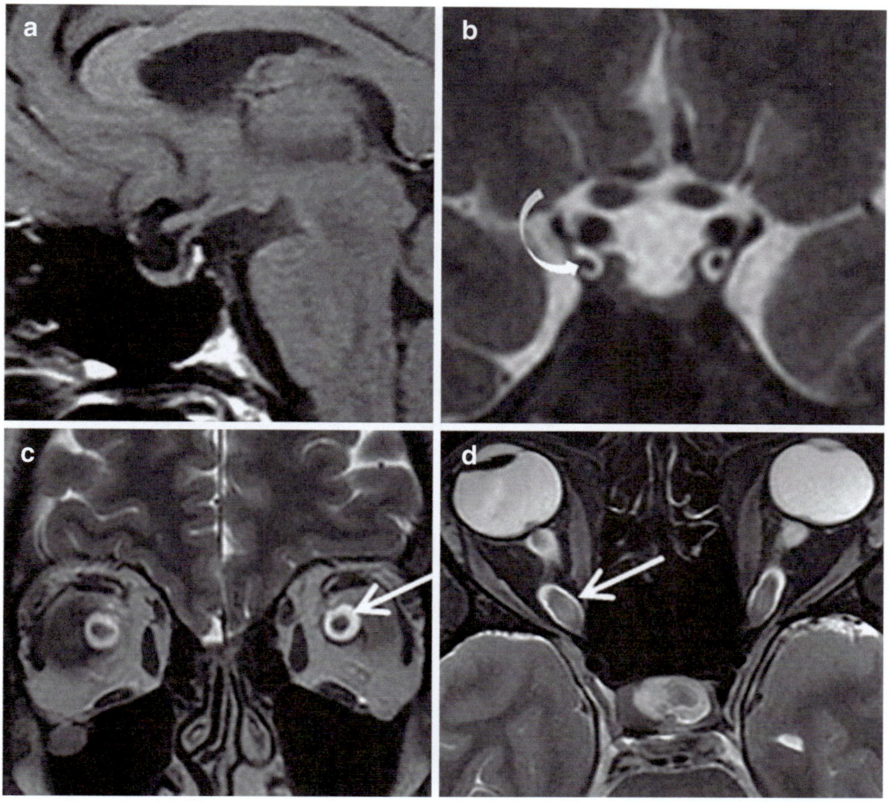

Fig. 30.2 Enlargement of oculomotor (curved arrow) and optic nerve sheaths (arrow) in a patient with benign intracranial hypertension. Partial empty sella. (**a**) Sagittal T1WI. (**b–d**) Coronal and axial T2WIs

with the more resistant cortical bone bordering the sphenoid sinus (Fig. 30.3). Indeed, a primary empty sella is usually observed with incomplete pneumatization of the sphenoid and is rarer if the pneumatization extends caudally to the level of the dorsum sellae.

A secondary empty sella occurs after pituitary surgery, radiotherapy, or Sheehan syndrome or as a result of a cyst or tumor shrinkage. A discrete V-shaped deformation of the optic chiasm may be an indicator of a pituitary adenoma or of a Rathke cleft cyst spontaneous shrinkage. Location of vasopressin can also help in showing an ectopic storage (Fig. 30.4).

A particular type of empty sella pattern is frequently observed in multiparous women in whom the pituitary gland—and consequently the sella turcica—has been enlarged by successive pregnancies (Fig. 30.5c, d).

Ptosis of the optic chiasm, optic nerves as well as the inferior part of the third ventricle can occur with secondary empty sella (Fig. 30.5a, b). A chiasmapexy has been rarely proposed in case of severe visual field defect. Bone erosion of the sellar floor and CSF leak can be observed in huge empty sella.

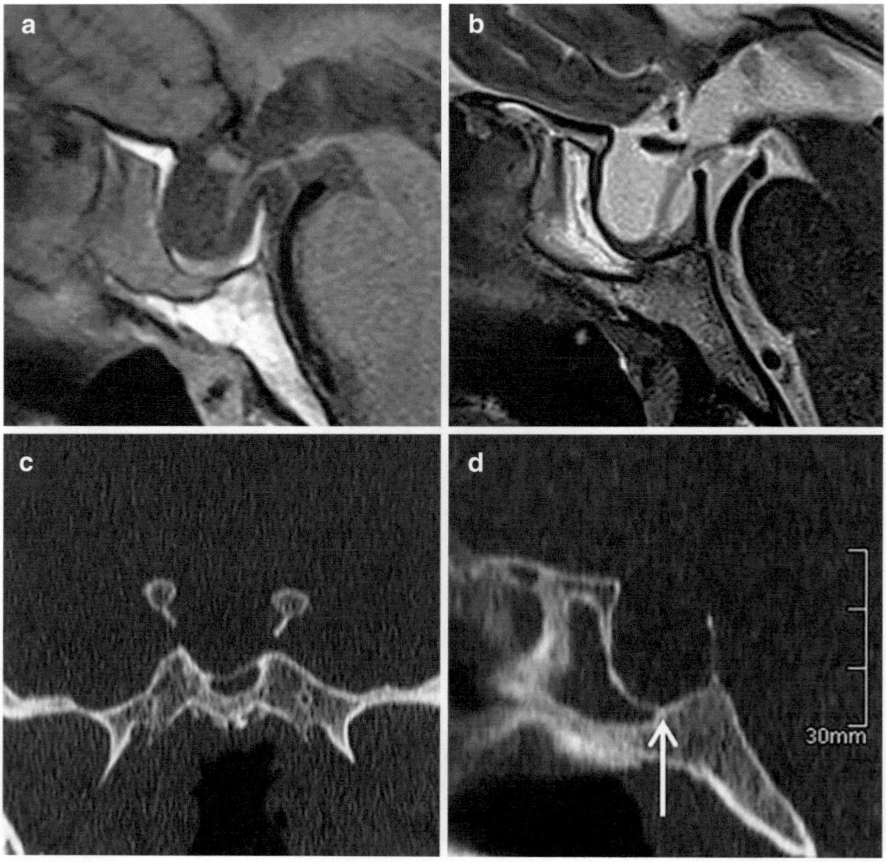

Fig. 30.3 Putative role of sphenoid pneumatization in empty sella syndrome. Pneumatization stops at the nadir of the sella level (arrow). (**a**, **b**) Sagittal T1 and T2WIs. (**c**, **d**) Coronal and sagittal CT (bone window)

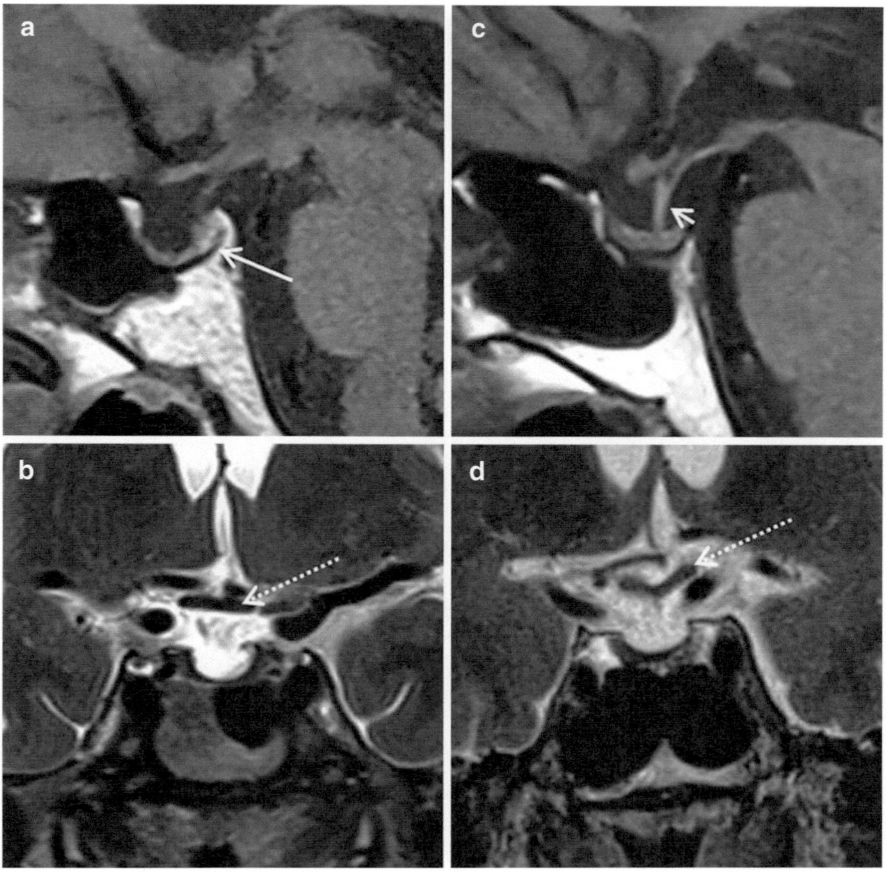

Fig. 30.4 Primary (**a**, **b**) versus secondary empty sella after spontaneous shrinkage of a Rathke cleft cyst. The optic chiasm is in place in b, distorted in **d** (dotted arrows). Vasopressin storage (straight arrows) is normal in **a** (confirmed by an axial T1WI, not shown); not seen intrasellarly in **c**. Spontaneous T1W hypersignal of the pituitary stalk indicating ectopic vasopressin storage (short arrow in **c**). Note that pneumatization of the sphenoid is incomplete in **a**, primary empty sella, complete in **c**, secondary empty sella. (**a**, **c**) Sagittal non-enhanced T1WIs. (**b**, **d**) Coronal T2WIs

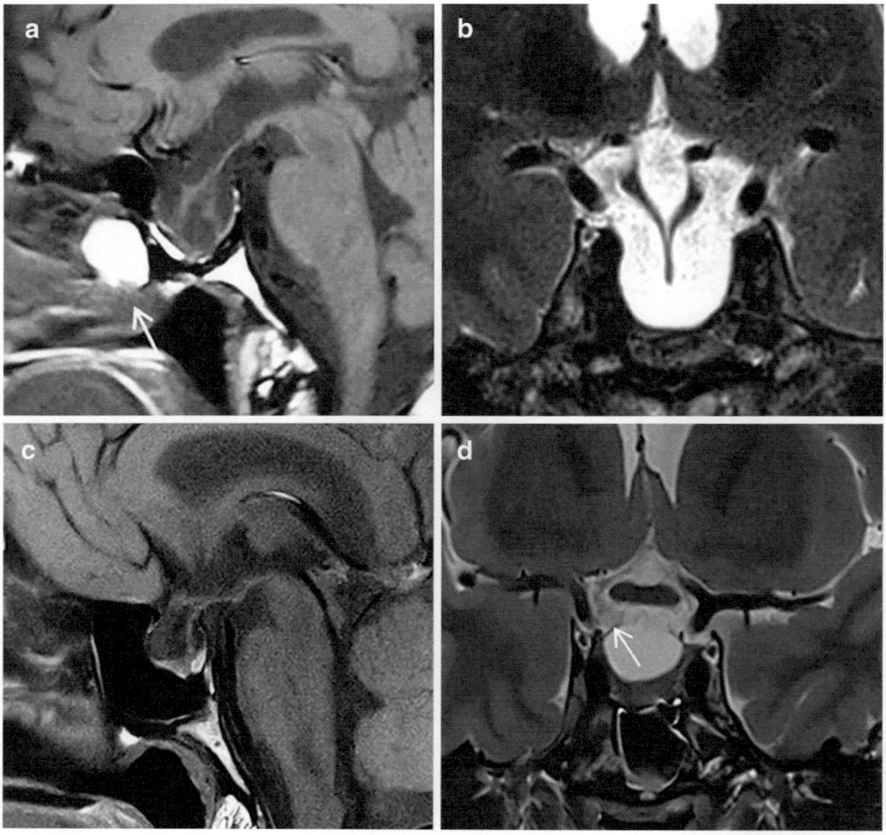

Fig. 30.5 Upper row. Post-operative secondary empty sella. Ptosis of the optic chiasm and optic nerves. Residual fat packing (arrow) (**a**, **b** sagittal T1 and coronal T2WIs). Lower row. Empty sella in a multiparous woman. Note the large opening of the sellar diaphragm (arrow). (**c**, **d** Sagittal T1 and coronal T2WIs)

Further Readings

Barkatullah AF, Leishangthem L, Moss HE. MRI findings as markers of idiopathic intracranial hypertension. Curr Opin Neurol. 2021;34(1):75–83. https://doi.org/10.1097/WCO.0000000000000885. PMID: 33230036; PMCID: PMC7856277.

Carosi G, Brunetti A, Mangone A, et al. Multicenter cohort study in patients with primary empty sella: hormonal and neuroradiological features over a long follow-up. Front Endocrinol (Lausanne). 2022;13:925378. https://doi.org/10.3389/fendo.2022.925378. PMID: 35813618; PMCID: PMC9259926.

Himes BT, Bhargav AG, Brown DA, et al. Does pituitary compression/empty sella syndrome contribute to MRI-negative Cushing's disease? A single-institution experience. Neurosurg Focus. 2020;48(6):E3. https://doi.org/10.3171/2020.3.FOCUS2084. PMID: 32480375.

31 Hypophysitis or PitNET?

Hypophysitis is defined as an inflammatory pituitary disease usually leading to pituitary deficiencies. It can be primary, the most frequent etiology being autoimmune or secondary as part of a systemic disease, such as sarcoidosis, histiocytosis, Crohn's disease, or granulomatosis with polyangiitis for instance (see Chap. 38).

Lymphocytic hypophysitis is the most common primary hypophysitis and affects preferentially young women, particularly during late pregnancy or postpartum. The first symptom of lymphocytic hypophysitis is headache which can occur in a dramatic fashion followed by nausea, vomiting, visual impairment, and various degrees of hypopituitarism.

It has been recently suggested that a significant number of cases of hypophysitis labeled lymphocytic hypophysitis could be in fact related to a previously unknown multifocal disease, the IgG4-related autoimmune disease which affects mainly middle-aged to elderly males. *IgG4 hypophysitis* could account for 30% of all cases of primary hypophysitis. The involvement of IgG4-related diseases elsewhere in the body can be a diagnostic indicator.

The specific inflammatory involvement of the pituitary stalk and posterior lobe, named *infundibuloneurohypophysitis,* represents the most frequent etiology of isolated AVP deficit (previously diabetes insipidus). The disease is most often of autoimmune origin. It affects preferentially young adults and children. Headache is frequently missing. Manifestations can be relapsing. Thickening of the pituitary stalk can be very discrete or even questionable but the absence of vasopressin storage on axial Fatsat T1 WI reinforces the diagnosis. A focal T2W hypointensity of the infundibulum can sometimes be observed. Secondary atrophy of the pituitary stalk is observed in a few months. The diagnosis of infundibuloneurohypophysitis must be retained only after elimination of a systemic disease (Fig. 31.1).

Hypophysitis related to immunomodulatory drugs such as ipilimumab may have low visible manifestation if MRI is not obtained in the acute phase of the disease since pituitary enlargement rapidly resolved. Later one, a mild pituitary atrophy and post-contrast delayed enhancement may be observed (Fig. 31.2).

J.-F. Bonneville, *Tricks and Traps in MRI of the Pituitary Region*,
https://doi.org/10.1007/978-3-031-64710-9_31

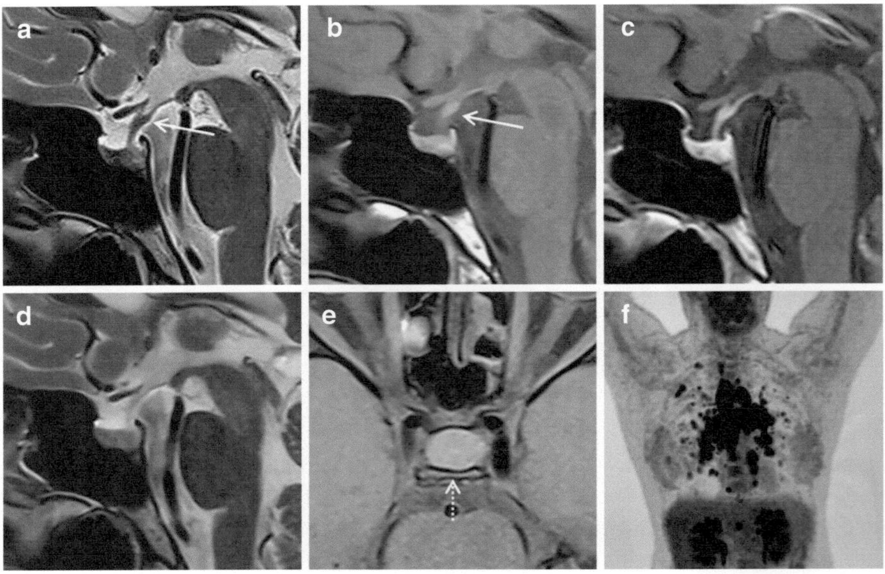

Fig. 31.1 Sudden onset of a polyuro-polydipsic syndrome in a 40-year-old woman 3 months ago. A diagnosis of infundibuloneurohypophysitis was initially proposed. Sarcoidosis was demonstrated later. Upper row. T1W hyperintense/T2W hypointense signal of the infundibulum without clear thickening of the pituitary stalk (arrows). The sagittal CE T1WI (**c**) is not informative. Lower row. Six months later, marked thinning of the pituitary stalk. The T1 and T2W signal abnormalities have gone. The bright spot corresponding to AVP storage is always missing on axial Fatsat T1WI (dotted arrow in **e**). (**a**, **d**) Sagittal T2WIs. (**b**) Sagittal T1WI. (**f**) Thoracic PET

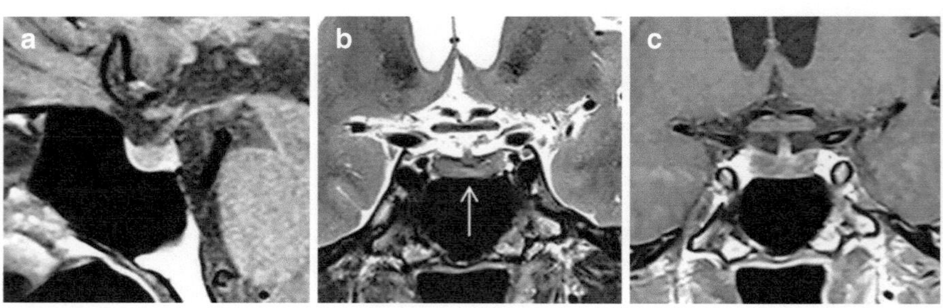

Fig. 31.2 Hypophysitis after immunotherapy, late stage. T2W heterogeneous hyperintensity (arrow) and lack of enhancement of the anterior pituitary in (**c**). (**a**) Sagittal CE T1WI. (**b**, **c**) Coronal T2W and CE T1WIs

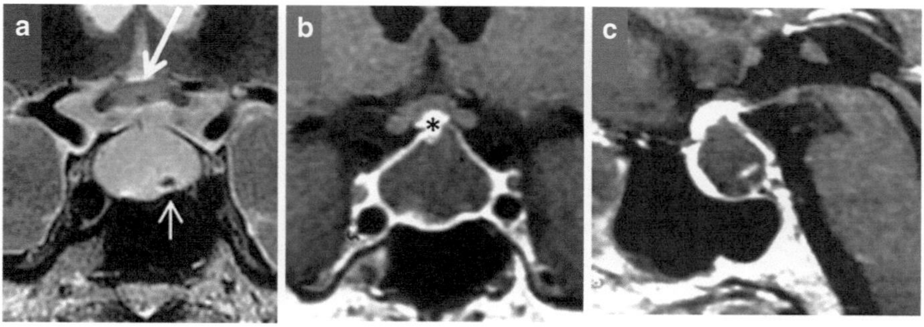

Fig. 31.3 Xanthomatous hypophysitis after RCC rupture. (**a**) Coronal T2WI. Intrasellar T2W hyperintense RCC. T2W hypointense hyperproteinic nodule (small arrow). Note an edema of the optic chiasm despite a limited suprasellar extension of the lesion (long arrow). (**b**, **c**) Coronal and sagittal CE T1WIs. Thick and intense enhancement of the cyst wall, reinforced at the infundibulum (*)

Xanthomatous hypophysitis is now generally considered secondary to an RCC leakage or rupture (Fig. 31.3).

Primary hypophysitis is sometimes mistaken radiologically with PitNET and this error may have unfortunately led to surgery. If MRI features of hypophysitis can vary with etiology, some findings are relatively constant and differ with what is observed with PitNET (Fig. 31.4).

- The pituitary gland is enlarged in hypophysitis, but this feature can be difficult to assess in the elderly whose anterior pituitary gland is physiologically shrunk. Importantly, the enlargement is symmetrical. It can present an upward tongue-like extension to the pituitary stalk and the infundibulum giving a pear-shaped appearance to the mass.
- The pituitary stalk is not deviated.
- The sella turcica is not enlarged and the sellar floor is not depressed.
- The normal pituitary tissue which is visible superiorly and/or laterally in pituitary adenoma is not demonstrated in hypophysitis on T2 or in CE T1WIs.
- Signal of hypophysitis is hyperintense on FLAIR
- The T2W signal is mostly slightly hyperintense on T2 WI with possible areas of necrosis evidenced by a marked T2 hyperintense signal.
- Classically, post-gadolinium enhancement is described as intense, but this feature depends on the gadolinium dosage and the time of the data acquisition. It is reinforced peripherally in xanthomatous hypophysitis.
- Dynamic MRI could show a slow and delayed enhancement (Fig. 9.3).
- The cavernous sinus is not invaded in hypophysitis, except in IgG4 hypophysitis where the involvement of both cavernous sinuses and the narrowed carotid arteries can remind an elephant-head (Fig. 31.5d, e).
- An edema and a T2 hyperintensity of the optic chiasm are evocative of hypophysitis (Figs. 31.3a and 31.4f).

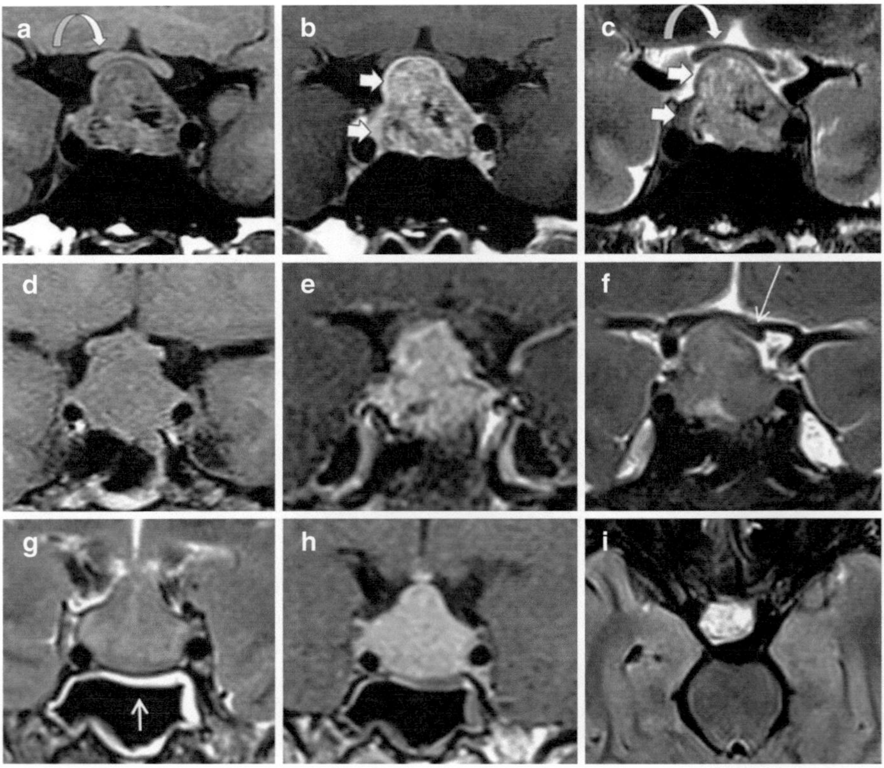

Fig. 31.4 Primary hypophysitis versus PitNET. Upper row. Non-secreting PitNET. The normal pituitary is demonstrated laterally and superiorly (double arrows). The optic chiasm is slightly raised but is not edematous (curved arrow). (**a**–**c**) Coronal T1, CE T1WI and T2WIs. Middle row. Lymphocytic hypophysitis. Intra and suprasellar mass of the same volume as the PitNET in the upper row. Marked heterogeneous enhancement without demonstration of the normal gland. Edematous optic chiasm (rail-like image, arrow in **f**). (**d**–**f**) Coronal T1, CET1 and T2WIs. Lower row. Lymphocytic hypophysitis during pregnancy. Reactional thickening of the sphenoid sinus mucosa (short arrow). The sella mass is hyperintense on T2WI (**g**), homogeneously enhanced on CE T1WI (**h**), and hyperintense on axial FLAIR (**i**)

- A dural tail, i.e., a thickening and post gadolinium enhancement of the perisellar dura mater is very suggestive of an inflammatory process but inconstant and nonspecific.
- Inconsistently, a thickening of the sphenoid sinus mucosa can be found as it is in pituitary apoplexy (Fig. 31.4g).
- The posterior pituitary bright spot is absent in infundibuloneurohypophysitis.
- Pituitary fibrosis, which is seen as a thick hypoT2W signaling of the border of the pituitary, can be observed at later stages, particularly in IgG4 hypophysitis (Fig. 31.5) and in xanthomatous hypophysitis.

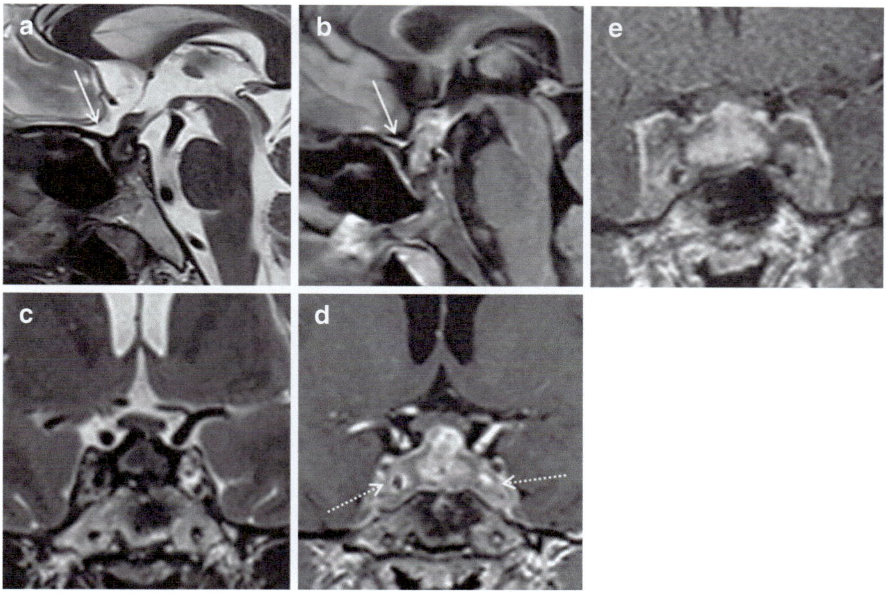

Fig. 31.5 IgG4 hypophysitis. Late phase. Sellar mass surrounded by a thick T2W hypointense ring extended anteriorly to the dura (arrows). Both cavernous sinuses are affected and internal carotid arteries are narrowed (dotted arrows). (**a**, **b**) Sagittal T2 and CE T1WIs. (**c**, **d**) Coronal T2 and CE T1WIs. (**e**) Coronal CE T1WI in in another patient with IgG4 hypophysitis: "elephant-head appearance" resulting from enlarged bilateral cavernous sinuses and narrowed internal carotid arteries

Further Readings

Carpenter KJ, Murtagh RD, Lilienfeld H, Weber J, Murtagh FR. Ipilimumab-induced hypophysitis: MR imaging findings. AJNR Am J Neuroradiol. 2009;30(9):1751–3. https://doi.org/10.3174/ajnr.A1623. Epub 2009 May 27.

Kyriacou A, Gnanalingham K, Kearney T. Lymphocytic hypophysitis: modern day management with limited role for surgery. Pituitary. 2017;20(2):241–50. https://doi.org/10.1007/s11102-016-0769-3.

Shikuma J, Kan K, Ito R, Hara K, Sakai H, Miwa T, Kanazawa A, Odawara M. Critical review of IgG4-related hypophysitis. Pituitary. 2017;20(2):282–91. https://doi.org/10.1007/s11102-016-0773-7.

Meningioma or Pituitary Adenoma? 32

Meningiomas of the sellar region are common and usually benign. A few display aggressive behavior and can be candidate for a targeted therapy. Recently, emphasis was placed on the occurrence of meningiomas in patients with long-term exposition to progestins for instance in women treated for severe hirsutism or in transgender women. In these situations, meningiomas may be multiple and they frequently shrink after drug discontinuation.

Several methods have been proposed to differentiate meningiomas and non-secreting adenomas: the apparent diffusion coefficient value could be higher in pituitary adenomas; quantitative dual-energy CT could be also discriminating. In fact, coronal T2WIs are quite always largely sufficient to achieve properly the diagnosis of meningioma.

The sites of insertion of sellar meningiomas are numerous and may affect the clinoid processes, the dorsum or the tuberculum sellae, and the planum sphenoidale (Fig. 32.1): at these levels, associated bony and dural changes—osteoma, thickening, erosion, blistering, and dural tail, even if they are not absolutely specific—make the diagnosis easy. Most meningiomas of the sellar region are T2W hyperintense. *Meningiomas of the planum or of the tuberculum sellae* may invade the sella turcica and simulate a pituitary macroadenoma with suprasellar extension: the recognition of the osseous changes which can be discrete is essential (Fig. 3.5). It should also be noted that the sella is either minimally or not enlarged in meningiomas. If very large, meningiomas can be circumscribed by a vasogenic edema. A ring of CSF delineates sometimes the tumor contours. Signal voids may attest a marked blood supply in some meningiomas (Fig. 31.1a, b). These observations are not seen in PitNETs.

The diagnosis of meningioma could be less easy in two other locations: at the sellar diaphragm level and in the cavernous sinus.

Meningiomas attached to the sellar diaphragm extend in the sella. Their signal is usually homogeneous and more or less hyperintense on T2WI and isointense on

J.-F. Bonneville, *Tricks and Traps in MRI of the Pituitary Region*,
https://doi.org/10.1007/978-3-031-64710-9_32

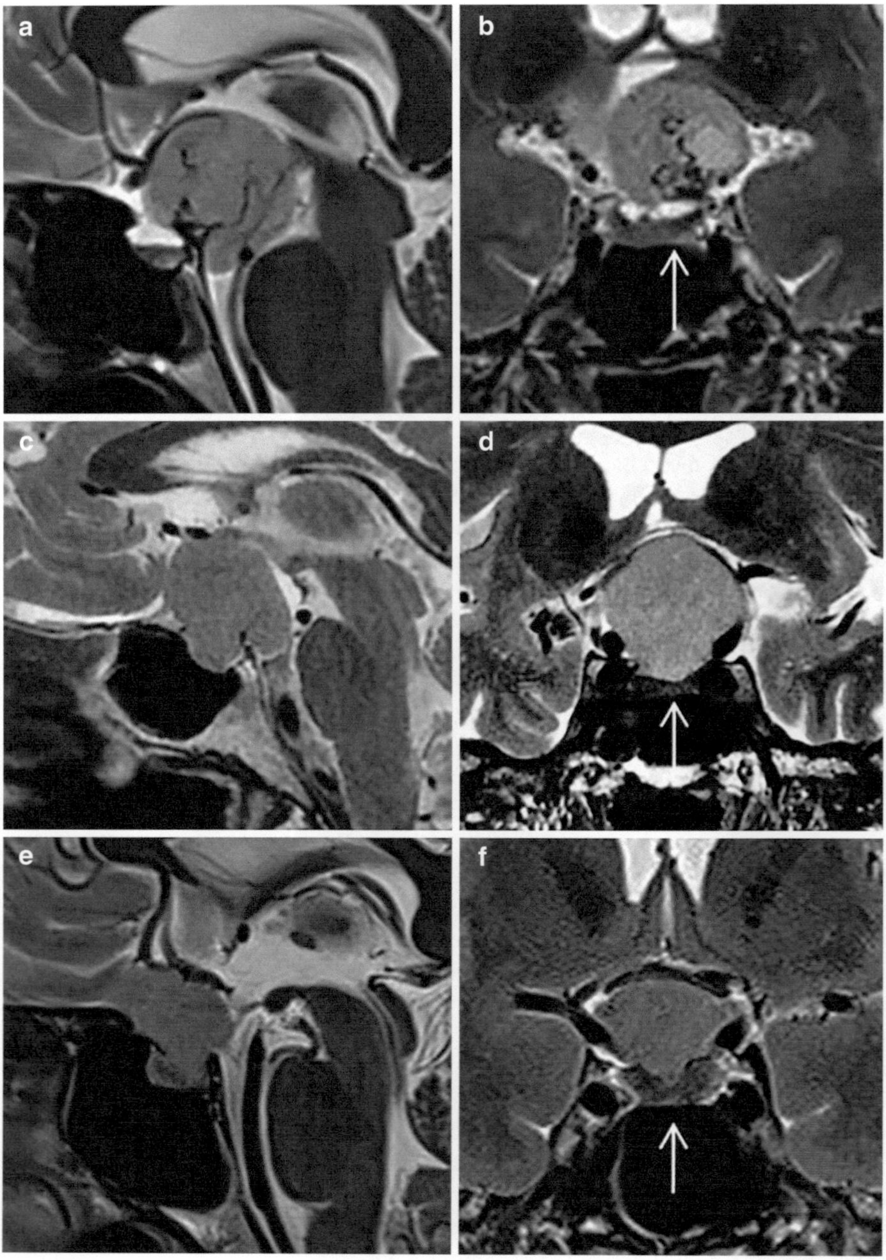

Fig. 32.1 Different insertions of sellar meningiomas. (**a**, **b**) Hypervascular meningioma of the dorsum sellae with signal voids. (**c**, **d**) Insertion at the tuberculum sellae. (**e**, **f**) At the planum sphenoidale. (**a**–**f**) Sagittal and coronal T2WIs The pituitary gland is shown below the tumor on coronal images (arrows)

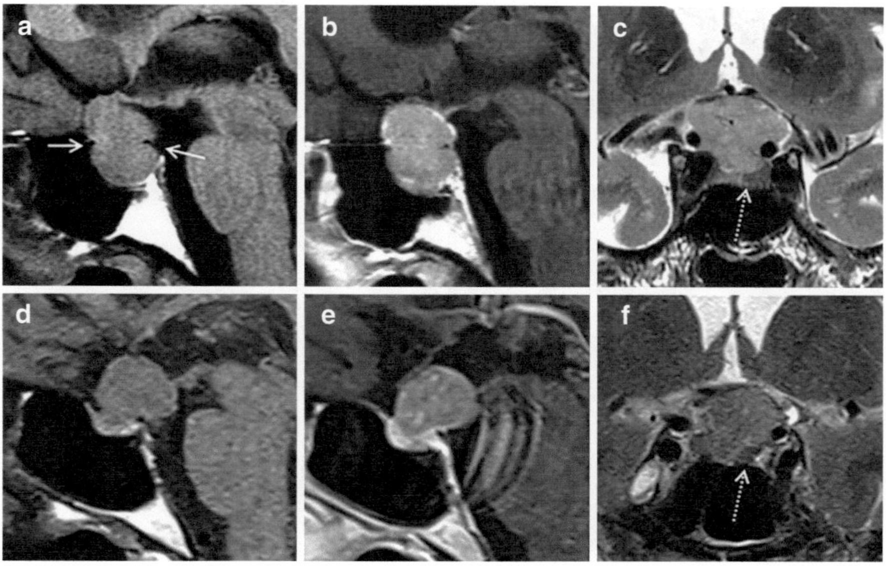

Fig. 32.2 Sellar diaphragm meningioma (upper row) versus pituitary macroadenoma (lower row). Normal pituitary gland (dotted arrows). The meningioma is clearly hyperintense on T2WI (**c**) if compared with the PitNET. Note in a and d the imprint of the sellar diaphragm on the tumor (small arrow). (**a**, **d**) Sagittal T1WIs. (**b**, **e**) Sagittal CE T1WIs. (**c**, **f**) Coronal T2WIs

T1WI. They may enhance after gadolinium injection with the same degree as the pituitary gland which can be severely compressed. Dynamic MRIs could show an early enhancement of the meningioma and can help if the T2W sequence is suboptimal. Inconsistently, the sellar diaphragm is thickened and becomes visible (Fig. 32.2).

A good trick to remember is that the pituitary gland is almost never located below a pituitary macroadenoma, at the difference of what is observed in meningiomas, in Rathke cleft cysts, or in craniopharyngiomas (Fig. 28.6).

Meningiomas of the cavernous sinus frequently invade the sella, mimicking an adenoma with extrasellar extension (Figs. 32.3 and 32.4). Indeed, specific patterns of meningioma, such as the thickening of the lateral wall of the cavernous sinus (Fig. 41.4), are frequently absent. Clinical symptoms rarely help: ophthalmoplegia is very rare in PitNETs with cavernous sinus invasion. In meningiomas, ophthalmoplegia is observed in large tumors or during pregnancy only. MR signal and enhancement can be similar in both conditions but meningiomas frequently exhibit a T2W hyperintensity if compared with the PitNET (Fig. 33.2). Stenosis of the intracavernous internal carotid artery seen in meningiomas is inconstant and not specific. It is the same for the dural tail which can be seen but rarely with PitNETs (Fig. 32.5).

The diagnosis may be challenging in the case of collision lesions, such as, for instance, double meningiomas (Fig. 34.3) or meningioma plus prolactinoma.

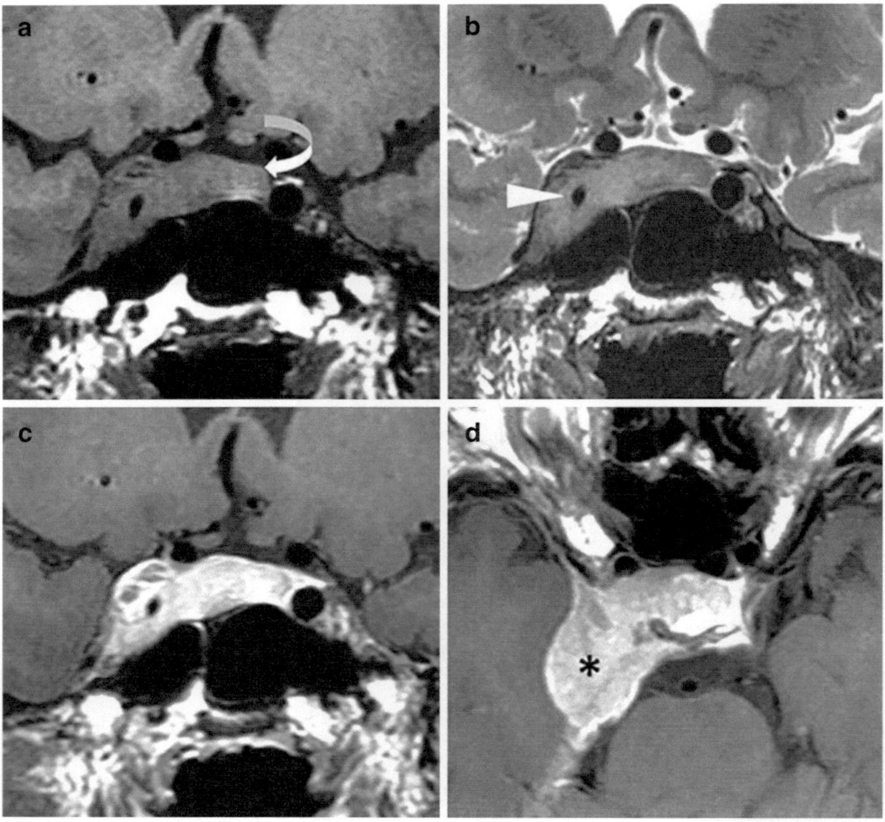

Fig. 32.3 Meningioma of the cavernous sinus with intrasellar extension. (**a–c**) Coronal T1, T2, and CE T1WIs. (**d**) Axial CE T1WI. Discrete T1 hypointensity, T2W hyperintensity of the meningioma. The pituitary gland is compressed (curved arrow). Stenosis of right internal carotid artery (arrowhead). Tumoral extension along the free edge of the tentorium (*)

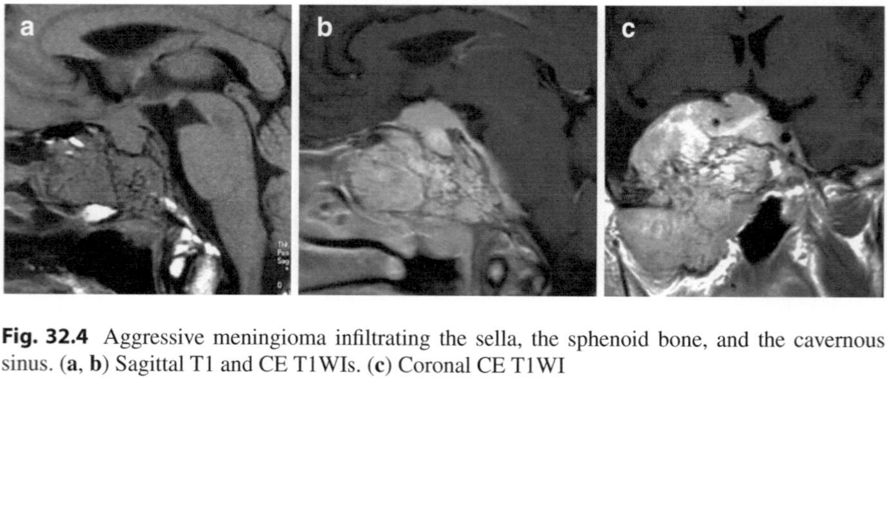

Fig. 32.4 Aggressive meningioma infiltrating the sella, the sphenoid bone, and the cavernous sinus. (**a**, **b**) Sagittal T1 and CE T1WIs. (**c**) Coronal CE T1WI

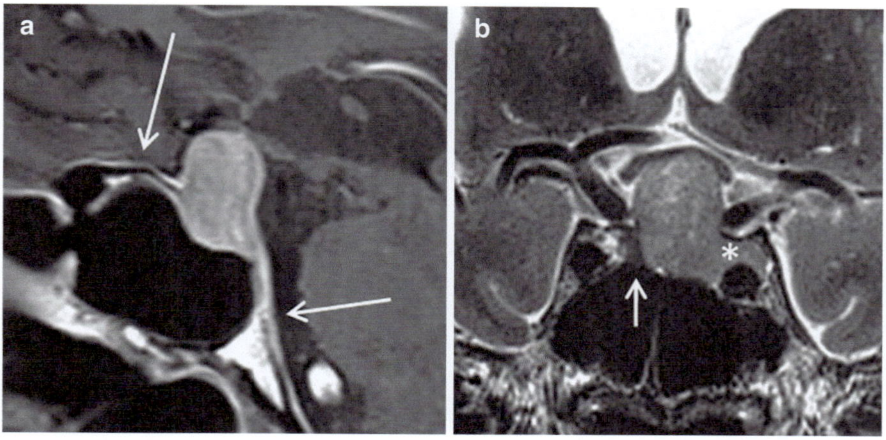

Fig. 32.5 Differential diagnosis. Non-secreting PitNET with cavernous sinus invasion (*). Nonspecific anterior and posterior dural tail (arrows). Normal pituitary pushed away by the adenoma (short arrow). (**a**) Sagittal CE T1WI. (**b**) Coronal T2WI

Further Readings

Buerki RA, Horbinski CM, Kruser T, Horowitz PM, James CD, Lukas RV. An overview of meningiomas. Future Oncol. 2018;14(21):2161–77. https://doi.org/10.2217/fon-2018-0006. Epub 2018 Aug 7.

Graillon T, Regis J, Barlier A, Brue T, Dufour H, Buchfelder M. Parasellar meningiomas. Neuroendocrinology. 2020;110(9–10):780–96. https://doi.org/10.1159/000509090. Epub 2020 Jun 3.

Graillon T, Boissonneau S, Appay R, Boucekine M, Peyrière H, Meyer M, Farah K, Albarel F, Morange I, Castinetti F, Brue T, Fuentes S, Figarella-Branger D, Cuny T, Du H. Meningiomas in patients with long-term exposition to progestins: characteristics and outcome. Neurochirurgie. 2021;67(6):556–63. https://doi.org/10.1016/j.neuchi.2021.04.018. Epub 2021 May 11.

The Jewel Box

33

The so-called cavernous sinus contains vital and precious anatomical structures and for this reason is also known as the "jewel box". It is a crowded hub full of nerves, arteries, and veins and it will not be a question here of drawing up a catalog of all the cavernous sinus lesions, but simply to illustrate the most frequent, the most characteristic, and the most trapping ones.

First, a few words on the term "cavernous sinus".

In anatomy, this term designates either a cavity containing air (such as the sphenoidal sinus) or a large vein (such as the transverse sinus), but "cavernous sinus" does not correspond to these definitions. Actually, the cavernous sinus contains many small veins which merge rarely into a true sinus. The famous neurosurgeon Dwight Parkinson proposed the more exact term of "laterosellar extradural space" but the term "cavernous sinus" remains the one universally used to refer not only to veins but also to the whole content of the cavernous sinus space, i.e., the internal carotid artery, the oculomotor and trigeminal nerves, and connective tissue.

The cavernous sinuses are almost always asymmetrical and this can constitute a first trap. Another trap is the "true cavernous sinus" present in about 5% of cases (Fig. 33.1): this large venous component that is responsible for a homogeneous T2W hyperintense signal can mimic an abnormality, for instance, an invasive pituitary adenoma (Fig. 7.2g), but a uniform enhancement after gadolinium injection makes the difference.

The meningioma of the cavernous sinus space is the most frequent lesion and can mimic *tumoral invasion from pituitary adenoma* when they extend into the sella (Fig. 32.3). They can originate from the cavernous space wall or from the nerve sheaths.

T2W signal is usually hyperintense if compared with that of the anterior pituitary gland (Fig. 33.2). Enhancement is usually but not always more intense in meningiomas than in PitNETs and its peak occurs earlier on dynamic MRI (Fig. 9.3). Inconsistently, a dural tail thickening of the free edge of the tentorium is observed on axial sequences (Fig. 32.3). The diameter of the internal carotid artery is frequently narrowed in meningiomas. The multiplicity of the meningiomas pleads in

J.-F. Bonneville, *Tricks and Traps in MRI of the Pituitary Region*,
https://doi.org/10.1007/978-3-031-64710-9_33

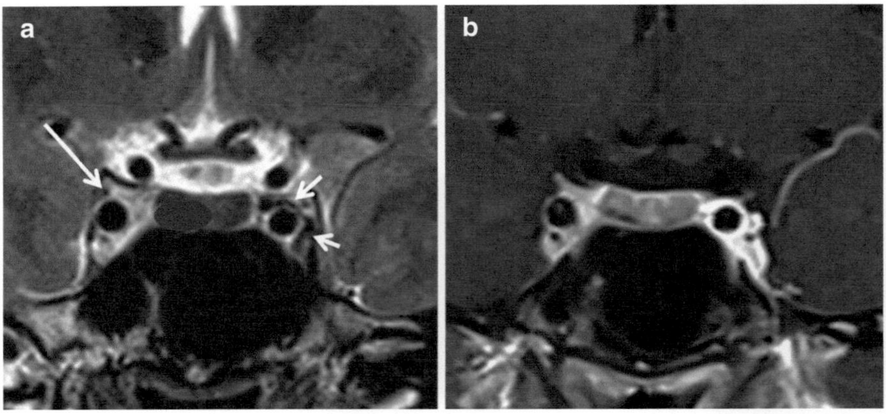

Fig. 33.1 Asymmetrical normal cavernous sinuses. "True" right cavernous sinus with slow flow exhibits a T2W hyperintensity (long arrow). On the left, veins are not confluent (small arrows). Their T2W hypointensity testifies of their more rapid flow. (**a**, **b**) Coronal T2 and CE T1WIs

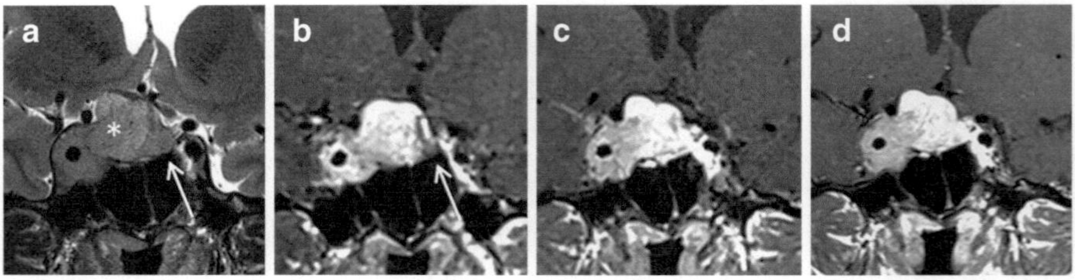

Fig. 33.2 Cavernous sinus meningioma with intrasellar extension. The tumor (*) is T2W hyperintense if compared with the pituitary gland (arrow). On dynamic imaging, meningioma enhancement occurs first (**b**) and decreases quickly (**d**). (**a**) Coronal T2WI. (**b**–**d**) Dynamic sequence

favor of the diagnosis. Obviously, a normal hormonal analysis eliminates a secreting PitNET. If most meningiomas are discovered by chance, some may become symptomatic during pregnancy, for instance, in the form of oculomotor nerve palsy.

Many vascular conditions can affect the cavernous sinus space.

Internal carotid aneurysms display a well-defined signal loss (Fig. 33.3a, b) or more frequently various signal intensities when partially thrombosed. In these last cases, circumferential layers of thrombus of different intensities and a central or eccentric flow void representing the patent central lumen are in favor of the diagnosis (Fig. 33.3).

Carotid-cavernous fistulas are responsible for chemosis and display dilated veins. The normal variability of cavernous sinus veins can make the diagnosis difficult in small fistulas. Concomitant T1W hyperintensity and bulging of the pituitary gland consecutive to impaired venous flow can help in high-flow fistulas (Fig. 39.5).

Cavernous sinus thrombosis can complicate regional infection, surgery or occur during pregnancy especially in the setting of a thrombophilic disorder (Fig. 33.4).

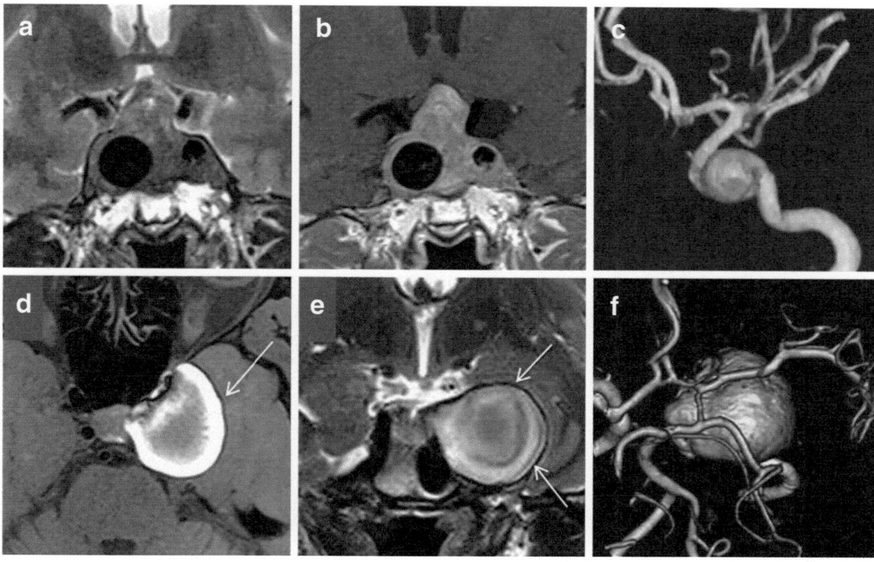

Fig. 33.3 Upper row. Aneurysm of the internal carotid artery with patent lumen and GH-secreting PitNET. Signal void on T2 and T1WIs (**a**, **b**). AngioMRI (**c**). Lower row. Partially thrombosed giant aneurysm with slow flow. Heterogeneous T1 and T2W signal with peripheral hyperintensity on both sequences and thin hypointense border corresponding to hemosiderin deposit (arrows). (**d**) Axial T1W Fatsat image. (**e**) Coronal T2WI. (**f**) Angiography, 3D reformat

The MR picture is that of an enlarged cavernous sinus with a delayed enhancement. T1W signal varies with time from isointense to heterogeneously hyperintense. T2W is more variable. The MR signal is quickly changing with anticoagulation therapy.

The *Tolosa-Hunt syndrome* is caused by non-specific inflammation of the cavernous sinus area. Its main manifestation is painful ophthalmoplegia. MRI displays a widened cavernous sinus with a strong enhancement. Due to the lack of specificity of this syndrome, several scholars have proposed to drop the term Tolosa-Hunt syndrome and use the term "cavernous sinus syndrome" as a replacement to design any tumor, infection, inflammation, trauma, or vascular abnormality affecting the cavernous sinus. It is one more example that most diseases still named after their discoverer will soon lose their original denomination.

Cavernous hemangioma, a rare vascular lesion usually discovered as an incidentaloma, must be recognized since accidental surgery would lead to severe hemorrhagic complications (Fig. 33.5). Fortunately, the MR pattern is characteristic. Cavernous hemangioma contains slow-flow blood, and may extend from the cavernous sinus toward the pituitary fossa and can mimic a meningioma or an invasive pituitary adenoma. The lesion displays a well-circumscribed rounded limit. The internal carotid artery diameter is never compromised. Its T2W signal is usually very hyperintense and homogeneous and its T1W signal is hypo- or isointense. T1W hyperintensity indicates focal thrombosis. After gadolinium injection a unique slow centripetal enhancement is pathognomonic (Fig. 9.5). While we generally

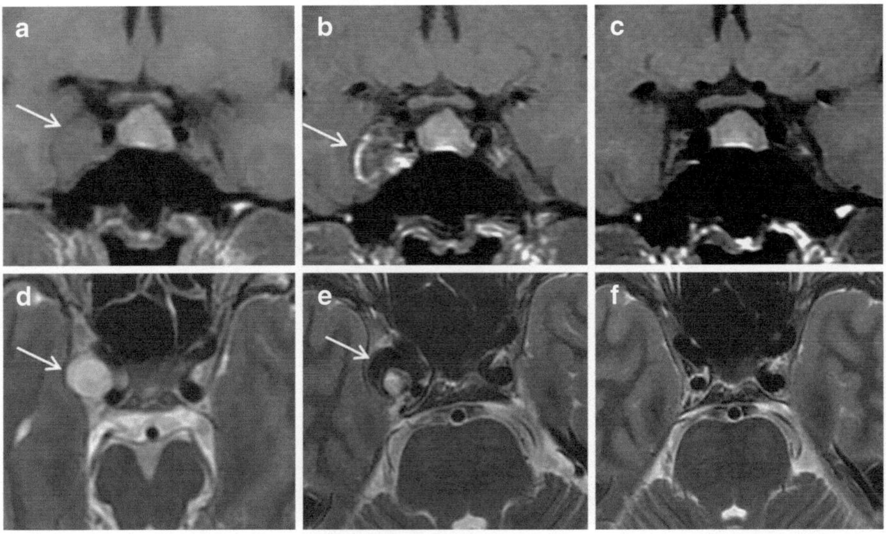

Fig. 33.4 Severe headache 2 weeks before delivery revealing a cavernous sinus thrombophlebitis in a 21-year-old pregnant woman. (**a**–**c**) Coronal T1WIs at diagnosis (**a**), 1 week (**b**), and 6 weeks later (**c**). (**d**–**f**) Corresponding axial T2WIs. Enlarged isointense T1W, hyperintense T2W cavernous sinus in (**a**, **d**) (arrow). Occurrence of a peripheral T1W hyper/T2W hypointensity at 1 week (**b**, **e**). Complete resolution of the abnormalities at 6 weeks with anticoagulation therapy (**c**, **f**)

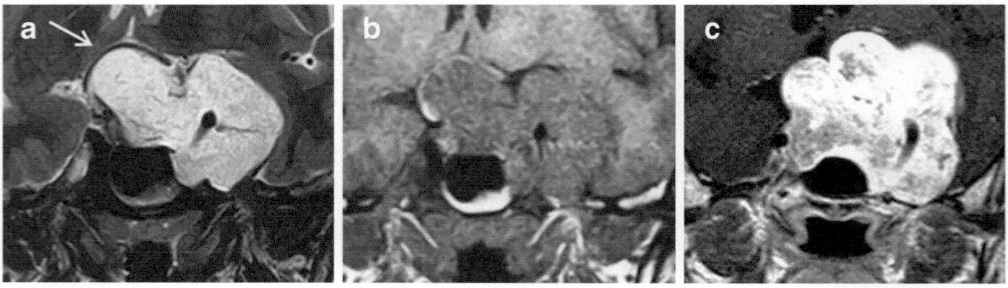

Fig. 33.5 Cavernous sinus hemangioma. Huge vascular lesion extended to the sella and suprasellar area with optic chiasm distortion (arrow). The hemangioma demonstrates T2 hyperintensity (**a**), T1 hypointensity (**b**), and is strongly enhanced (**c**). Dynamic MRI should have shown a slow centripetal enhancement

consider dynamic MRI useless or even misleading for the diagnosis of pituitary microadenomas, it is here a rare case where this modality is critical for the diagnosis of cavernous hemangiomas. At the distance of the injection, enhancement is intense and homogeneous.

Further Readings

He K, Chen L, Zhu W, et al. Magnetic resonance standard for cavernous sinus hemangiomas: proposal for a diagnostic test. Eur Neurol. 2014;72:116–24.

He W, Zhu Y, Zhang Y, Dong L, Zhou Z, Zhou J. A case report on recurrent alternating Tolosa-Hunt syndrome due to bacterial sphenoid sinusitis: rediscussing the diagnostic terminology and classification. BMC Neurol. 2023;23(1):25. https://doi.org/10.1186/s12883-023-03067-z.

Press CA, Lindsay A, Stence NV, et al. Cavernous sinus thrombosis in children: imaging characteristics and clinical outcomes. Stroke. 2015;46:2657–60.

34 Collision Lesions

Anomalies, malformations, cysts, and tumors of the sellar region are so frequent that the concomitant presence of two (or more) lesions in the sellar area named collision lesions is not rare and may complicate the diagnosis. Most are pituitary adenomas coexisting with Rathke cleft cysts and this is not surprising since both lesions share the same ancestry and are separately the most frequently found at autopsy. In the very dense list of sellar collision lesions, meningiomas, and carotid artery aneurysms emerge next.

Intrasellar Rathke cleft cysts are usually easily recognizable through their MR signal and by their midline position. But things are not so simple if RCCs are pushed off-midline by a pituitary adenoma (Fig. 34.1). Axial T1W images are very informative in such cases (Fig. 34.2). It is noticeable that a pituitary adenoma exerts pressure on a cyst and distorts its wall, and not the reverse. Not infrequently, RCCs are multiple, for instance located at the base of the pituitary stalk and in front of the posterior lobe (Fig. 27.4a, b).

Perisellar meningiomas are not infrequently associated with pituitary adenomas. They are located in the cavernous sinus, or attached to the clinoid process, the dorsum sellae, the tuberculum, the planum sphenoidale, or the sellar diaphragm and can be multiple (Fig. 34.3). Meningiomas of the sellar diaphragm may be difficult to identify since they are not associated with any bony change but a T2W hypointense thickened sellar diaphragm may be observed (Fig. 34.3a). A prolactinoma invading the cavernous sinus or an intrasellar extension of a cavernous sinus meningioma may mimic collision lesions (Fig. 32.3).

An intracavernous internal carotid aneurism may coexist with a pituitary adenoma, particularly in acromegaly, making surgery hazardous (Fig. 33.3).

In addition, each of the collision lesions cited above may be multiple. The challenge is higher in Cushing's disease where a non-secreting microadenoma and a corticotropic microadenoma may coexist. A delayed post-gadolinium 3D Flair has been proposed to try to demonstrate a different wash-out profile between both adenomas.

J.-F. Bonneville, *Tricks and Traps in MRI of the Pituitary Region*,
https://doi.org/10.1007/978-3-031-64710-9_34

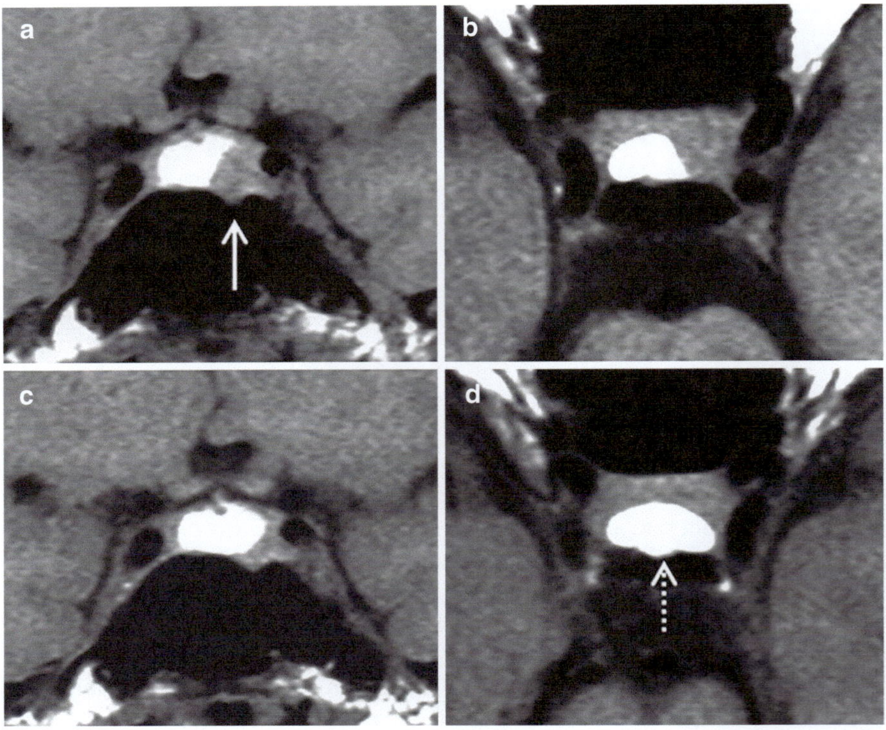

Fig. 34.1 RCC and prolactinoma. Upper row. Left-sided T1W isointense prolactinoma slightly distorting the sellar floor (arrow) and making its mark onto a right-sided T1W hyperintense RCC. Lower row. After 6 months of cabergoline treatment, shrinkage of the prolactinoma results in expansion of the RCC which regains its usual kidney-like shape and its location on midline as demonstrated at the best on axial T1WI (**d**). Note that the T1W hyperintense signal of the posterior lobe (dotted arrow) is partly masked by the RCC. (**a**, **c**) Coronal and (**b**, **d**) Axial T1WIs

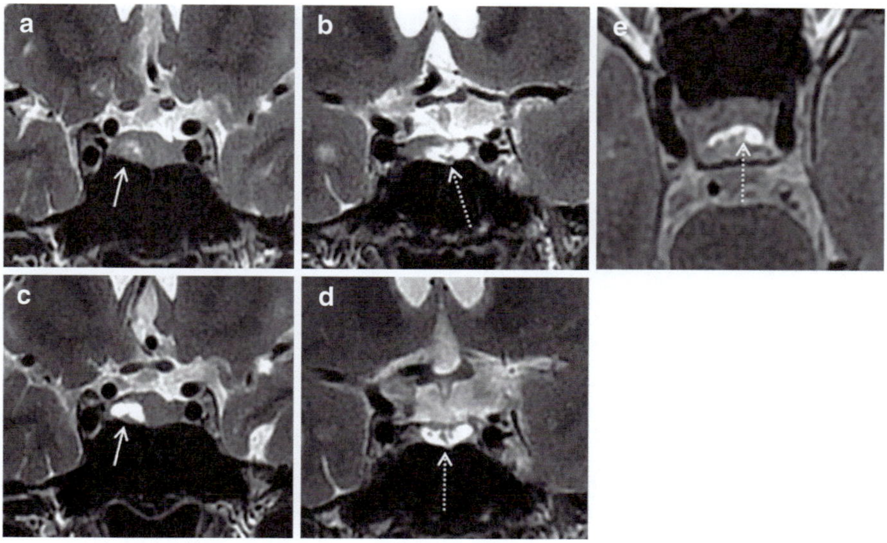

Fig. 34.2 RCC (dotted arrow) and microprolactinoma (arrow). Prolactin is 47 μG/L. Upper row. Right-sided T2W hyperintense lesion with poorly defined contours (**a**). On a more posterior coronal section, oval T2W hyperintense lesion slightly off midline (**b**). Several tiny T2W hypointense nodules favor the diagnosis of RCC (dotted arrow). Lower row. After 6 months of cabergoline treatment, the T2W hyperintensity of the prolactinoma is now very marked and the lesion is presumably softer. The RCC is strictly on midline. The axial T2WI confirms the presence of a serous RCC located between anterior and posterior lobes of the pituitary gland with its characteristic anteriorly convex shape. (**a**–**d**) Coronal T2WIs. (**e**) Axial T2WI. This is one more example that the use of T2WIs associated here with axial projection as well as a perfect reproducibility of the images make, as in many cases, gadolinium injection unnecessary, particularly for follow-up of sellar lesions

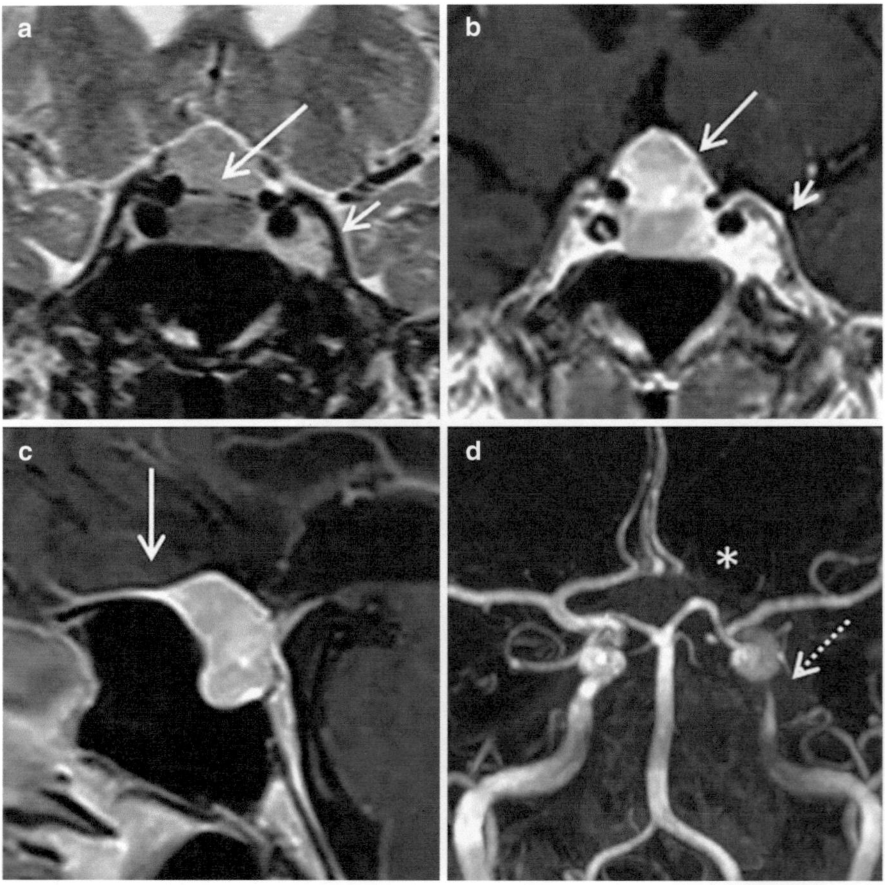

Fig. 34.3 Cavernous sinus meningioma and sellar diaphragm meningioma. Suprasellar lesion with anterior dural tail (arrow in **c**) and presumed attachment to an unusually well visible T2W hypointense sellar diaphragm (arrow in **a**). Meningioma of the left cavernous sinus with thickening of the T2W hypointense lateral wall (short arrows). Narrowing of the lumen of the internal carotid artery (dotted arrow in **d**). Agenesis of the A1 segment of the left anterior cerebral artery (*) constitutes here an additional neurological risk. Note that both meningiomas are T2W hyperintense if compared with the pituitary gland. (**a, b**) Coronal T2 and CE T1WIs. (**c**) Sagittal CE T1WI. (**d**) MRA

Further Readings

Noh SJ, Ahn JY, Lee KS, Kim SH. Pituitary adenoma and concomitant Rathke's cleft cyst. Acta Neurochir. 2007;149(12):1223–8. https://doi.org/10.1007/s00701-007-1295-x. Epub 2007 Oct 3.

Wang M, Fu Q, Song M, Zhao Z, Wang R, Zhang J, Ma W, Wang Z. A potential concomitant sellar embryonic remnant-associated collision tumor: systematic review. Front Oncol. 2021;11:649958. https://doi.org/10.3389/fonc.2021.649958.

Wu W, Jia G, Jia W, Li G, Zhang J, Zhang L. Pituitary adenoma associated with Rathke's cleft cyst: report of 15 cases. Can J Neurol Sci. 2018;45(1):68–75. https://doi.org/10.1017/cjn.2017.252. Epub 2017 Nov 6.

A Spiny Diagnosis

35

The sellar spine is a osseous spur arising horizontally from the dorsum sellae and protruding forward into the pituitary fossa. It corresponds to an ossified remnant of the cephalic tip of the notochord. Its incidence is said very low, occurring in one in every 5000 people, but certainly underevaluated. Described initially by the anatomist J. Lang, it has been recognized radiologically for the first time by J.L.Dietemann. If the sellar spine is not seen, it can lead to misinterpretation, because its presence may result in an upper extension of the upper surface of the pituitary gland simulating a pituitary mass.

On CT, the sellar spine is easily recognized as a bony spur of variable length (Figs. 8.4 and 35.1) arising from the anterior surface of the dorsum sellae.

Its demonstration is much more challenging on MRI and even impossible on sagittal views. On coronal T2 and especially on T1W images, it realizes a complex target-like image corresponding to the piercing of the posterior lobe and mimicking a susceptibility artifact (Fig. 35.2). It is also sometimes possible to recognize two components made of cortical bone and spongious bone (Fig. 35.2a). Incidental presence of a Rathke cleft cyst (Fig. 10.3) may make the diagnosis even more harder. Axial images are frequently the key of the diagnosis. If necessary, the ultimate proof of the presence of a sellar spine can be given by CT.

A sellar spine is frequently discovered incidentally or after a first diagnosis of a "sellar mass" (Fig. 35.3). It is most of the time non-symptomatic but several cases of pituitary deficit or precocious puberty have been published. A recent paper has shown an increased size of a sellar spine with time in a child.

J.-F. Bonneville, *Tricks and Traps in MRI of the Pituitary Region*,
https://doi.org/10.1007/978-3-031-64710-9_35

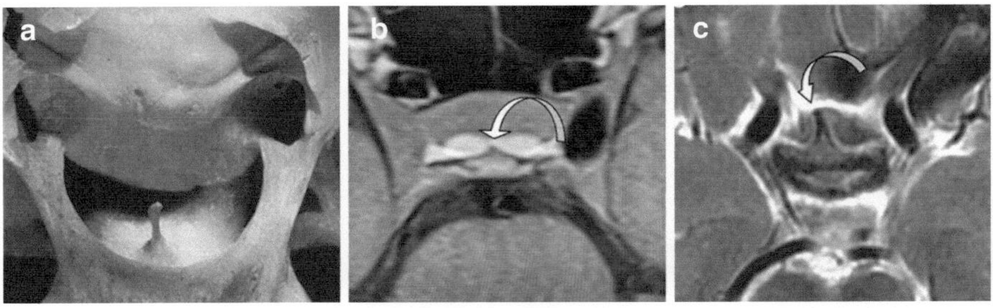

Fig. 35.1 Sellar spine. (**a**) Anatomic specimen (courtesy J. Lang). (**b**) Small sellar spine piercing the posterior lobe on axial T1WI; (**c**) Long sellar spine on axial T2WI

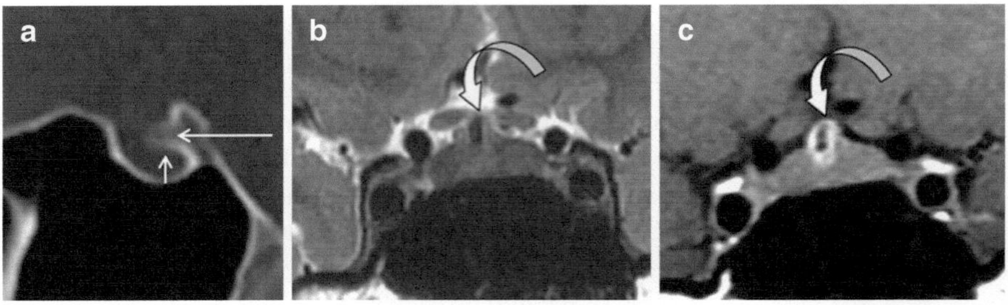

Fig. 35.2 Sellar spine. The structure of the sellar spine with its cortical (short arrow) and spongious (long arrow) compartments is well seen on CT (**a**). In (**b**), coronal T2WI, the spongious bone of the spine is surrounded by its T2W hypointense cortical bone. In (**c**), coronal T1WI, the sellar spine is surrounded by the pierced posterior lobe

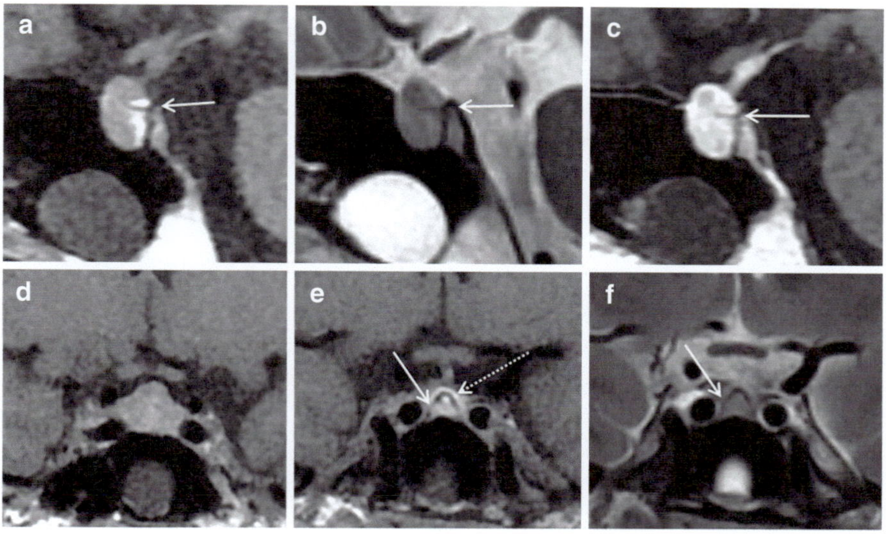

Fig. 35.3 Initial diagnosis of "sellar mass" in a 16-year-old adolescent presenting with migraine. (**a**–**c**) Barely visible sellar spine on sagittal T1, T2, and CE T1WIs. The posterior lobe is transfixed by the spine. (**d**) Coronal T1WI. Normal pituitary gland given a narrow and short sella in this adolescent. On coronal T1 and T2W posterior sections (**e**, **f**), a complex image shows a T1 and T2W hypointense arch (arrows) representing the cortical bone of the sellar spine. The transfixed posterior lobe is T1 hyperintense (dotted arrow in **e**)

Further Readings

Dietemann JL, Lang J, Francke JP, Bonneville JF, Clarisse J, Wackenheim A. Anatomy and radiology of the sellar spine. Neuroradiology. 1981;21(1):5–7. https://doi.org/10.1007/BF00518787.

Hosokawa T, Yamada Y, Sato Y, Tanami Y, Kurihara J, Oguma E. Postnatal sellar spine growth: a case report and literature review. Medicine (Baltimore). 2016;95(33):e4579. https://doi.org/10.1097/MD.0000000000004579.

Metelo-Liquito LD, Buthelezi TE. Sellar spine: a rare Bony variant of the Sella Turcica. SA J Radiol. 2022;26(1):2371. https://doi.org/10.4102/sajr.v26i1.2371.

After Surgery

36

A pituitary MRI is usually obtained between 3 and 6 months after surgery of the sellar region and then every year for 3 or 5 years or more. Some neurosurgeons ask for an early control the day after the procedure to rule out any complications. In case of massive postoperative hemorrhage, an angio MRI must be obtained to exclude an internal carotid artery false aneurysm which will be cured by embolization. Indications for immediate reintervention are rare, but can occur because of a massive hemorrhage or in the case of a visible secreting pituitary adenoma remnant seemingly accessible by surgery. Generally speaking, MRI obtained in the immediate post-operative period is often not reliable for the search of a tumoral remnant which can be masked by packing material (Fig. 36.1) and/or serohematic suffusion (Fig. 36.2).

The goal of post-operative MRIs differs according to the type of pituitary adenomas.

After surgery of non-secreting PitNETs, MRI will check for the presence and possible growth of a tumoral remnant, usually laterally located, opposite to the normal residual pituitary tissue. Small changes of the remnant are demonstrated very early if strictly comparable images are obtained (Fig. 36.3a). Sophisticated calculated volume changes are unuseful in daily practice. If radiotherapy of an adenoma regrowth has been given, signal changes namely foci of T2 hyperintensity, precede volume changes by months (Fig. 36.3d, e).

In our practice, few sequences are enough. We particularly like coronal T2WIs. Gadolinium injection can be spared. Over 6 months post-op, the surgical bed is clean. Only fat grafts can persist for decades. A frequent mistake is the confusion between the normal pituitary tissue and a pituitary adenoma remnant but it is easily avoidable. Indeed, the T2W signal of the normal residual pituitary tissue is very similar to that of the temporal cortex. Moreover, the pituitary stalk is oriented towards the normal pituitary, which is located laterally, against the cavernous sinus (Fig. 36.4). At last, in case of persistent doubt, it will be recalled that most pituitary

J.-F. Bonneville, *Tricks and Traps in MRI of the Pituitary Region*,
https://doi.org/10.1007/978-3-031-64710-9_36

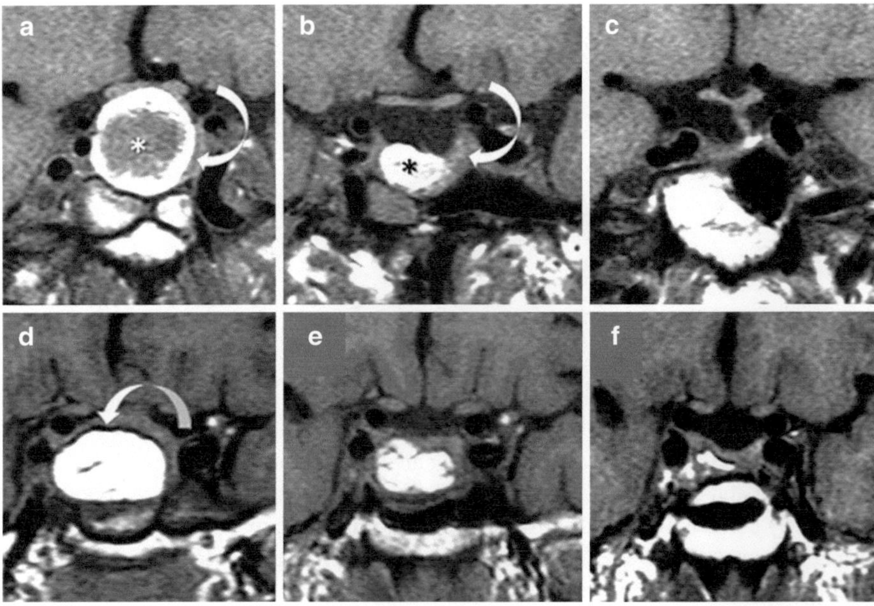

Fig. 36.1 Evolution of packing material after PitNET surgery. Upper row. Characteristic pattern of Gelfoam. (**a**) In the early post-operative phase: T1W hypointense signal related to deoxyhemoglobin and peripheral T1W hyperintensity related to methemoglobin. (**b**) At 2 months; (**c**): At 1 year. Lower row: Characteristic pattern of fat packing. (**d**) In the early post-operative phase. Chemical shift artifact (curved arrow) bordering the hemmed fat T1W hyperintensity. (**e**) At 1 year. (**f**) At 10 years

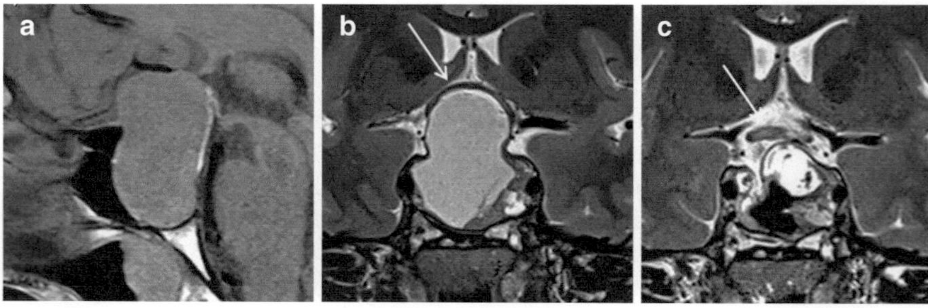

Fig. 36.2 Pituitary macroadenoma raising the optic chiasm before (**a**, **b**) and 3 days (**c**) after surgery. Partial shrinkage of the mass which is heterogeneous. The optic chiasm is now in place but is still edematous: Note its rail-like image in c (arrow). Presence and size of a potential remnant cannot be specified at this time. (**a**) Sagittal T1WI. (**b**, **c**) Coronal T2WIs

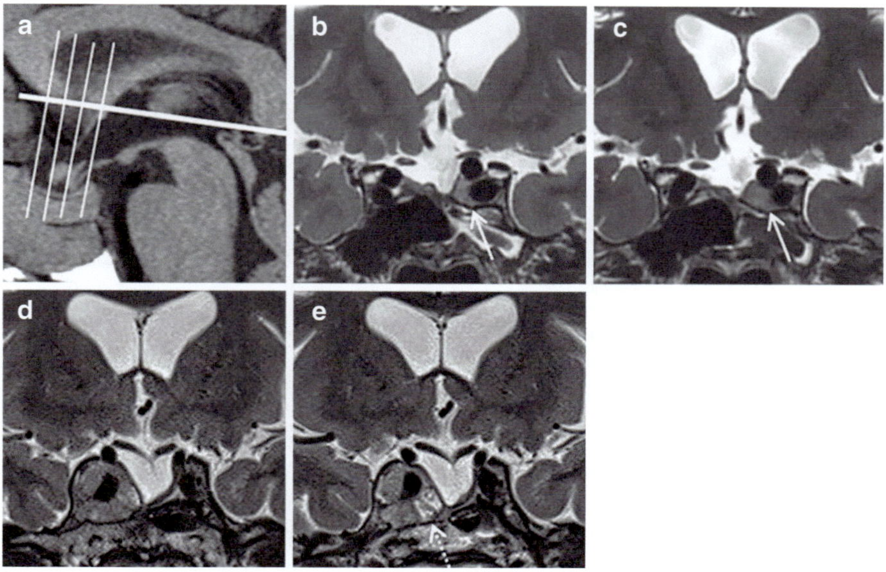

Fig. 36.3 All T2W Coronal images are obtained perpendicularly to the subcallosal line (**a**). Upper row: Small increase in size of a corticotropic pituitary adenoma remnant 6 months (**b**) and 2 years (**c**) after surgery (arrows). Lower row. Intrasellar and intracavernous remnant of a non-secreting PitNET (**d**). T2W hyperintense intratumoral foci are shown as early as 6 months after radiotherapy without noticeable volume change (dotted arrow in **e**)

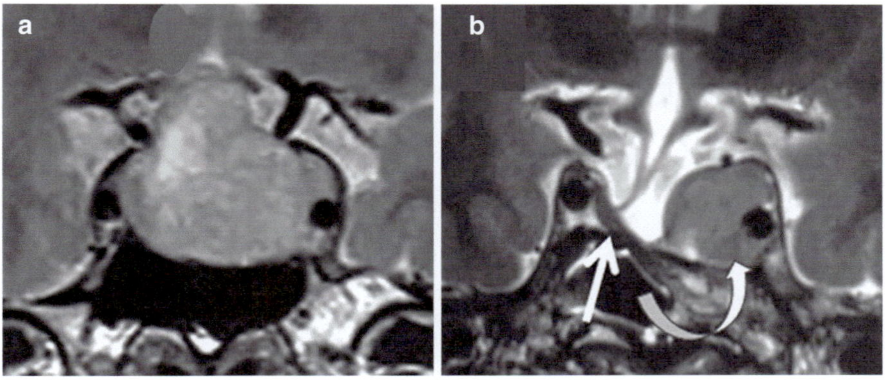

Fig. 36.4 Delineation of a pituitary adenoma regrow (curved arrow in **b**, coronal T2WI) and of the residual normal pituitary tissue (arrow) on coronal T2WIs. Gadolinium injection is not necessary. Note that the pituitary stalk is directed toward the normal pituitary. (**a**) Coronal T2WI is before surgery

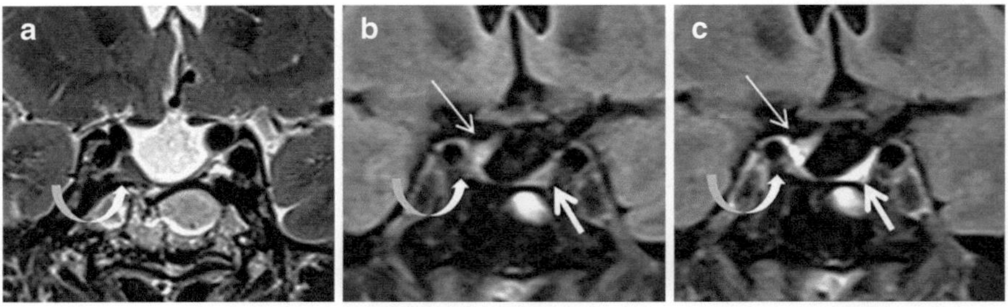

Fig. 36.5 Left-sided pituitary adenoma remnant (thick arrows) long after surgery. Enhancement of the remnant on 3D CE FLAIR (**c**) but not of the pituitary (curved arrow). Ectopic vasopressin storage (small arrow in **b**), enhanced in (**c**). (**a**) Coronal T2WI. (**b**, **c**) 3D and 3D CE FLAIR

tumor remnants enhanced but not the normal pituitary tissue on FLAIR when a dose of 0.03 mmol/kg of gadolinium is injected (Fig. 36.5).

Beyond the sixth post-operative month and the following years, the most cost-effective follow-up must be taken into consideration. The monitoring of a possible remnant is simply solved with non-contrast sagittal T1 and coronal T2WIs obtained as we proposed, perpendicularly to the line joining genu and splenium of corpus callosum. Of course, a 3D MRI would be indicated if radiation therapy is considered.

After surgery of secreting adenomas in non-cured acromegalic or Cushing's patients, the issue is to detect a small or tiny remnant which can change radically the patient management. A full MRI must be performed with T2WIs and CE 3D SE or CE 3D GE T1WIs (Fig. 36.6). Dynamic MRI is not useful and can be misleading. The tumoral remnant or regrow, when present, displays the same T2W signal as the one observed on the preoperative MRI. Thus, a comparison with the pre-operative MRI is essential.

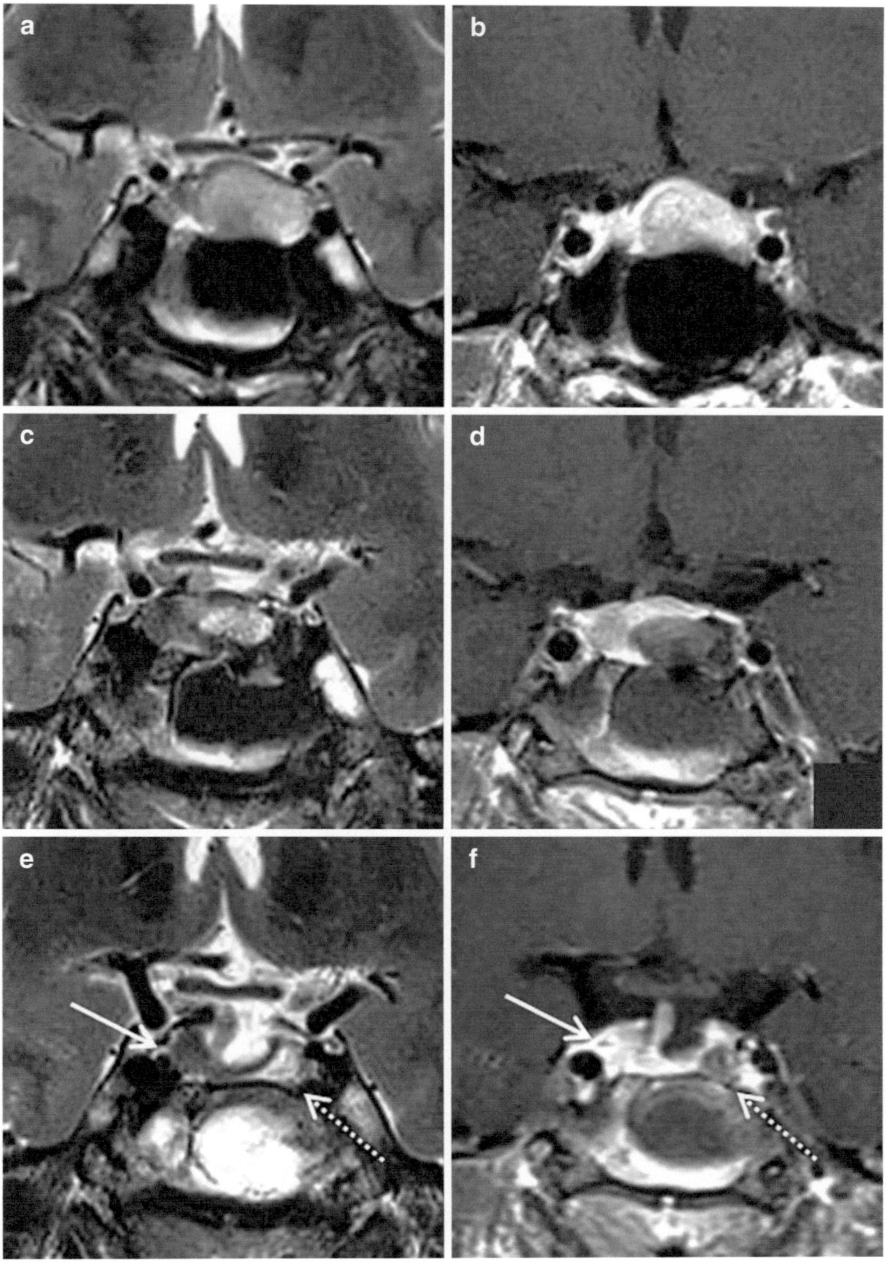

Fig. 36.6 Resistant prolactinoma (**a**, **b**) 3 months (**c**, **d**) and 1 year after surgery (**e**, **f**). The size of the adenoma remnant cannot be evaluated at 3 months but is clearly shown at 1 year as well on T2 and on CE T1WIs. The T2 signal of the remnant (dotted arrow) is identical to that observed initially. Normal pituitary gland (arrow). (**a**, **c**, **e**) Coronal T2WIs. (**b**, **d**, **f**) Coronal CE T1WIs

Further Readings

Alali AA, Hanagandi PB, Maralani PJ. Do we need gadolinium-based contrast agents for routine MRI surveillance of unoperated pituitary macroadenoma? AJNR Am J Neuroradiol. 2022;43(7):1024–8. https://doi.org/10.3174/ajnr.A7554. Epub 2022 Jun 23.

Alhilali LM, Little AS, Yuen KCJ, Lee J, Ho TK, Fakhran S, White WL. Early postoperative MRI and detection of residual adenoma after transsphenoidal pituitary surgery. J Neurosurg. 2020;134(3):761–70. https://doi.org/10.3171/2019.11.JNS191845.

Connor SE, Wilson F, Hogarth K. Magnetic resonance imaging criteria to predict complete excision of parasellar pituitary macroadenoma on postoperative imaging. J Neurol Surg B Skull Base. 2014;75(1):41–6. https://doi.org/10.1055/s-0033-1353362. Epub 2013 Aug 21.

37 Ectopic Posterior Lobe or Ectopic AVP Storage?

Some erroneous medical terms remain largely used, such as "ectopic posterior lobe", even though "ectopic vasopressin storage" would be more appropriate. Indeed, when this condition is acquired, the posterior lobe is in place contiguous to the anterior surface of the dorsum sellae but does not contain antidiuretic hormone (or arginine vasopressin, AVP) anymore and consequently does not demonstrate T1 hyperintensity. Nevertheless, "ectopic posterior lobe" is time-honored and will probably permanently persist. When the normal road of AVP from the hypothalamic nuclei—where it is synthesized—to the posterior part of the sella turcica is missing or cut, AVP is blocked and accumulates on the way, at the infundibulum level or in the pituitary stalk.

In the setting of growth hormone deficit in <u>children, an</u> ectopic posterior lobe is part of the classical triad with pituitary stalk abnormality and hypoplastic anterior pituitary. There is some correlation between the level of AVP accumulation along the pituitary stalk and the severity of the prognosis (Fig. 11.3).

Delayed skeletal maturation is objectivized through a delayed closure of the spheno-occipital synchondrosis and delayed aeration of the sphenoid bone. Sphenoid sinus pneumatization increases quickly with growth hormone treatment. Other midline malformations can be associated.

The diagnosis of GH deficiency can also be made later in children with growth deceleration or in adults of short stature: MRI demonstrates the same pattern of a nonfunctional pituitary stalk, ectopic AVP storage, and usually a small sella and a small anterior pituitary gland (Fig. 37.1a, b). A large ectopic posterior lobe in an adult can be confusing if the malformation is unknown or has been forgotten since childhood (Fig. 37.1c, d).

<u>Acquired ectopic AVP storage</u> may occur in three main situations: with sellar tumors, after transsphenoidal surgery, or more rarely after head trauma. It appears when a stress is exerted on the pituitary stalk. AVP storage is demonstrated at the infundibulum level with macroadenomas more than 18–20 mm high (Fig. 37.2a, b) but may be observed with smaller tumors if they are firm such as meningiomas or when the pituitary stalk is brutally compressed, for instance, in the case of pituitary

J.-F. Bonneville, *Tricks and Traps in MRI of the Pituitary Region*,
https://doi.org/10.1007/978-3-031-64710-9_37

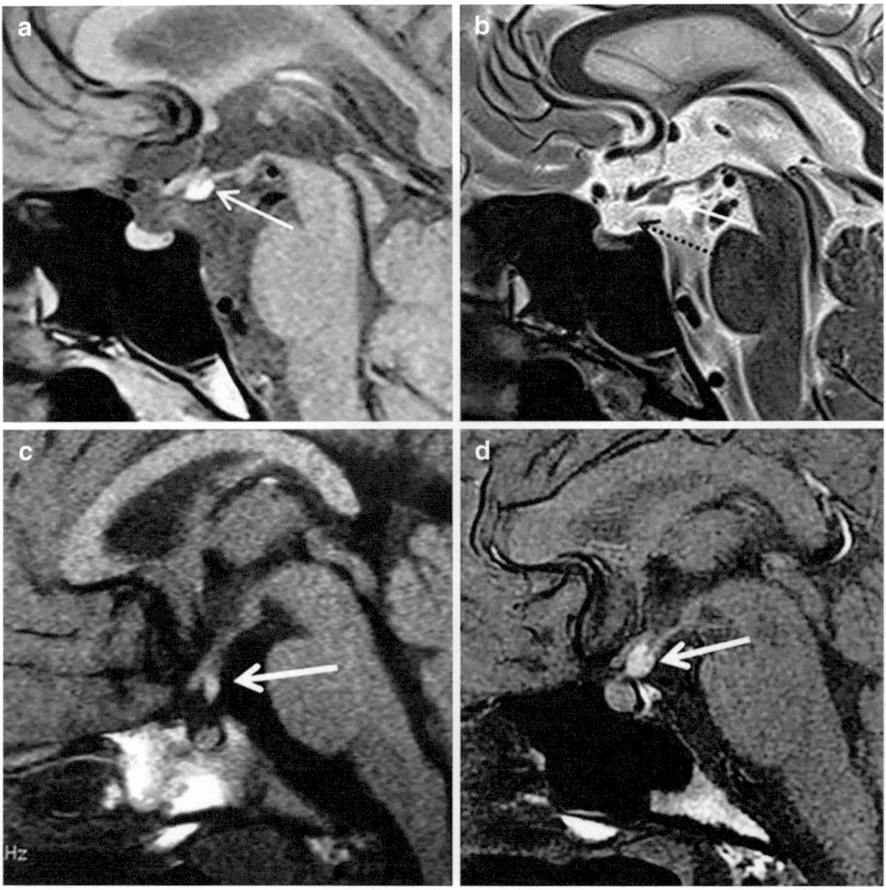

Fig. 37.1 Upper row. Pituitary stalk interruption syndrome (PSIS) in an adult. Classical triad: ectopic posterior lobe (arrow), very thin pituitary stalk visible on T2WI only (dotted arrow), small anterior pituitary. Lower row. PSIS from childhood to adulthood. Classical triad. Delayed pneumatization of the sphenoid in childhood (**c**). Increased size of the anterior pituitary and rounded enlargement of the ectopic posterior lobe in adult (short arrow in **d**). Note in both cases treated with GH a complete pneumatization of the sphenoid. (**a**, **c**, **d**) Sagittal T1WIs. (**b**) Sagittal T2WI

apoplexia, hemorrhage, traumatic brain injury, or with tumoral recurrency. In practice, demonstration of an ectopic AVP storage above an incidentaloma makes the diagnosis of pituitary adenoma unlikely if the mass is less than 18–20 mm (Fig. 37.2d–f). Rarely, when the pituitary stalk is moderately compressed, the AVP storage may be visible together in ectopic position and eutopic position against the dorsum sellae (Fig. 37.2c).

After pituitary surgery, ectopic AVP storage is observed with a variable delay. It tends to grow with time because of the slow accumulation of AVP. Sometimes, AVP storage is large enough to mimic a tumoral process in the suprasellar cistern or in the post-operative empty sella. The diagnostic difficulty can be high if the T1W

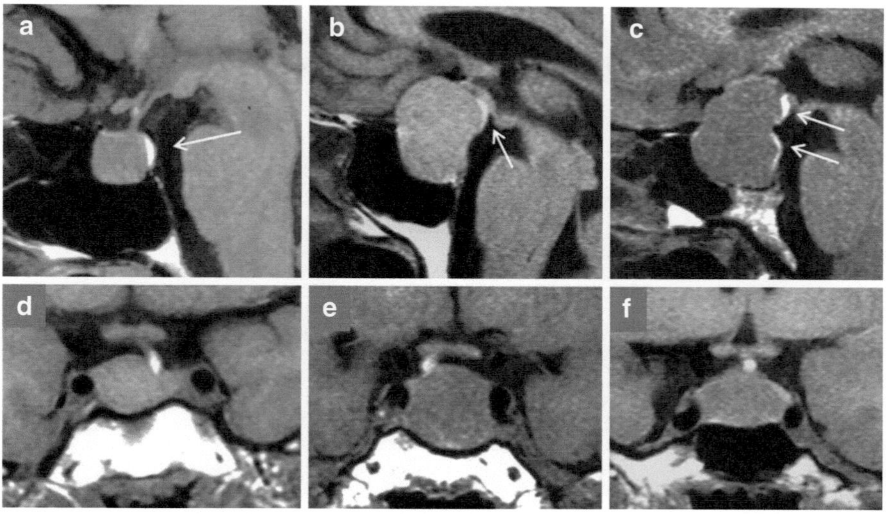

Fig. 37.2 Acquired AVP storage (arrows) above a 20 mm high PitNET (**b**) versus a compressed posterior lobe with an intrasellar PitNET (**a**). Rare ectopic and eutopic AVP storage (**c**). Lower row. Ectopic AVP storage with pituitary masses less than 18 mm high. (**d**) Hemorrhagic PitNET. (**e**) Sellar diaphragm meningioma. (**f**) PitNET recurrency after surgery. (**a–c**) Sagittal T1WIs. (**d–f**) Coronal T1WIs

hyperintense signal of AVP is low or missing such as in the elderly (Fig. 37.3a–c). Exceptionally, a T1W hypointense–T2W hyperintense microcyst may be observed within the AVP storage (Fig. 37.3d–f).

The differential diagnosis of ectopic AVP storage includes the rare asymptomatic lipoma in contact with the tuber cinereum. Characteristic location, chemical shift artifact, T2W signal, and fat suppression sequence make the diagnosis easy (Figs. 37.4 and 39.2).

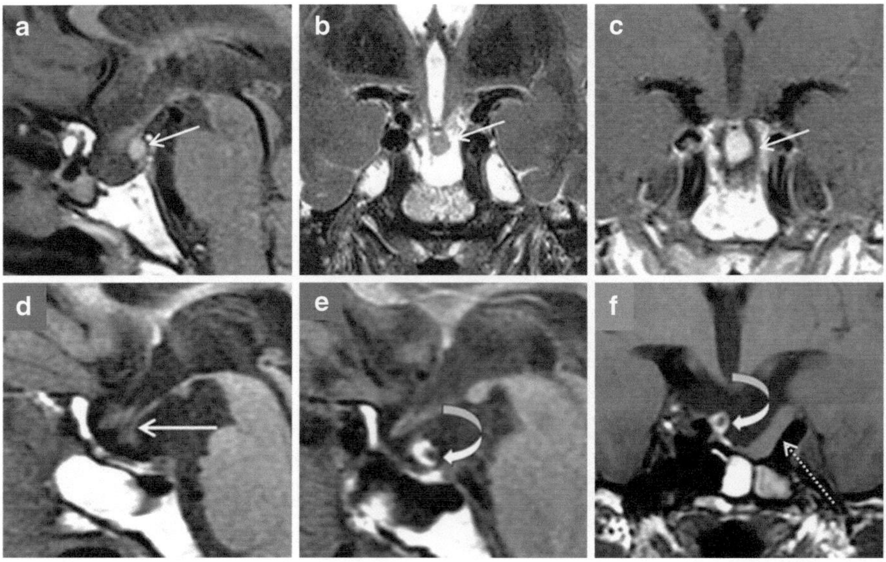

Fig. 37.3 Upper row. T1W slightly hyperintense ectopic AVP storage in a 78-year-old man 20 years after pituitary surgery. The mass enhances after gadolinium injection (**c**). Lower row. Isointense AVP ectopic storage in a 65-year-old man 12 years after pituitary surgery (**d**). Visualization of a microcyst within the enhanced ectopic posterior lobe (curved arrows) in (**e**, **f**). Tumoral remnant (dotted arrow). (**a**, **d**) Sagittal T1WIs. (**b**) Coronal T2WI. (**e**) Sagittal CE T1WI. (**c**, **f**) Coronal CE T1WIs

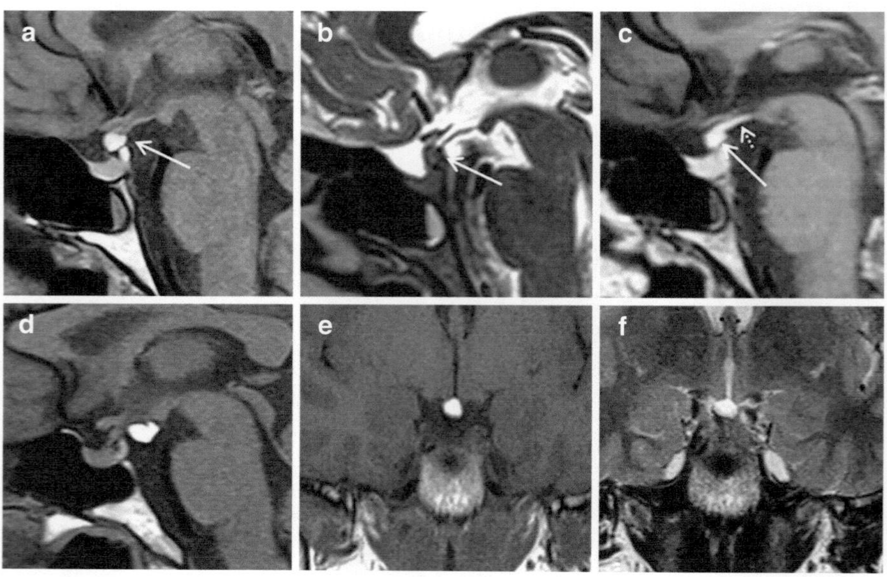

Fig. 37.4 Ectopic posterior lobe (upper row) versus lipoma (lower row). The ectopic posterior lobe is slightly T2W hypointense (**b**) while the more posteriorly located lipoma is hyperintense on T2WI (**f**). Note the normal enhancement of the tuber cinereum in (**c**) (short arrow). (**a**, **d**) Sagittal T1WIs. (**b**, **f**) Sagittal and coronal T2WIs. (**c**) Sagittal CE T1WI. (**e**) Coronal T1WI

Further Readings

Bonneville F, Narboux Y, Cattin F, Rodière E, Jacquet G, Bonneville JF. Preoperative location of the pituitary bright spot in patients with pituitary macroadenomas. AJNR Am J Neuroradiol. 2002;23(4):528–32.

Fujisawa I. Magnetic resonance imaging of the hypothalamic-neurohypophyseal system. J Neuroendocrinol. 2004;16(4):297–302. https://doi.org/10.1111/j.0953-8194.2004.01183.x.

Takahashi T, Miki Y, Takahashi JA, Kanagaki M, Yamamoto A, Fushimi Y, Okada T, Haque TL, Hashimoto N, Konishi J, Togashi K. Ectopic posterior pituitary high signal in preoperative and postoperative macroadenomas: dynamic MR imaging. Eur J Radiol. 2005;55(1):84–91. https://doi.org/10.1016/j.ejrad.2004.10.003. Epub 2004 Dec 7.

38 Goodbye Diabetes Insipidus

There are good reasons to change the name of some diseases. It is particularly the case of diseases named after their discoverers who, at a distance from their publication, were considered unworthy because of their unethical behavior. Thus, “Wegener’s granulomatosis” has become “granulomatosis with polyangiitis”. For the same reasons, statues of some public persons are today unbolted.

For diabetes insipidus, the reason is different, but it was high time for a change: the term diabetes insipidus was introduced in the seventeenth century to differentiate patients whose urine was sweet—i.e., with diabetes mellitus—from those whose urine was not. Above all, recent understanding of pathophysiology fully justifies a renaming. It is now well known that polyuria and secondary polydipsia may be of central origin, relating to the inability to produce, transfer, or secrete arginine vasopressin (AVP) at the hypothalamus, pituitary stalk or posterior pituitary level, rarely nephrogenic due to resistance to the action of AVP on the kidney or due to an excess of vasopressinase. It is therefore fortunate that central diabetes insipidus has changed for <u>AVP deficiency</u> and nephrogenic diabetes insipidus for <u>AVP resistance</u>. But time will tell which term will ultimately prevail.

The biological diagnosis of primary polyuria-polydipsia has been improved by the adjunct of plasma copeptin dosage after hypertonic saline perfusion to the classic water deprivation test. At the same time, the radiological diagnosis of former central diabetes insipidus is today severely contested in the endocrinological literature which tries to dismantle the statue of the posterior pituitary bright spot. Here, our goal will be to restore the role of pituitary MRI in the diagnosis of AVP deficiency. The opponents of the radiological diagnosis of AVP deficiency argue that a large percentage of patients with AVP deficiency have a normal posterior pituitary high signal in T1W and conversely that a substantial percentage of normal volunteers have not. But all these issues result from the demonstration of the posterior pituitary on sagittal T1W MRI: in this projection, the posterior pituitary—which is normally much narrower than its representation in anatomical textbooks (Fig. 5.3)—is easily mistaken for the dorsum sellae or for a mucinous Rathke’s cleft cyst (Fig. 38.1). The only way to distinguish these T1W hyperintense structures is to

J.-F. Bonneville, *Tricks and Traps in MRI of the Pituitary Region*,
https://doi.org/10.1007/978-3-031-64710-9_38

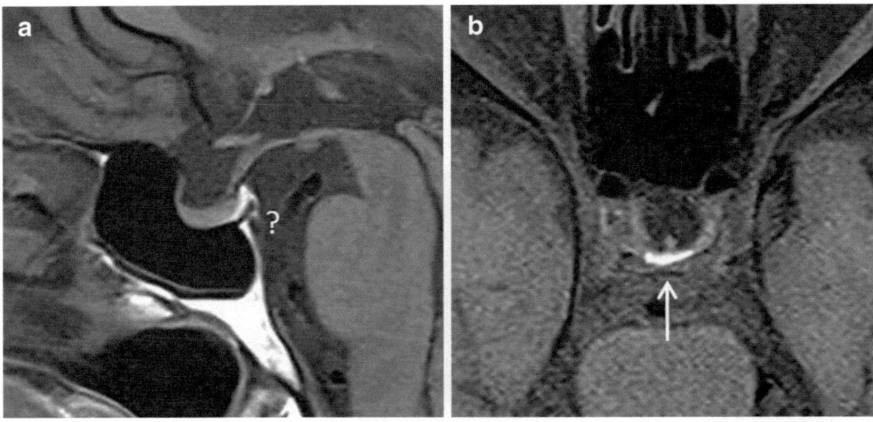

Fig. 38.1 Demonstration of the posterior lobe (arrow) is equivocal in (**a**), sagittal T1WI, formal in (**b**), axial Fatsat T1WI

perform an axial non-contrast T1W MR sequence, preferably with fat saturation to avoid a chemical shift from a fatty dorsum sellae. In this projection, the posterior pituitary is clearly identified and easily separated from the dorsum sellae or Rathke's cleft cyst (Figs. 3.3 and 23.3).

Another argument of the opponents is that the pituitary bright spot can be invisible in the absence of any polyuro-polydipsic syndrome, for instance in the elderly. What is true is that osmolality changes in diabetics or in pregnant women make the posterior pituitary less bright and the same in seniors. But a recent cohort study of AVP deficiency—formerly central diabetes insipidus—has shown that the mean age of diagnosis of this condition is 35 years and even before 20 years in almost three out of four cases, that is at an age where the posterior lobe is constantly brilliant, particularly on axial MRI in volunteers.

Thus, we still think that MRI performed in proper conditions is a useful tool in the diagnosis of polyuria-polydipsia. If the bright spot is not demonstrated, this will orient to AVP deficiency; if demonstrated, to potomania or AVP resistance.

The role of MRI is less controversial for the research of etiologies. Unfortunately, the common link, i.e., the pituitary stalk changes, is weakly specific at least at the onset of the disease.

- Diabetes insipidus can develop with Langerhans cell histiocytosis, neurosarcoidosis, Hodgkin's lymphoma, hypophysitis, craniopharyngioma, complicated Rathke cleft cyst, metastases, germinoma, head trauma, or after surgery. Diabetes insipidus is so rare with pituitary adenomas that its presence practically eliminates the diagnosis of PitNET in front of an incidentaloma.
- In children, the spectrum of germinoma has always to be kept in mind in the presence of a so-called idiopathic vasopressin deficiency and MRI follow-up must be close in time.
- In histiocytosis, seborrheic lesions of the scalp and folds are frequently observed and make the diagnosis much easier.

- Sarcoidosis is rare in children. In adults, lesions are usually multiple and may affect the meninges, the brain, the optic chiasm, and the cranial nerves. They can shrink rapidly with corticotherapy but may recur (Fig. 38.2). In histiocytosis as well as in sarcoidosis, nodular lesions such as those of the optic chiasm appear with an evocative T2 hypo- or isointensity (Fig. 38.3).
- During pregnancy, a usually transient polyuro-polydipsic syndrome, may be observed. It is caused by an increased placenta production of vasopressinase that inactivates vasopressin. High-quality MRI has not been reported in this situation but should demonstrate the bright spot even if less brilliant than in non-pregnant women because of the osmotic changes related to pregnancy. The differential diagnosis must be made with infundibuloneurohypophysitis which may also occur during pregnancy or early postpartum (see below).

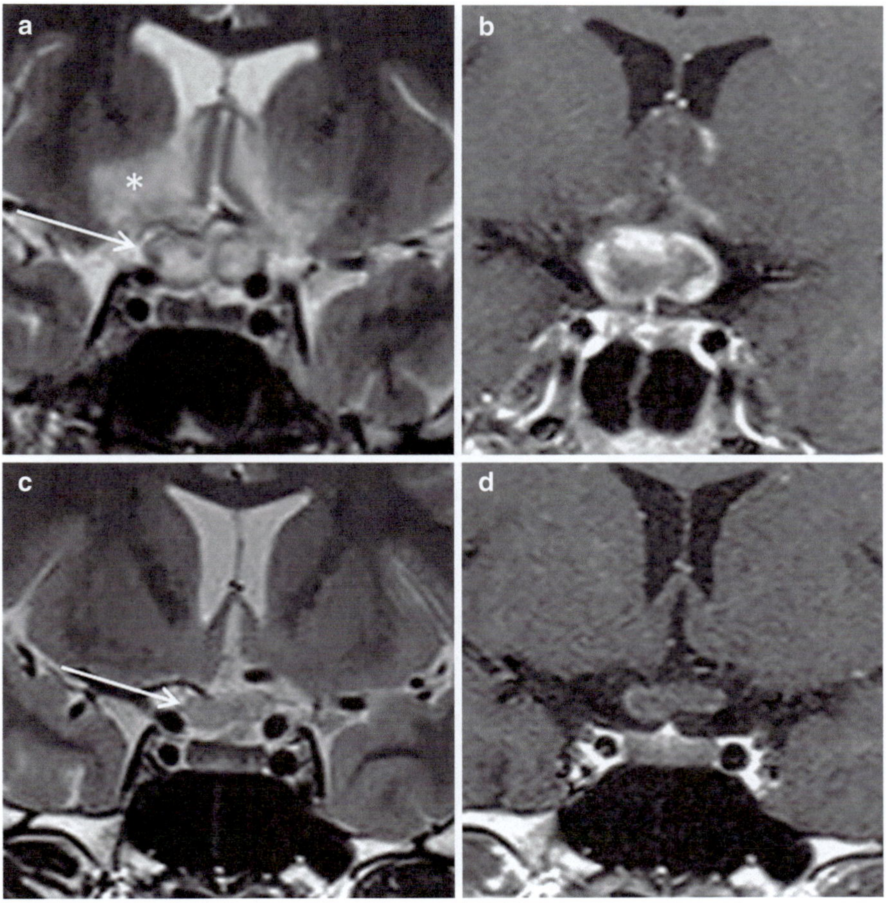

Fig. 38.2 Sarcoidosis. (**a**, **b**) Massive enlargement of the optic chiasm (arrow) with T2W hyperintensity and enhancement. Diffuse edema (*). (**c**, **d**) Rapid focal changes 1 month after corticotherapy. (**a**, **c**) Coronal T2WIs. (**b**, **d**) Coronal CE T1WIs

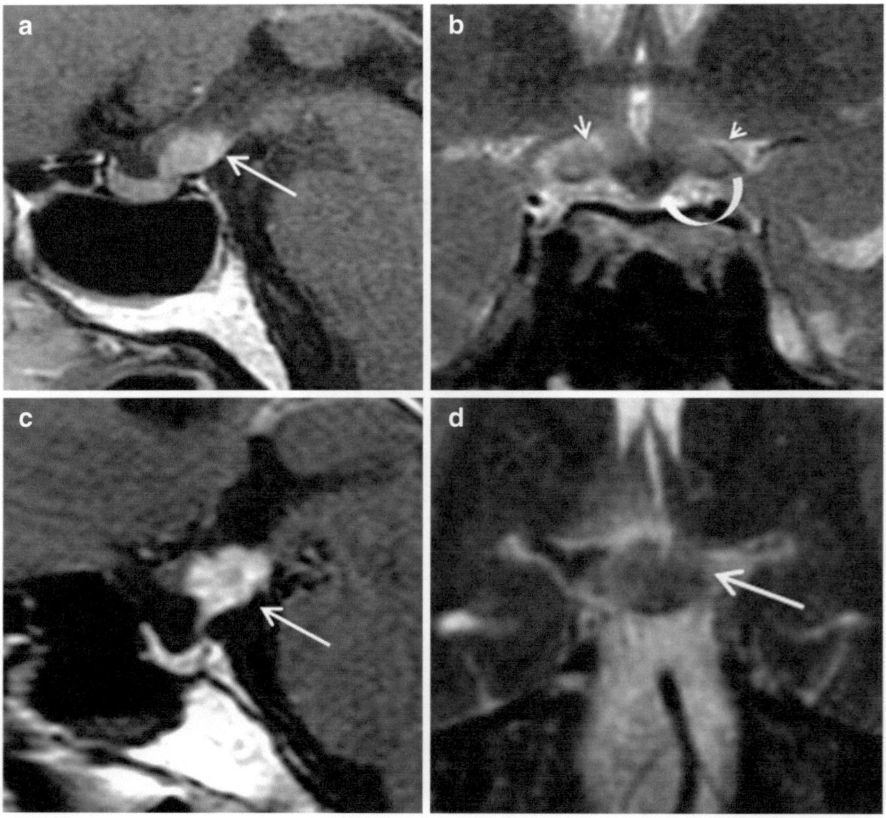

Fig. 38.3 Upper row: sarcoidosis. Lower row: histiocytosis. In both cases, thickening and T2W hypointensity of the infundibulum and optic chiasm. (**a**, **c**) Sagittal CE T1WIs. (**b**, **d**) Coronal T2WIs

- The precise etiology of AVP deficiency is undiscovered in a large proportion of cases, probably more than half of them and this is referred to as idiopathic diabetes insipidus and infundibuloneurohypophysitis. These patients may have an autoimmune disease such as Hashimoto thyroiditis or rheumatoid arthritis but this assertion is now disputed. Young adults and females are preferentially affected. The pituitary bright spot is missing. Thickening of the pituitary stalk is frequently discrete. A moderate T1W hyperintensity–T2W hypointensity of the infundibulum can draw attention (Fig. 31.1). Recurrences can be seen with episodes of thickening and shrinkage of the pituitary stalk. Finally, an atrophy of the distal pituitary stalk occurs. A T2W hypointense nodular expansion of the infundibulum may persist for years possibly associated with a FLAIR hyperintensity (Fig. 38.4). A shrinkage of the anterior pituitary gland is inconsistently observed with or without anterior pituitary deficit (Fig. 38.5). Vasopressin deficiency is usually isolated but anterior pituitary hormone deficits can develop during follow-up.

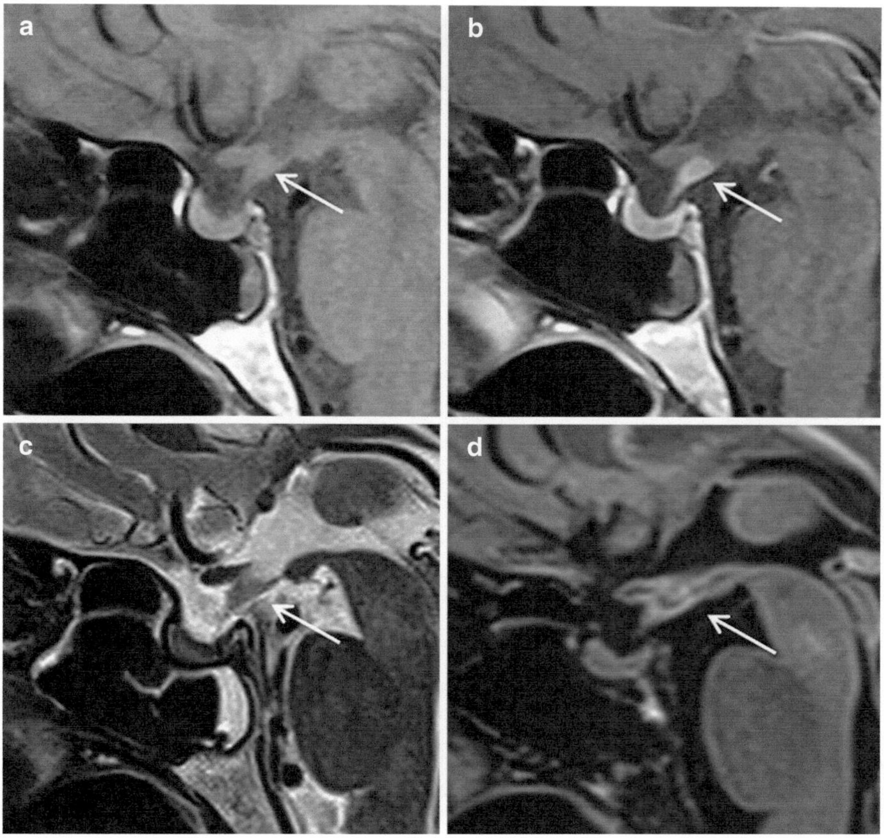

Fig. 38.4 Infundibulohypophysitis. The diagnosis is made 6 years after the onset of a polyuro-polydipsic syndrome. Thickening of the infundibulum with T2W hypointensity and FLAIR hyperintensity extended to the tuber cinereum (arrows). Atrophy of the distal pituitary stalk. No pituitary bright spot, confirmed on axial T1WIs (not shown). (**a–d**) Sagittal T1, CE T1, T2WIs, and FLAIR

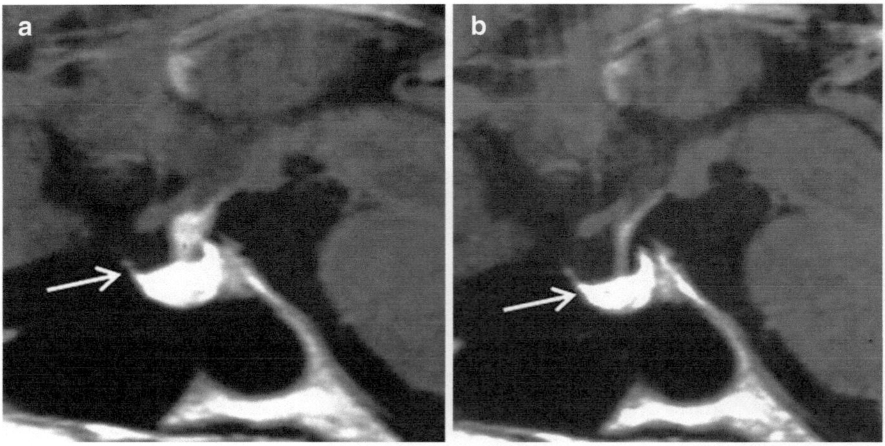

Fig. 38.5 Infundibuloneurohypophysitis. At the acute phase (**a**), isolated enlargement of the pituitary stalk. In the sequelae phase (**b**), atrophy of the pituitary stalk and discrete shrinkage of the anterior pituitary (arrows) without anterior pituitary deficit. (**a**, **b**) Sagittal CE T1WIs

Further Readings

Angelousi A, Alexandraki KI, Mytareli C, Grossman AB, Kaltsas G. New developments and concepts in the diagnosis and management of diabetes insipidus (AVP-deficiency and resistance). J Neuroendocrinol. 2023;35(1):e13233. https://doi.org/10.1111/jne.13233. Epub 2023 Jan 22.

Christ-Crain M, Winzeler B, Refardt J. Diagnosis and management of diabetes insipidus for the internist: an update. J Intern Med. 2021;290(1):73–87. https://doi.org/10.1111/joim.13261. Epub 2021 Mar 13.

Tomkins M, Lawless S, Martin-Grace J, Sherlock M, Thompson CJ. Diagnosis and management of central diabetes insipidus in adults. J Clin Endocrinol Metab. 2022;107(10):2701–15. https://doi.org/10.1210/clinem/dgac381.

What Is Bright on T1W?

39

T1 hyperintensity of the anterior pituitary gland is defined as a signal brighter than that of the normal anterior lobe or brighter than that of the pons on sagittal views or that of the temporal white matter on coronal views. In every case, a correlation with the T2W sequence may be needed to approach the diagnosis.

A T1W hyperintensity of the sellar region has many different sources and we illustrate here the most frequent or the most intriguing. It may result from the presence of blood such as in hemorrhagic pituitary adenomas, proteins such as in craniopharyngiomas, Rathke cleft cysts or fat such as in lipomas, dermoid cysts, or lipiodol remnants (Fig. 39.1).

Brain lipomas are rare and develop in the midline, preferentially at the corpus callosum level or in the sellar area. They are specifically recognized in the interpeduncular cistern, in contact with the tuber cinereum. These are easily differentiated from an ectopic posterior lobe which lies more anteriorly from the infundibulum. If necessary, an additional T1W fat-saturation sequence will confirm the fatty nature of the lipoma (Fig. 39.2).

Fat can be used by neurosurgeons to close a CSF fistula in the sella. A fat implant is easily recognized by its polycyclic contour and a chemical shift artifact (Fig. 39.3e).

A T1W hyperintensity of the anterior pituitary gland itself can be related to increased hormonal synthesis, as seen in newborns and pregnant and lactating women (Fig. 39.1).

After pituitary surgery, the residual normal pituitary tissue may exceptionally demonstrate some degree of T1 hyperintensity, which could reflect a temporary focal increase of hormonal activity (Fig. 39.1f).

T1W hyperintensity of the anterior pituitary gland can also be related to the deposition of paramagnetic substances in acute (Fig. 39.4) or chronic liver diseases (Fig. 39.1b) or of manganese in patients on long-term parenteral nutrition (Fig. 39.1i) or some drug abusers. In these different conditions, T1 hyperintensity of the basal ganglia may be also noted.

J.-F. Bonneville, *Tricks and Traps in MRI of the Pituitary Region*,
https://doi.org/10.1007/978-3-031-64710-9_39

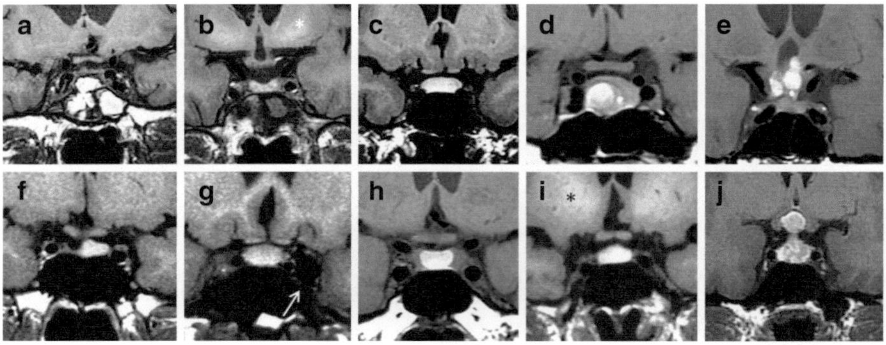

Fig. 39.1 Hyperintensities of the anterior pituitary. (**a–j**) Coronal non-enhanced T1WIs. (**a**) Fat packing after surgery. (**b**) Chronic hepatic failure. (**c**) Pregnancy, third trimester. (**d**) Hemorrhagic prolactinoma. (**e**) Craniopharyngioma. (**f**) Transitory T1 hyperintensity of the normal pituitary gland after pituitary microadenoma removal. (**g**) Cavernous sinus fistula (arrow). (**h**) Rathke cleft cyst. (**i**) Manganese deposit in a patient on parenteral nutrition. (**j**) Melanocytic tumor. Associated T1 hyperintensity of the basal ganglia in (**b**) and (**i**) (*)

Another rare cause of T1 hyperintensity is melanin in pituitary primary or metastatic melanocytic tumors (Fig. 39.1j).

T1 hyperintensity and associated bulging of the pituitary gland are observed in high-flow carotid-cavernous fistulae (Fig. 39.1g and 39.5). This pattern is related to the altered venous outflow of the pituitary gland. After embolization of the fistula, shrinkage of the pituitary occurs in a few days while T1 hyperintensity can persist for some weeks.

The same mechanism may explain the enlargement and the T1 hyperintensity of the anterior pituitary gland which can be seen in contact with a giant internal carotid aneurysm and resolves after treatment (Fig. 39.6).

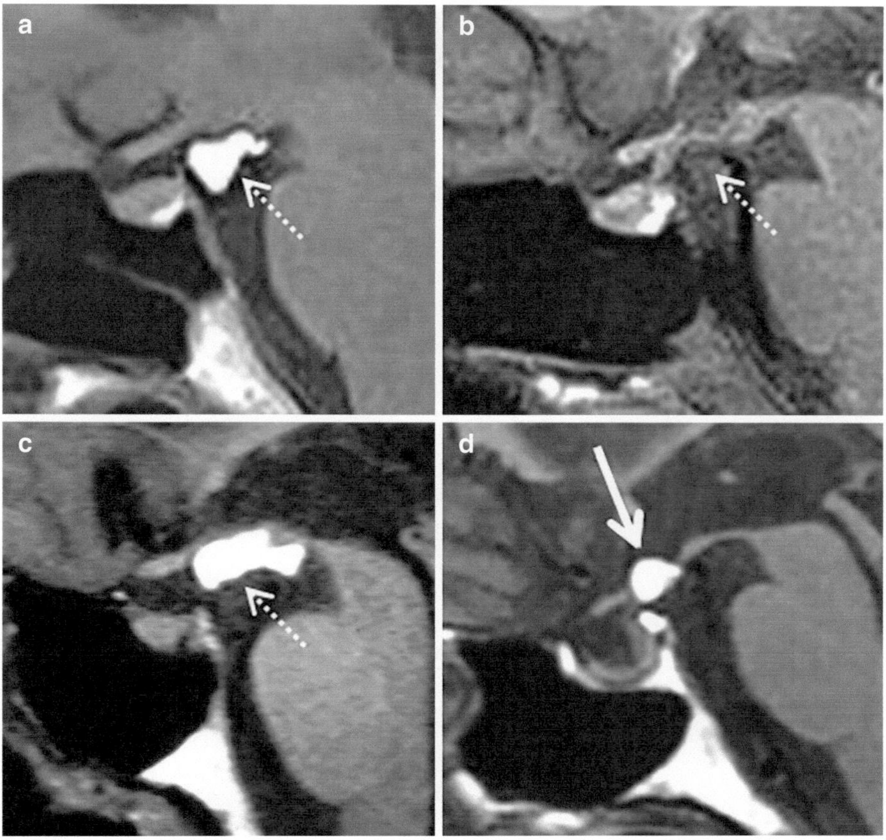

Fig. 39.2 Lipomas (**a**, **c**) versus ectopic posterior lobe (**d**) on sagittal T1WIS. (**b**) T1W Fatsat sequence

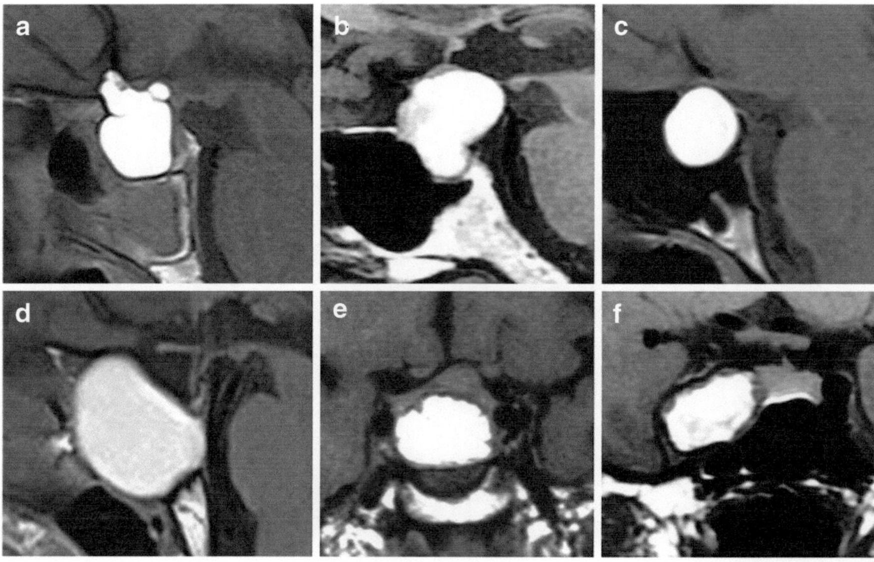

Fig. 39.3 T1W hyperintensity on sagittal (**a**–**d**) and coronal (**e**, **f**) T1WIs. (**a**) Recurrent Rathke cleft cyst. (**b**) Craniopharyngioma. (**c**) Hemorrhagic pituitary adenoma. (**d**) Sphenoid mucocele. (**e**) Surgical fat graft. (**f**) Thrombosed internal carotid aneurysm

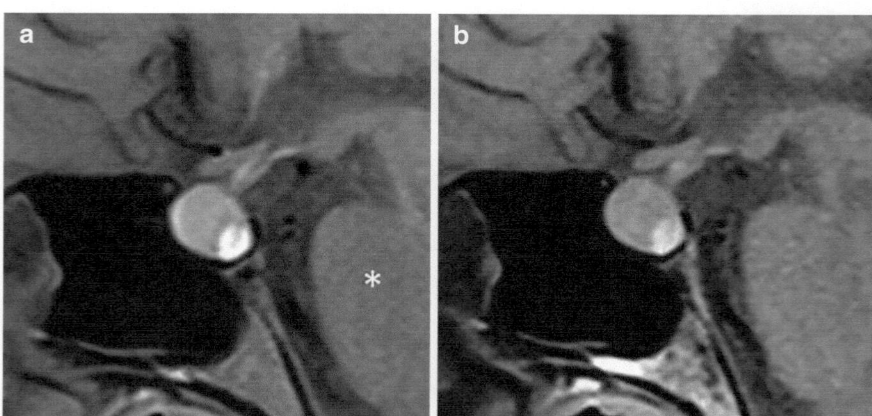

Fig. 39.4 Severe post-Covid hepatic failure in a 21-year-old woman. T1 hyperintensity of the pituitary gland (**a**) which partially regresses at 1 year (**b**). Compare in a the signal of the pituitary gland with that of the pons (*). Sagittal TIWIs

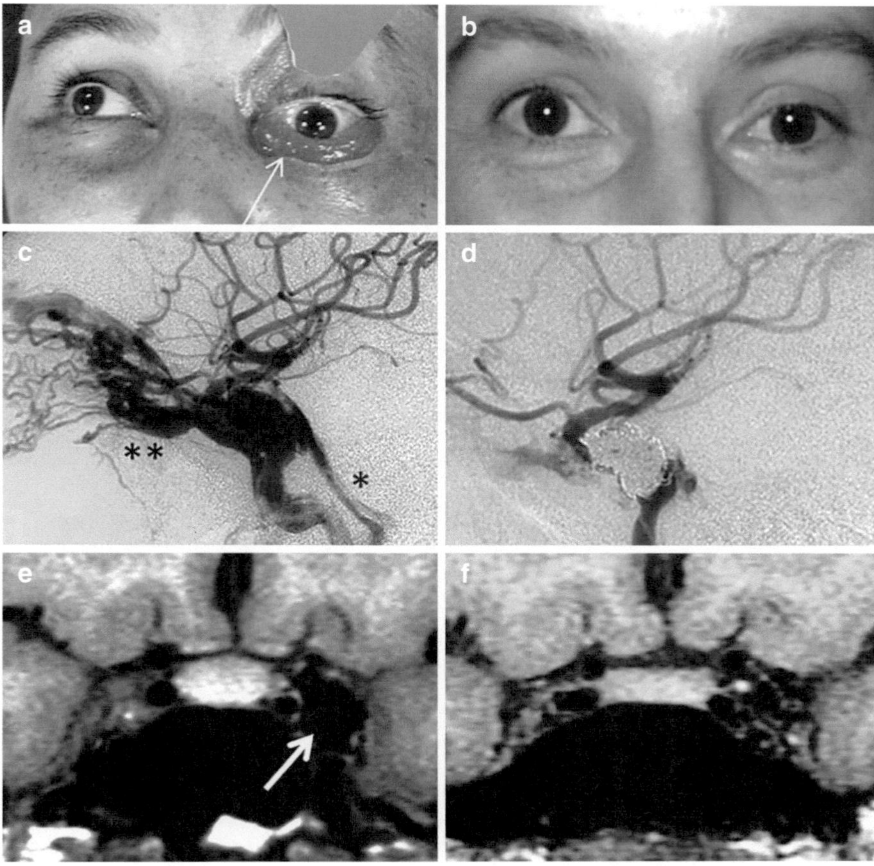

Fig. 39.5 Carodido-cavernous fistula and chemosis. Upper row: Photographs before and 6 months after treatment (**a**, **b**). Middle row (**c**, **d**): Selective internal carotid artery angiography showing the engorged veins draining anteriorly in the ophthalmic veins (**) and posteriorly in the inferior petrosal sinus (*). Almost complete closure of the fistula 6 months after coil embolization (**d**). Lower row (**e**, **f**): Coronal T1WIs. The whole cavernous sinus is occupied high flow confluent veins (arrow). The pituitary gland is bulging and T1W hyperintense. Six months after treatment (**f**), veins of the cavernous sinus are barely enlarged. The pituitary gland has returned to normal size and almost normal T1W signal

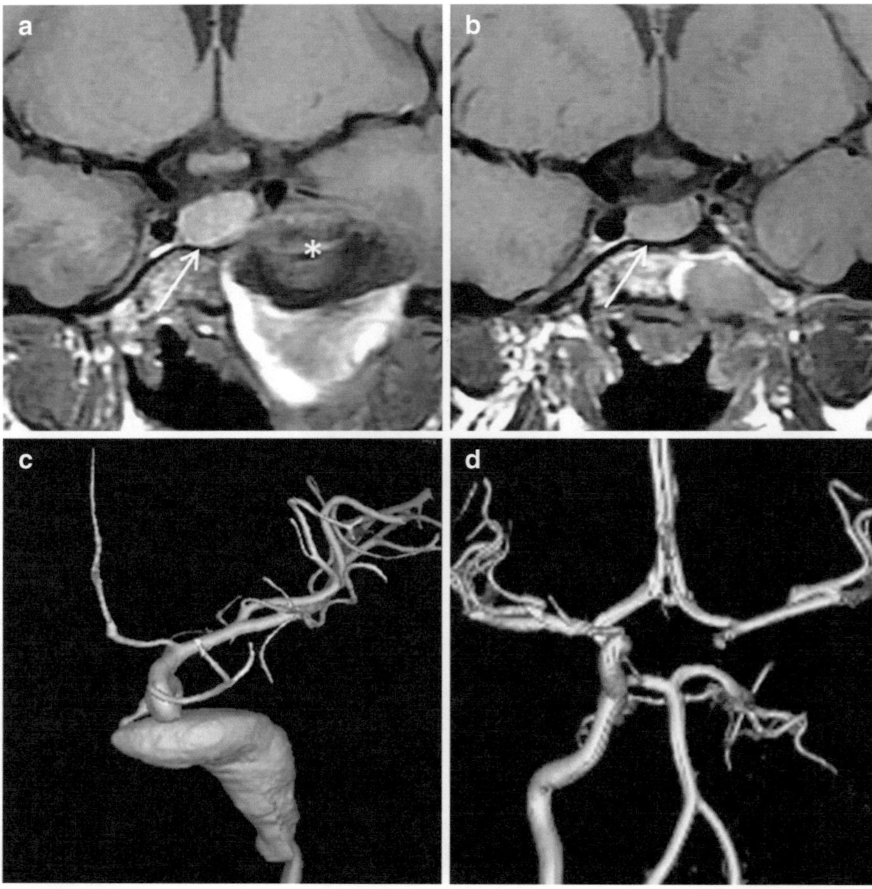

Fig. 39.6 (**a**) Swelling and T1 hyperintensity of the pituitary gland in a patient presenting a giant partially thrombosed aneurism of the internal carotid artery (*). (**b**) Shrinkage of the pituitary gland and disappearance of the T1 hyperintense signal after occlusion of the internal carotid artery. (**a**, **b**) Coronal T1WIs. (**c**, **d**) 3D reformatted angiography before (**c**) and after treatment (**d**)

Further Readings

Bonneville F, Cattin F, Barrali E, Lucas X, Narboux Y, Bonneville J. Hypersignal T1 de l'antéhypophyse saine résiduelle après traitement médical des adénomes à prolactine [Increased T1 signal of the residual normal anterior pituitary gland following medical treatment of pituitary prolactinoma]. J Radiol. 2001;82(4):501–5. French.

Bonneville F, Cattin F, Marsot-Dupuch K, Dormont D, Bonneville JF, Chiras J. T1 signal hyperintensity in the sellar region: spectrum of findings. Radiographics. 2006;26(1):93–113. https://doi.org/10.1148/rg.261055045. Erratum in: Radiographics. 2021 Nov–Dec;41(7):E210.

What Is Dark on T2?

40

A T2W hypointense signal of the pituitary gland can be defined conveniently as a signal darker than that of the normal pituitary gland or alternatively, that of the cortex of the temporal lobe. It must of course be interpreted in correlation with the T1W signal. The most common causes are hemorrhage, protein, and calcification (Fig. 40.1). Hemochromatosis and amyloidosis are rare. Signal voids are another cause of a dark pituitary gland.

We will describe and illustrate first the conditions where T2W hypointense signals are limited within the pituitary gland, then those where the whole gland or a large part of the gland is concerned.

- Hemorrhagic pituitary PitNETs usually display a mixture of T1W hyperintensity and T2W hypointensity and their signals vary a lot with time.
- Prolactinomas frequently present an asymptomatic bleeding as well before or after medical treatment (Figs. 12.2 and 12.3). This bleeding can be perceived very late as a thin peripheral T2W hypointense ring surrounding the lesion (Fig. 12.4).
- T2W hypointense hyperproteinic nodules are characteristic of RCC. These nodules can be large or very tiny but always pathognomonic of RCC (Fig. 24.1).
- Focal T2W hypointense areas in a pituitary mass can be related to calcification in a craniopharyngioma (Fig. 28.2), or in a TSH-secreting PitNET (Fig. 17.4).
- Teeth present in some teratomas express an intense hypointense signal in T2 and T1WIs (Fig. 29.4).
- A T2W hypointense ring encircling the pituitary content may be observed long after hypophysitis (Fig. 31.5).
- T2WIs millimetric hypointense foci corresponding to hemosiderin deposits are described in oncocytomas (Fig. 5.4).
- Parasellar signal voids may reveal vascular abnormalities such as a trigeminal artery or an intracavernous fistula. An aneurysm must be evoked in front of any rounded T2W hypointense image of the sellar region (Fig. 40.2).

J.-F. Bonneville, *Tricks and Traps in MRI of the Pituitary Region*,
https://doi.org/10.1007/978-3-031-64710-9_40

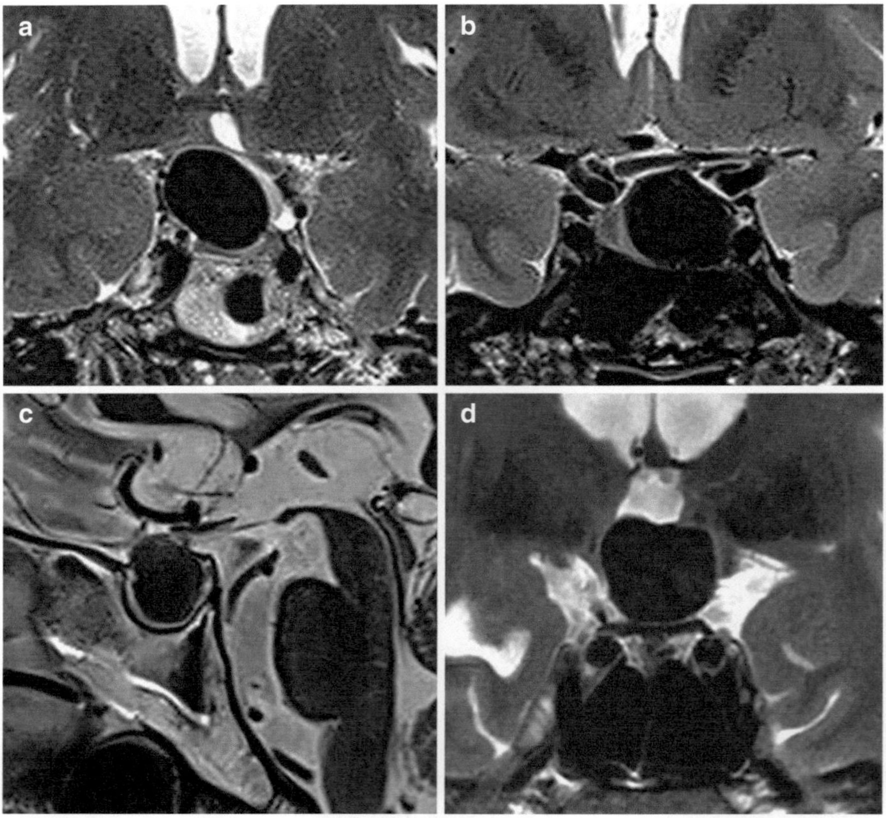

Fig. 40.1 T2W hypointense/signal void sellar masses. (**a**) Internal carotid artery intrasellar aneurysm. (**b**) Hemorrhagic prolactinoma. (**c**) Rathke cleft cyst. (**d**) Craniopharyngioma. (**a**, **b**, **d**) Coronal T2WIs. (**c**) Sagittal T2WI

A T2W hypointense signal of the whole pituitary gland can be difficult to perceive if the contrast resolution is not optimal. The T2W signal of the cortex of the temporal lobe is a practical referential tissue.

- In acromegaly, a T2W hypointense signal evokes a densely granulated growth-hormone PitNET which may respond to somatostatin analogs treatment better than sparsely granulated ones (Fig. 14.6).
- Prolactinomas may display a T2 hypointense signal in men (Fig. 13.3), much more rarely in women in whom they can behave more aggressively (Fig. 22.2).
- Hemochromatosis is a systemic disease characterized by increased iron deposition in the body. A distinction is made between primary or genetic hemochromatosis or hemosiderosis and secondary hemochromatosis caused principally by chronic transfusions. The diagnosis is confirmed by the dosage of ferritin and the transferrin saturation level. The pituitary gland appears hypointense on T2 or

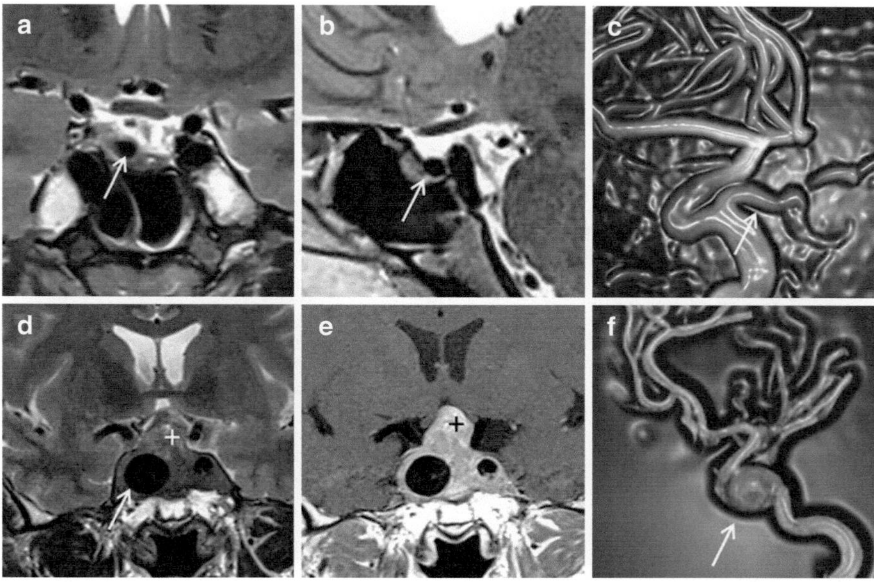

Fig. 40.2 Upper row. Trigeminal artery. Supplementary vascular anastomosis of the Willis circle (arrow). (**a**, **b**) Coronal and sagittal T2WIs. Lower row. Internal carotid artery intrasellar aneurysm (arrow) in a patient presenting a GH-secreting PitNET (+). (**d**, **e**) Coronal T2 and CE T1WIs. (**c**, **f**) 3D reformatted angiography

T2*WIs without contrast enhancement and with preservation of the bright spot of the posterior pituitary (Fig. 40.3c, d).

- The expression of the transferrin receptor is said to be confined to gonadotrophinomas, this explaining the frequency of hypogonadotropic hypogonadism in this disease (Fig. 40.4a–c). Nevertheless, iron deposits have been described in lactotrophs and we have observed a progressive T2W very hypointense signal of a prolactinoma in a man developing a siderosis (Fig. 40.4d–f).
- Amyloidosis is another infiltrative disorder frequently triggered by a chronic bowel inflammation and possibly leading to renal failure. In the brain, T2W hypointense amyloid deposits may be found in regions where the blood-brain barrier is insufficient such as the infundibulum, the pineal gland, or the pituitary gland. The anterior pituitary gland is hypointense on T2WIs (Fig. 40.3e, f). The bright spot of the posterior pituitary is preserved. Pituitary insufficiency is rare.
- Two histological types of amyloid deposits have been described in pituitary adenomas, the stellate, and the spherical patterns. Stellate amyloid is found perivascularly and small amounts may be encountered in pituitary adenomas. They are too small to be detected in MRI. Spherical amyloid is characterized by amorphous spheres. Spherical amyloid deposits have rarely been described in PitNETs, mainly in prolactinomas either under the form of a large T2W hypointense mass or as characteristic stippled calcifications (Fig. 40.5).

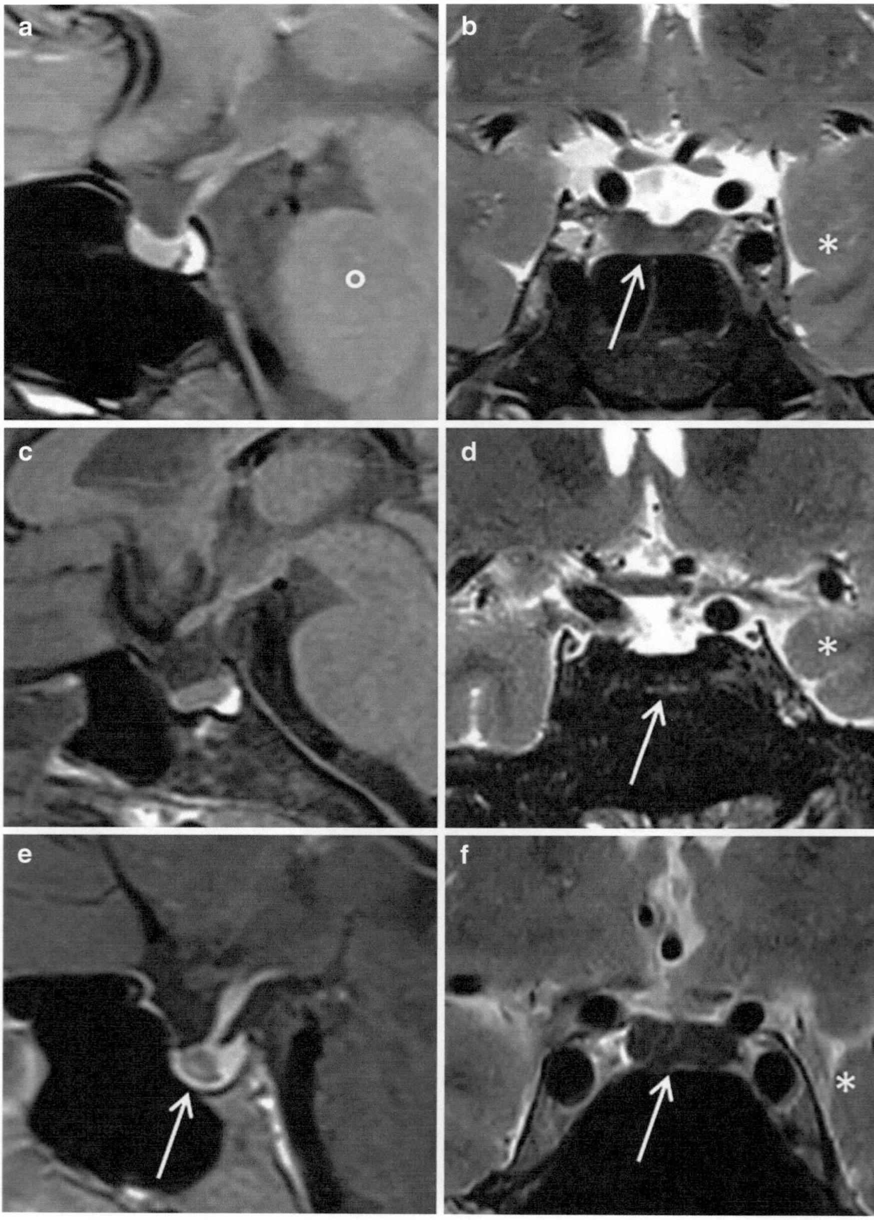

Fig. 40.3 T2W hypointense pituitary gland in different conditions. Compare with the T2W signal of the temporal cortex (*). Upper row: Patient under chronic dialysis. Note the T1W hyperintense signal of the anterior pituitary gland if compared with that of the brain stem (°). Middle row. Hemosiderosis. The T1W signal of the posterior lobe is preserved (as in **a**). Lower row. Amyloidosis. T2W hypointense non-enhanced anterior pituitary (**a**, **c**) Sagittal non-enhanced T1WIs. (**e**) Sagittal CE T1WI. (**b**, **d**, **f**) Coronal T2WIs

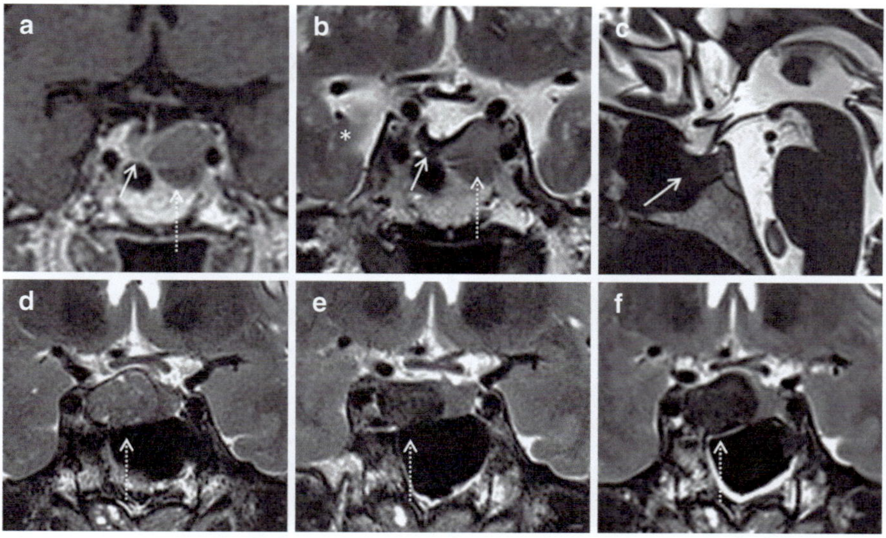

Fig. 40.4 Hemochromatosis in two patients presenting a PITNET. Upper row. High ferritin and high transferrin saturation levels in a 70-year-old female presenting a non-secreting PitNET followed for 7 years. The T2W hypointense anterior pituitary gland (arrow) is compressed by the adenoma (dotted arrow). Compare with the T2W signal of the grey matter of the temporal lobe (*). Lower row. Development of a hemochromatosis confirmed by genetic tests in a 42-year-old male patient presenting a prolactinoma (dotted arrow). Prolactin is 5600 mUI/L (280 μG/L). Ferritin is 1800 μG/L. Transferrin saturation is 53%. (**d**) Right-sided T2W hyperintense prolactinoma. (**e**) 3 years later with dopamine agonist irregular treatment, partial shrinkage of the lesion which is now T2W hypointense. (**f**) Five more years later. The treatment has been stopped. Regrow of the adenoma and increase of its T2W hypointense signal. (**a**) Coronal CE T1WI. (**c**) Sagittal T2 WI through the normal anterior pituitary. (**b**, **d**, **e**, **f**) Coronal T2WIs

– T2W hypointensity associated with T1W hyperintensity attributed to manganese accumulation may be observed in the pituitary gland and in the basal ganglia of patients undergoing hemodialysis (Fig. 40.3a, b).

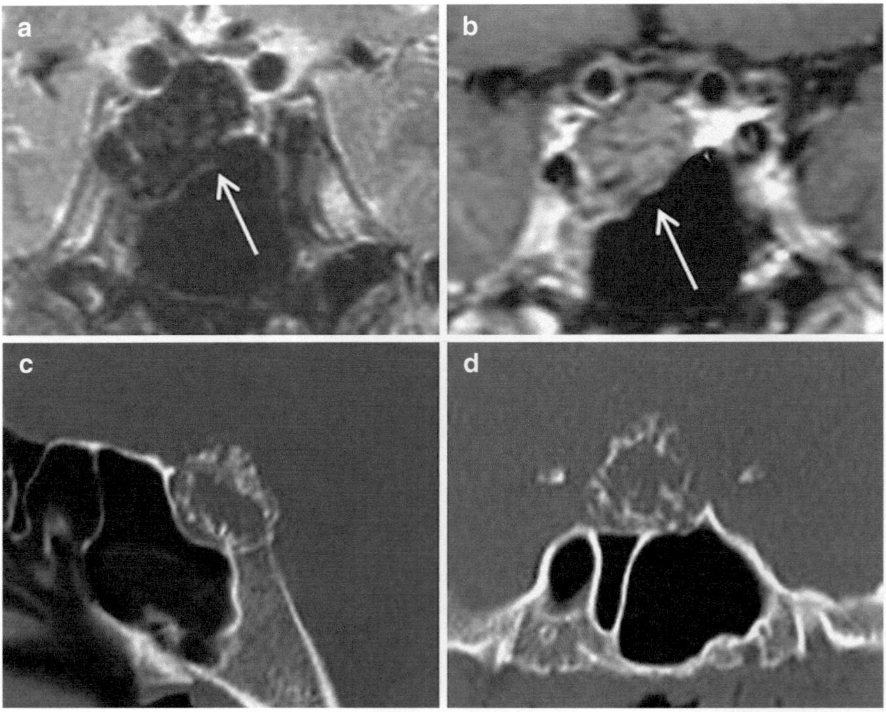

Fig. 40.5 Upper row. Amyloidosis. Right-sided T2W hypointense non-enhanced mass (arrows). (**a**) Coronal T2WI. (**b**) Coronal CE T1WI (from Wiesli, P., Brändle, M., Brandner, S. et al., Extensive spherical amyloid deposition presenting as a pituitary tumor. *J Endocrinol Invest* **26**, 552–555 (2003), Springer Nature, with permission). Lower row. Characteristic stippled sellar calcifications in another patient presenting amyloidosis on sagittal and coronal reformatted CT (**c**, **d**). (Courtesy F. Bonneville)

Further Readings

Martin SW, Lefton DR, Pinto RS, Rosenblum M, Elowitz E. MR imaging characteristics of amyloid deposits in pituitary adenoma. AJNR Am J Neuroradiol. 2002;23(3):368–70.

Rousset P, Cattin F, Chiras J, Bonneville JF, Bonneville F. Valeur diagnostique d'un hyposignal T2 de la région sellaire. J Radiol. 2009;90:693–705.

Verberckmoes B, Dekeyzer S, Decaestecker K. The dark pituitary: hemochromatosis as a lesser-known cause of pituitary dysfunction. J Belg Soc Radiol. 2022;106(1):63. https://doi.org/10.5334/jbsr.2771.

Do You Have FLAIR?

41

The FLAIR (fluid-attenuated inversion recovery) sequence is not commonly used for the evaluation of the sellar region. It is traditionally performed to characterize arachnoid cysts (Fig. 41.1) or, for instance, to demonstrate a vasogenic oedema of the optic tract. Contrast-enhanced three-dimensional T2 fluid-attenuated inversion recovery (CE 3D T2 FLAIR) has recently emerged as a useful sequence to evaluate several conditions of the pituitary region. In our hands, CE 3D FLAIR has recently become a useful tool (Figs. 7.3, 9.1, 10.1, 11.2, 12.5, 16.4, 17.4, 25.4, 25.5, 26.1, 26.3, 26.6, 27.1, 27.4, 31.4, 36.5, and 38.4). 2D FLAIR can also help but CE 3D FLAIR has the advantages to suppress flow artifacts from the CSF, to provide ultra-thin sections in any plane and to minimize partial volume effect.

Although FLAIR is considered a T2W sequence, it also shows a mild T1W effect responsible of some contrast enhancement, much less intense than that on CE T1WIs. Such an enhancement in CE 3D FLAIR may be visible in normal intracranial structures and particularly in the circumventricular organs of the brain. These small structures lining the cavity of the third and fourth ventricles are thought to be an important link in the regulation of metabolic and endocrine functions. Among them, the median eminence, the tuber cinereum and in part the lamina terminalis and the pineal gland are frequently enhanced (Fig. 41.2). The secondary hypophyseal capillary bed, a potential landmark located at the end of the pituitary stalk, previously named the pituitary tuft, may be visible as the pituitary stalk itself (Fig. 41.6). Generally, it must be recognized that the enhancement of these different structures is variable and inconstant and that a fine semiology remains to be specified. Arteries are not enhanced. Laterosellar veins are more intensely enhanced on CE 2D FLAIR than on CE 3D FLAIR (Fig. 41.6f).

Pituitary gland and pituitary tumors enhancement depends on various factors, an important factor being the gadolinium concentration in the tissues. *3D CE T2 FLAIR is more highly sensitive to low gadolinium concentrations* and less sensitive to high gadolinium concentrations than are T1-weighted sequences.

The enhancement pattern of meningiomas offers a clear demonstration of the relationship between gadolinium concentration and degree of enhancement in CE

J.-F. Bonneville, *Tricks and Traps in MRI of the Pituitary Region*,
https://doi.org/10.1007/978-3-031-64710-9_41

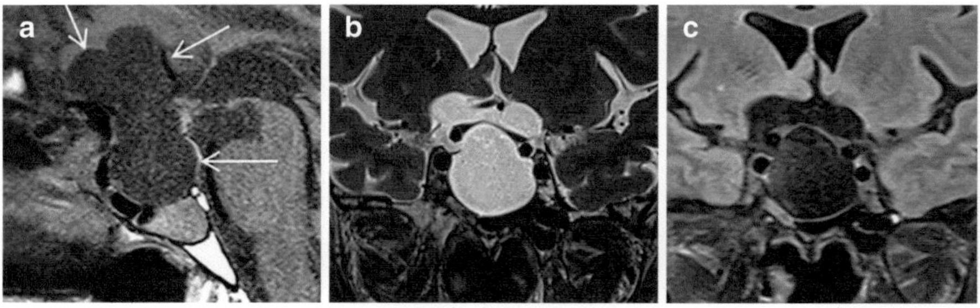

Fig. 41.1 Huge non-symptomatic arachnoid cyst extended from the sella to the subfrontal area. (**a**) Sagittal T1W. (**b**, **c**) Coronal T2WI and FLAIR. The signal of the cyst is similar to that of CSF in all sequences

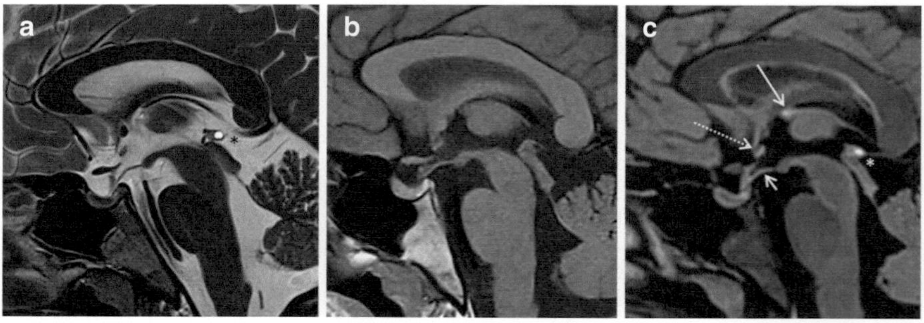

Fig. 41.2 Sagittal 3D CE FLAIR in a normal individual (**c**). The pituitary stalk, the infundibulum and the tuber cinereum (short arrow) are constantly enhanced. The lamina terminalis (in part, dotted arrow) and the fornix (long arrow) are frequently partially enhanced as well as the pineal gland (*). (**a**, **b**) Sagittal T2 and T1W are for comparison

FLAIR. In large meningiomas, the central part of the tumor which is richly supplied by meningeal arteries and is strongly enhanced on T1W sequence is unenhanced on CE FLAIR imaging, a high concentration of gadolinium inducing signal loss. On the contrary, the meningioma capsule which is more weakly supplied by pial arteries present contrast enhancement (Fig. 41.3).

Enhancement of the pituitary gland is variable on 3D CE FLAIR. The normal pituitary gland appears poorly enhanced at the usual gadolinium dose of 0.1 mmol/kg of body weight. Its signal decreases when the gadolinium concentration increases. At 0.3 mmol/kg, the pituitary gland appears totally dark, this observation being probably attributable to T2 shortening (Fig. 41.4).

Generally speaking, CE 3D FLAIR is not the panacea for the diagnosis of microadenomas but may sometimes help, particularly when T2 and CE T1WIs are not sufficiently informative (Fig. 41.5a–c). Solid PitNETS are slightly enhanced on CE 3D FLAIR images. Cystic tumors are frankly enhanced in CE 3D FLAIR as well as in 2D FLAIR (Fig. 41.6d–f). Tumors with high T2W hyperintense signal demonstrate a high degree of contrast enhancement while T2W hypointense lesions are unenhanced (Fig. 41.6a–d).

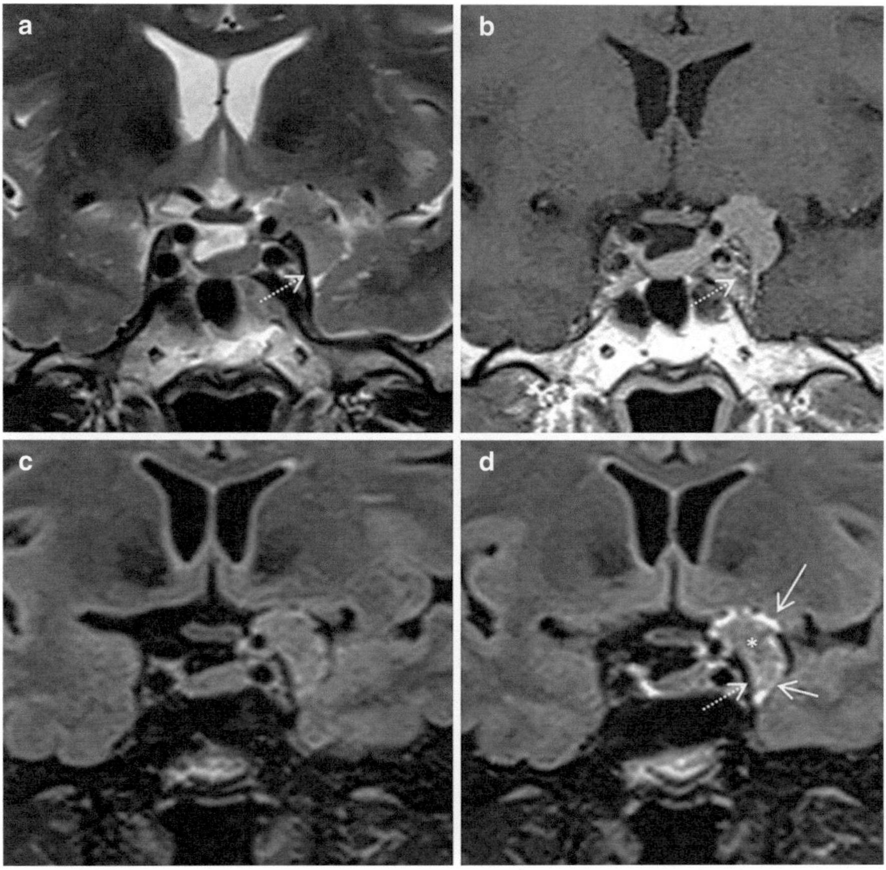

Fig. 41.3 (**a–c**) Meningioma inserted on the lateral thickened wall of the left cavernous sinus (dotted arrow). The external capsule of the tumor (arrows) which is less supplied (by pial arteries) is strongly enhanced in (**d**), 3D CE FLAIR. The central part of the tumor (*) which is richly vascularized by meningeal arteries is less enhanced

Microadenomas with a weak T2W hyperintense signal may demonstrate a sufficient enhancement on CE FLAIR to be depicted on the dark field of the anterior pituitary gland with a 0.3 mmol gadolinium dose (Fig. 41.6g–i). Unfortunately, these benefits are inconstant (Fig. 41.5c–e).

Delayed CE 3D FLAIR has been proposed for the research of microcorticotropinomas which could present a late washout if compared with non-secreting PitNETs. This assertion has not be proven in large series yet.

CE 3D FLAIR offers a better delineation of intrasellar RCCs or RCC remnants by erasing the normal pituitary gland (Fig. 41.4d–f).

CE 3D FLAIR may also help to differentiate uncomplicated versus complicated RCCs. Indeed, the peripheral ring which frequently surrounds a non-symptomatic RCC is in fact normal pituitary tissue displaced by the cyst and therefore does not

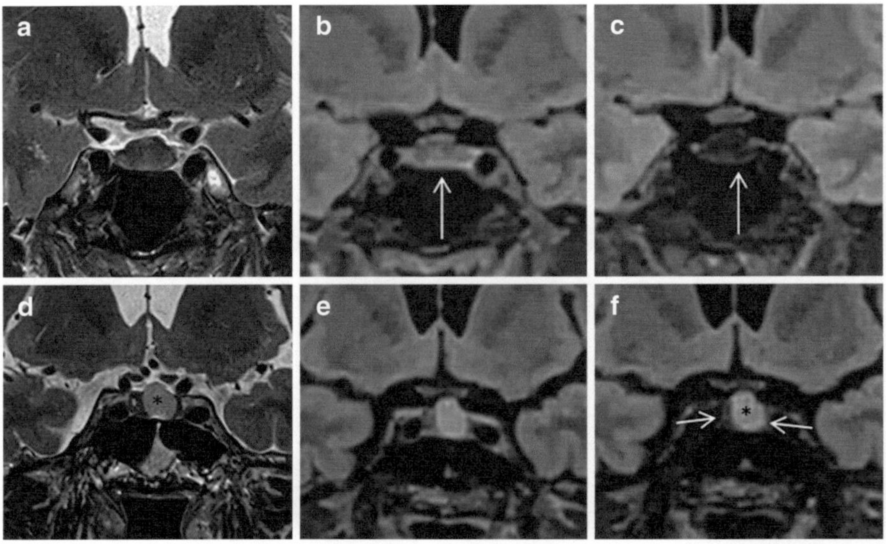

Fig. 41.4 High concentration of gadolinium (0.3 mmol/kg) induces a signal loss of the pituitary gland in 3D CE FLAIR (**c**, **f**). Upper row. Normal pituitary gland (arrow). Lower row. Rathke cleft cyst (*). The normal pituitary gland which surrounds the cyst has lost its signal after gadolinium injection (**f**). (**a**, **d**) Coronal T2WIs. (**b**, **e**) 3D enhanced FLAIR

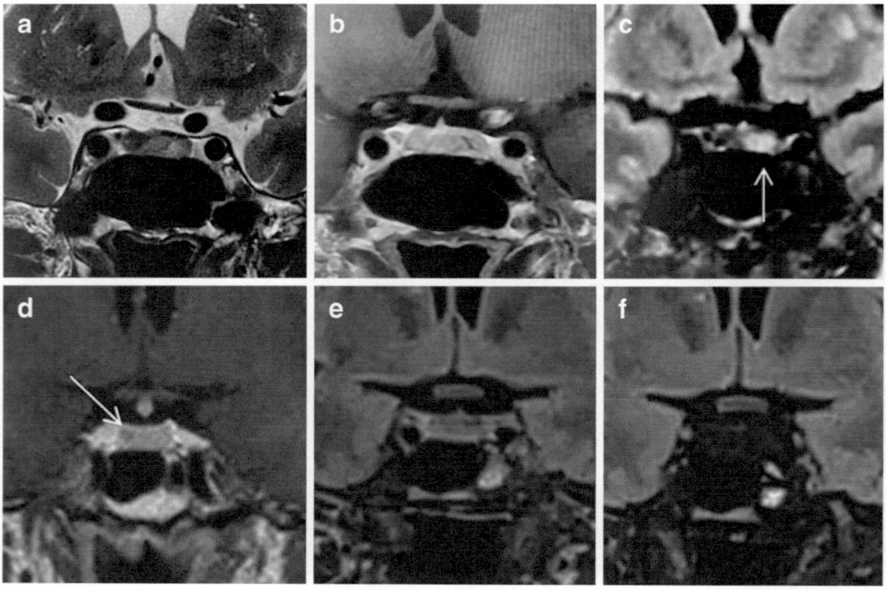

Fig. 41.5 Upper row. CE FLAIR can help for the diagnosis of PitNETS when T2 and CE T1WIs are not diagnostic. Cushing disease in a 42-year-old woman. Somatotropic PitNET (arrow). (**a**) Coronal T2WI. (**b**) Coronal CE 2D SE T1WI. (**c**) CE 2D coronal FLAIR. Lower row. CE 3D FLAIR failure. Picoprolactinoma in a 29-year-old woman. Prolactin is 117 µG/L. (**c**) Coronal CE T1WI. 3 mm right-sided non enhanced lesion (arrow) not demonstrated on 3D FLAIR (**d**) and CE 3D FLAIR (**e**)

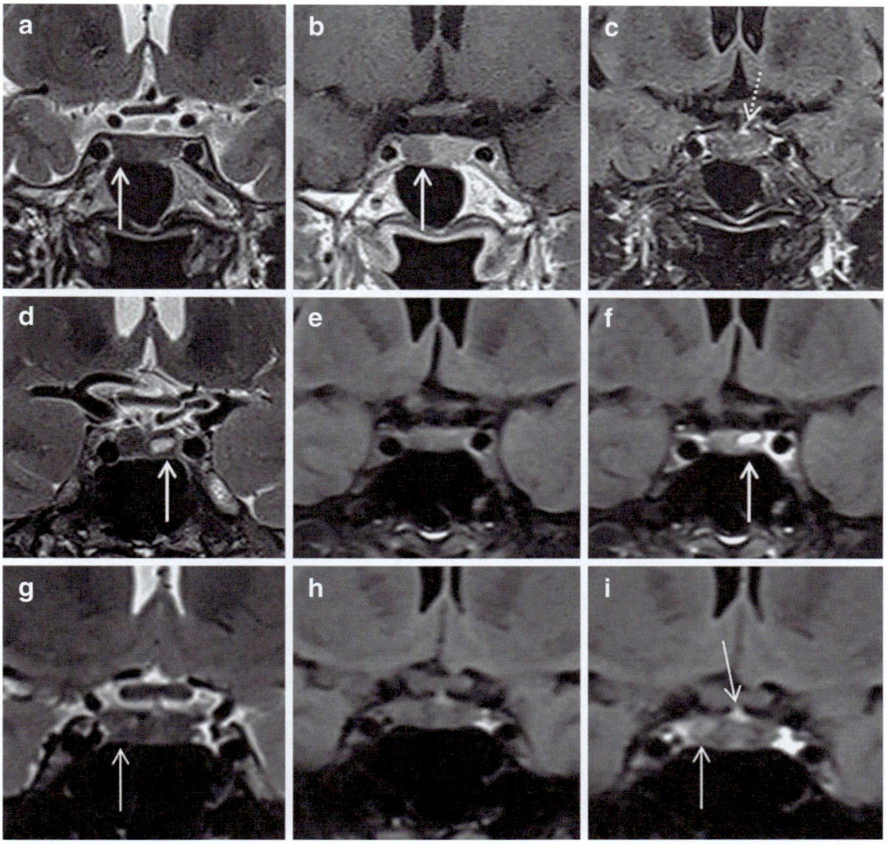

Fig. 41.6 Upper row. T2W hypointense PitNET not enhanced on 3D CE FLAIR (**c**). (**a**, **b**) Coronal T2 and CE T1WIs. Note that the pituitary "tuft" is displaced off midline (dotted arrow). Middle row. T2W hyperintense PitNET not seen on FLAIR (**e**) but intensively enhanced in a CE 2D 3 mm FLAIR (**f**). Note the enhancement of parasellar veins. Coronal T2WI (**d**) and 2D FLAIR (**e**). Lower row. T2W hypo-isointense PitNET confirmed in CE 2D FLAIR (**i**). The pituitary tuft is displaced (long arrow). (**g**) Coronal T2WI. (**h**) Coronal FLAIR

enhance on CE 3D FLAIR particularly with a 0.3 mmol/kg gadolinium dosage. By contrast, the thickened wall of a complicated RCC enhances (Fig. 24.5).

Lastly, in craniopharyngiomas, CE 3D FLAIR permits to separate liquid from solid tumoral compartments (Fig. 41.7).

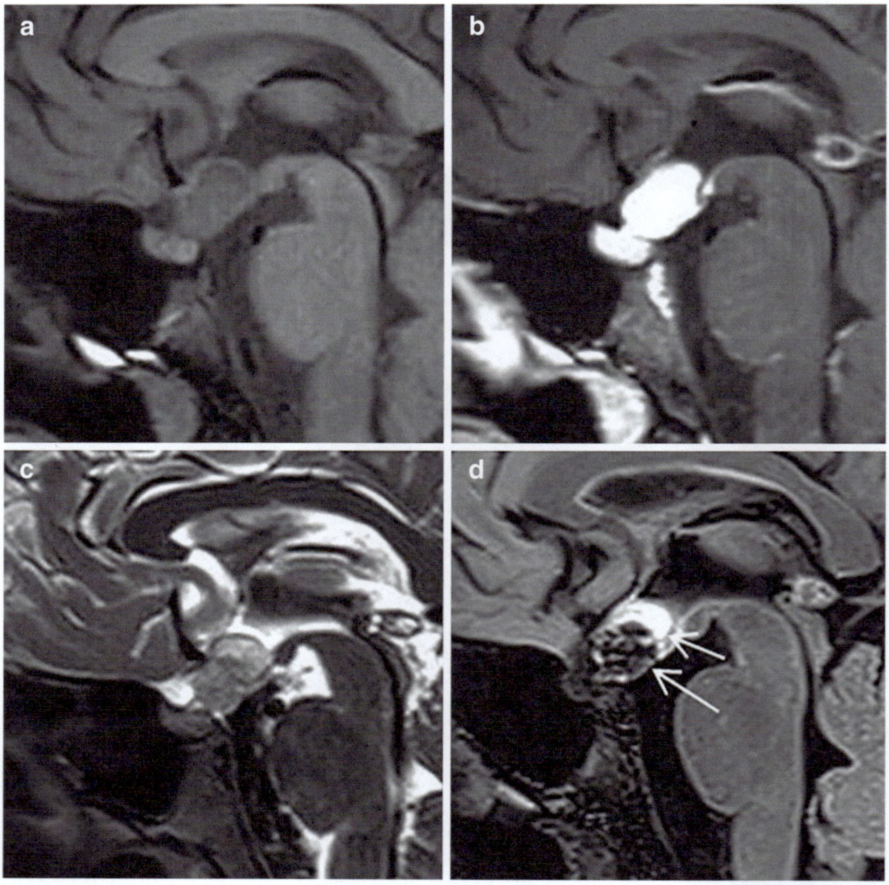

Fig. 41.7 Papillary craniopharyngioma revealed by a hypogonadotropic hypogonadism in a 44-year-old man. CE 3D FLAIR (**d**) helps to differentiate cystic (short arrow) from solid (long arrow) tumoral compartments better than T1WI (**a**), CE T1WI (**b**) and T2WI (**c**)

Further Readings

Azuma M, Hirai T, Kadota Y, Khant ZA, Hattori Y, Kitajima M, Uetani H, Yamashita Y. Circumventricular organs of human brain visualized on post-contrast 3D fluid-attenuated inversion recovery imaging. Neuroradiology. 2018;60(6):583–90. https://doi.org/10.1007/s00234-018-2023-3. Epub 2018 May 2.

Azuma M, Khant ZA, Kadota Y, Takeishi G, Watanabe T, Yokogami K, Takeshima H, Hirai T. Added value of contrast-enhanced 3D-FLAIR MR imaging for differentiating cystic pituitary adenoma from Rathke's cleft cyst. Magn Reson Med Sci. 2021;20(4):404–9. https://doi.org/10.2463/mrms.mp.2020-0127. Epub 2021 Jan 25.

Kubota T, Yamada K, Kizu O, Hirota T, Ito H, Ishihara K, Nishimura T. Relationship between contrast enhancement on fluid-attenuated inversion recovery MR sequences and signal intensity on T2-weighted MR images: visual evaluation of brain tumors. J Magn Reson Imaging. 2005;21(6):694–700. https://doi.org/10.1002/jmri.20331.

Osawa I, Nagawa K, Hara Y, Shimizu H, Tanaka S, Kozawa E. Utility of contrast-enhanced 3D STIR FLAIR imaging for evaluating pituitary adenomas at 3 Tesla. Eur J Radiol Open. 2023;11:100500. https://doi.org/10.1016/j.ejro.2023.100500.

42 Incidentaloma, a Plea for Clarification

When the term incidentaloma appeared in the medical literature in reference to any adrenal mass detected on imaging in the early 1980s, the same term started to be applied to an incidentally discovered pituitary mass in the early 1990s, i.e., with the advent of MRI. It was unemployed during the CT era. If the term could be acceptable for adrenal lesions—which are very frequent, of very different natures, and whose imaging patterns are poorly specific—its use for calling a pituitary lesion discovered by chance may be discussed.

Indeed, unlike adrenal masses, the nature of "pituitary incidentalomas" is almost always either a non-secreting pituitary adenoma (in more than 80% of the cases) or a Rathke cleft cyst. The imaging features of both lesions are easily distinguishable with optimal MR parameters and minimum knowledge. Yet, the term pituitary incidentaloma is flourishing and appears more and more often in the endocrinological literature. Particularly, the number of papers dealing with the management of pituitary incidentalomas continues to grow when such management is obviously different in adenomas and Rathke cleft cysts. Furthermore, some authors reserve this term exclusively to asymptomatic non-secreting adenomas while others include silent or whispering adenomas or even subclinical apoplexy.

Ultimately, if patients with incidentaloma are, as is strongly recommended, screened for pituitary hypersecretion or hypopituitarism, a certain number will be diagnosed as affected by a pituitary adenoma and not an incidentaloma, and this term will be erased from their medical file.

Then, the term "incidentalomas"—which has been described as a "by-product of modern imaging"—may cause confusion and, from a practical point of view, is not justified.

About one out of three non-secreting pituitary adenomas ("incidentalomas") grows and patients must be followed by periodic MRIs, generally 6 months after their discovery, and then every year for several years. It is useful to recall here the importance of strictly superimposable examinations over time, to catch a growth as early as possible. In these circumstances, contrast injection is unnecessary and must be prohibited.

J.-F. Bonneville, *Tricks and Traps in MRI of the Pituitary Region*,
https://doi.org/10.1007/978-3-031-64710-9_42

A group of pituitary pathologists has tried to impose a new word to design pituitary adenomas: PitNETs, for pituitary neuroendocrine tumors, arguing that these lesions affect the neuroendocrine system and are true tumors, which, even if quite always benign, may present an invasive or aggressive behavior with exceptional metastases. This term is widely used in the medical literature nowadays, although the ancient designation and the newly recommended term appear together here and there. The future will tell us if PitNET will replace pituitary adenoma in the current language and if the term incidentaloma will sink slowly.

Further Readings

Asa SL, Asioli S, Bozkurt S, Casar-Borota O, Chinezu L, Comunoglu N, Cossu G, Cusimano M, Delgrange E, Earls P, Ezzat S, Gazioglu N, Grossman A, Guaraldi F, Hickman RA, Ikeda H, Jaffrain-Rea ML, Karavitaki N, Kraljević I, La Rosa S, Manojlović-Gačić E, Maartens N, McCutcheon IE, Messerer M, Mete O, Nishioka H, Oz B, Pakbaz S, Pekmezci M, Perry A, Reiniger L, Roncaroli F, Saeger W, Söylemezoğlu F, Tachibana O, Trouillas J, Turchini J, Uccella S, Villa C, Yamada S, Yarman S. Pituitary neuroendocrine tumors (PitNETs): nomenclature evolution, not clinical revolution. Pituitary. 2020;23(3):322–5. https://doi.org/10.1007/s11102-019-01015-0.

Molitch ME. Pituitary tumours: pituitary incidentalomas. Best Pract Res Clin Endocrinol Metab. 2009;23(5):667–75. https://doi.org/10.1016/j.beem.2009.05.001.

Vasilev V, Rostomyan L, Daly AF, Potorac I, Zacharieva S, Bonneville JF, Beckers A. Management of endocrine disease: pituitary 'incidentaloma': neuroradiological assessment and differential diagnosis. Eur J Endocrinol. 2016;175(4):R171–84. https://doi.org/10.1530/EJE-15-1272. Epub 2016 Apr 11.

MIX
Papier aus verantwortungsvollen Quellen
Paper from responsible sources
FSC® C105338

If you have any concerns about our products,
you can contact us on
ProductSafety@springernature.com

In case Publisher is established outside the EU,
the EU authorized representative is:
Springer Nature Customer Service Center GmbH
Europaplatz 3, 69115 Heidelberg, Germany

Printed by Libri Plureos GmbH
in Hamburg, Germany